Plasma-Based Synthesis and Modification of Nanomaterials

Plasma-Based Synthesis and Modification of Nanomaterials

Special Issue Editor
Pawel Pohl

MDPI • Basel • Beijing • Wuhan • Barcelona • Belgrade

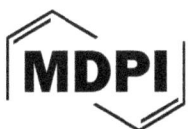

Special Issue Editor
Pawel Pohl
Wroclaw University of Science and Technology
Poland

Editorial Office
MDPI
St. Alban-Anlage 66
4052 Basel, Switzerland

This is a reprint of articles from the Special Issue published online in the open access journal *Nanomaterials* (ISSN 2079-4991) from 2018 to 2019 (available at: https://www.mdpi.com/journal/nanomaterials/special_issues/plasma_based_nano)

For citation purposes, cite each article independently as indicated on the article page online and as indicated below:

LastName, A.A.; LastName, B.B.; LastName, C.C. Article Title. *Journal Name* **Year**, *Article Number*, Page Range.

ISBN 978-3-03921-395-5 (Pbk)
ISBN 978-3-03921-396-2 (PDF)

© 2020 by the authors. Articles in this book are Open Access and distributed under the Creative Commons Attribution (CC BY) license, which allows users to download, copy and build upon published articles, as long as the author and publisher are properly credited, which ensures maximum dissemination and a wider impact of our publications.

The book as a whole is distributed by MDPI under the terms and conditions of the Creative Commons license CC BY-NC-ND.

Contents

About the Special Issue Editor vii

Preface to "Plasma-Based Synthesis and Modification of Nanomaterials" ix

Pawel Pohl
Plasma-Based Synthesis and Modification of Nanomaterials
Reprinted from: *Nanomaterials* 2019, 9, 278, doi:10.3390/nano9020278 1

Heon Lee, Won-June Lee, Young-Kwon Park, Seo Jin Ki, Byung-Joo Kim and Sang-Chul Jung
Liquid Phase Plasma Synthesis of Iron Oxide Nanoparticles on Nitrogen-Doped Activated Carbon Resulting in Nanocomposite for Supercapacitor Applications
Reprinted from: *Nanomaterials* 2018, 8, 190, doi:10.3390/nano8040190 3

Genki Saito, Hitoshi Sasaki, Heishichiro Takahashi and Norihito Sakaguchi
Solution-Plasma-Mediated Synthesis of Si Nanoparticles for Anode Material of Lithium-Ion Batteries
Reprinted from: *Nanomaterials* 2018, 8, 286, doi:10.3390/nano8050286 16

Ching-Bin Ke, Te-Ling Lu and Jian-Lian Chen
Capacitively Coupled Plasma Discharge of Ionic Liquid Solutions to Synthesize Carbon Dots as Fluorescent Sensors
Reprinted from: *Nanomaterials* 2018, 8, 372, doi:10.3390/nano8060372 26

Anna Dzimitrowicz, Aleksandra Bielawska-Pohl, George C. diCenzo, Piotr Jamroz, Jan Macioszczyk, Aleksandra Klimczak and Pawel Pohl
Pulse-Modulated Radio-Frequency Alternating-Current-Driven Atmospheric-Pressure Glow Discharge for Continuous-Flow Synthesis of Silver Nanoparticles and Evaluation of Their Cytotoxicity toward Human Melanoma Cells
Reprinted from: *Nanomaterials* 2018, 8, 398, doi:10.3390/nano8060398 38

Denis Mihaela Panaitescu, Sorin Vizireanu, Cristian Andi Nicolae, Adriana Nicoleta Frone, Angela Casarica, Lavinia Gabriela Carpen and Gheorghe Dinescu
Treatment of Nanocellulose by Submerged Liquid Plasma for Surface Functionalization
Reprinted from: *Nanomaterials* 2018, 8, 467, doi:10.3390/nano8070467 58

Anna Dzimitrowicz, Piotr Cyganowski, Pawel Pohl, Dorota Jermakowicz-Bartkowiak, Dominik Terefinko and Piotr Jamroz
Atmospheric Pressure Plasma-Mediated Synthesis of Platinum Nanoparticles Stabilized by Poly(vinylpyrrolidone) with Application in Heat Management Systems for Internal Combustion Chambers
Reprinted from: *Nanomaterials* 2018, 8, 619, doi:10.3390/nano8080619 76

Anna Dzimitrowicz, Agata Motyka-Pomagruk, Piotr Cyganowski, Weronika Babinska, Dominik Terefinko, Piotr Jamroz, Ewa Lojkowska, Pawel Pohl and Wojciech Sledz
Antibacterial Activity of Fructose-Stabilized Silver Nanoparticles Produced by Direct Current Atmospheric Pressure Glow Discharge towards Quarantine Pests
Reprinted from: *Nanomaterials* 2018, 8, 751, doi:10.3390/nano8100751 91

James Aluha, Stéphane Gutierrez, François Gitzhofer and Nicolas Abatzoglou
Use of Plasma-Synthesized Nano-Catalysts for CO Hydrogenation in Low-Temperature Fischer–Tropsch Synthesis: Effect of Catalyst Pre-Treatment
Reprinted from: *Nanomaterials* 2018, 8, 822, doi:10.3390/nano8100822 107

Shota Tamura, Tsutomu Mashimo, Kenta Yamamoto, Zhazgul Kelgenbaeva, Weijan Ma,
Xuesong Kang, Michio Koinuma, Hiroshi Isobe and Akira Yoshiasa
Synthesis of Pd-Fe System Alloy Nanoparticles by Pulsed Plasma in Liquid
Reprinted from: *Nanomaterials* **2018**, *8*, 1068, doi:10.3390/nano8121068 . . . . **138**

About the Special Issue Editor

Pawel Pohl received his PhD and DSc degrees in chemistry from the Faculty of Chemistry, Wroclaw University of Science and Technology (WUST) in Poland in 2002 and 2009, respectively. Since 2017, he has been a professor of chemistry at the same university. He is currently the head of the Analytical Chemistry and Chemical Metallurgy Division at the Faculty of Chemistry of WUST. His research and scientific interests focus on i) the hyphenation of the chromatographic separation and pre-concentration techniques (LC, HPLC, CE, SPE) with the spectrometric methods of detection (ICP-OES, ICP-MS, FAAS, ETAAS, MS/MS) for the speciation and fractionation analysis of metals and metalloids, ii) the development and application of chemical vapor generation (CVG) techniques for the analytical atomic and mass spectrometry, as well as iii) the analytical and spectroscopic characteristics of the cold atmospheric pressure plasmas (CAPPs) and their applications in analytical chemistry, biology, medicine and technology. He has published 175 JCR articles and five book chapters. The h-index of these works is 30 and they have already been cited over 3200 times.

Preface to "Plasma-Based Synthesis and Modification of Nanomaterials"

This book, entitled "Plasma-Based Synthesis and Modification of Nanomaterials", is a collection of nine original research articles [1–9] devoted to the application of different atmospheric pressure (APPs) and low-pressure (LPPs) plasmas for the synthesis or modification of various nanomaterials (NMs) of exceptional properties. The contributing works [1–9] also show the structural and morphological characterization of the synthesized NMs and their further interesting and unique applications in different areas of science and technology. The readers interested in the capabilities of plasma-based treatments will quickly be convinced that APPs and LPPs enable one to efficiently synthesize or modify differentiated NMs using a minimal number of operations. Indeed, the procedures described in the collected articles [1–9] are eco-friendly and usually involve single-step processes, thus considerably lowering the labor investment and costs. As a result, the production of new NMs and their functionalization is more straightforward and can be carried out on a much larger scale, compared to other methods and procedures involving complex chemical treatments and processes. The size and morphology, as well as the structural and optical properties of the resulting NMs are tunable and tailorable. In addition to leading to the desirable and reproducible physical dimensions, crystallinity, functionality, and spectral properties of the resultant NMs, another benefit of the plasma-based synthesis and modification is that the fabricated NMs are ready to be used prior to their specific applications, without any initial pre-treatments.

The full text of the Editorial of the Nanomaterials Special Issue "Plasma based Synthesis and Modification of Nanomaterials" with a concise description of all the contributing articles can be found at https://www.mdpi.com/2079-4991/9/2/278.

Pawel Pohl
Special Issue Editor

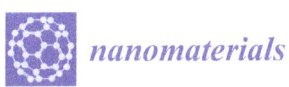

Editorial

Plasma-Based Synthesis and Modification of Nanomaterials

Pawel Pohl

Division of Analytical Chemistry and Chemical Metallurgy, Faculty of Chemistry, Wroclaw University of Science and Technology, Wyspianskiego 27, 50370 Wroclaw, Poland; pawel.pohl@pwr.edu.pl; Tel./Fax: +48-72-3202494

Received: 17 January 2019; Accepted: 14 February 2019; Published: 16 February 2019

This Special Issue of Nanomaterials, including nine original research works [1–9], is devoted to the application of different atmospheric pressure (APP) and low-pressure (LPP) plasmas for synthesis or modification of various nanomaterials (NMs) of exceptional properties. This is followed by their structural and morphological characterization and further interesting and unique applications in different areas of science and technology. All readers interested in the capabilities of plasma-based treatments will quickly be convinced that APPs and LPPs enable one to efficiently synthesize or modify differentiated NMs using a minimal number of operations. Indeed, the procedures described in the collected articles are eco-friendly and usually involve single-step processes, thus considerably lowering labor investment and costs. As a result, the production of new NMs and their functionalization is more straightforward and can be carried out on a much larger scale, compared to other methods and procedures involving complex chemical treatments and processes. The size and morphology, as well as structural and optical properties, of resulting NMs are tunable and tailorable. In addition to leading to desirable and reproducible physical dimensions, crystallinity, functionality, and spectral properties of the resultant NMs, another benefit of plasma-based synthesis and modification is that fabricated NMs are ready-to-use prior to their specific applications, without any initial pre-treatments.

Among the discharges and plasmas applied for plasma-mediated synthesis or modification of NMs, the readers can find, for example: impulse plasma in a solution initiated by spark discharge between two metallic electrodes immersed in this solution [1]; atmospheric pressure plasma jets provided by dielectric barrier discharge (DBD) operated in Ar–H_2 [2] or Ar–O_2, Ar–N_2, and Ar–NH_3 [5] mixtures; atmospheric pressure glow discharges (APGDs) generated in air between solid metallic electrodes and flowing solutions [3,4,6]; low-pressure capacitively coupled plasma (CCP) sustained in O_2 or N_2 between two electrodes, one being at the end of a chamber field with ionic liquids or low boiling point solvents [7]; and contact glow discharge electrolysis (CGDE) [8] or liquid phase plasma (LPP) [9], operated in both cases between two electrodes immersed in solutions of different compositions. Plasma-chemical processes and reactions occurring directly in plasmas or at interfacial zones between gaseous phases of these plasmas and liquids led to the fabrication of various metal-, nonmetal- and carbon-based NMs, including bimetallic Pd–Fe nanoparticles (NPs) formed by melting and eroding Pd–Fe electrodes [1], fructose-functionalized AgNPs [3], PVP-stabilized PtNPs [4], and pectin-stabilized AgNPs [6] (all synthesized by the reduction of appropriate ions of these metals dissolved in solutions), carbon dots (CDs) formed by irradiation of aliphatic acids dispersed in viscous media, SiNPs fabricated by melting and eroding Si electrodes under plasma heat [8], and nanocomposites supported by Fe_3O_4 NPs on N-doped activated carbon [9]. Interestingly, NMs were also synthesized by introducing suspensions of substrates into a plasma torch (suspension-plasma spray, SPS) [2] to form Co/C, Fe/C, and Co–Fe/C NMs, containing a nanometallic phase in addition to carbide and oxide phases of Co and Fe. Immersing plasma jets in liquid suspensions, it was possible to modify the surface of dispersed nanocellulose (NC) fibers [5].

The morphological, structural, and functional properties of NMs result in their having a wide variety of applications, e.g., as catalysts for the Fischer–Tropsch synthesis of CH_4 from H_2 and

CO [2], antimicrobial agents against different phytopathogenic bacteria [3], heat conductive media in heat management systems [4], necrotic agents toward cancerous cells of the human melanoma cell line [6], fluorescence sensors for detecting and measuring metal ions and flavonoids in solutions [7], and materials for the production of anodes in lithium-ion batteries [8] or electrochemical capacitor electrodes [9].

I sincerely thank all of the authors who sent their valuable works to this Special Issue on Plasma-Based Synthesis and Modification of Nanomaterials. All interested readers are encouraged to become familiar with these works and use discharges and plasmas in their future research on plasma-mediated synthesis or functionalization of nanomaterials.

Acknowledgments: This work was funded by a statutory activity subsidy from the Polish Ministry of Science and Higher Education for the Faculty of Chemistry of Wroclaw University of Science and Technology (Poland).

References

1. Tamura, S.; Mashimo, T.; Yamamoto, K.; Kelgenbaeva, Z.; Ma, W.; Kang, X.; Koinuma, M.; Isobe, H.; Yoshiasa, A. Synthesis of Pd-Fe System Alloy Nanoparticles by Pulsed Plasma in Liquid. *Nanomaterials* **2018**, *8*, 1068. [CrossRef] [PubMed]
2. Aluha, J.; Gutierrez, S.; Gitzhofer, F.; Abatzoglou, N. Use of Plasma-Synthesized Nano-Catalysts for CO Hydrogenation in Low-Temperature Fischer–Tropsch Synthesis: Effect of Catalyst Pre-Treatment. *Nanomaterials* **2018**, *8*, 822. [CrossRef] [PubMed]
3. Dzimitrowicz, A.; Motyka-Pomagruk, A.; Cyganowski, P.; Babinska, W.; Terefinko, D.; Jamroz, P.; Lojkowska, E.; Pohl, P.; Sledz, W. Antibacterial Activity of Fructose-Stabilized Silver Nanoparticles Produced by Direct Current Atmospheric Pressure Glow Discharge towards Quarantine Pests. *Nanomaterials* **2018**, *8*, 751. [CrossRef] [PubMed]
4. Dzimitrowicz, A.; Cyganowski, P.; Pohl, P.; Jermakowicz-Bartkowiak, D.; Terefinko, D.; Jamroz, P. Atmospheric Pressure Plasma-Mediated Synthesis of Platinum Nanoparticles Stabilized by Poly(vinylpyrrolidone) with Application in Heat Management Systems for Internal Combustion Chambers. *Nanomaterials* **2018**, *8*, 619. [CrossRef] [PubMed]
5. Panaitescu, D.M.; Vizireanu, S.; Nicolae, C.A.; Frone, A.N.; Casarica, A.; Carpen, L.G.; Dinescu, G. Treatment of Nanocellulose by Submerged Liquid Plasma for Surface Functionalization. *Nanomaterials* **2018**, *8*, 467. [CrossRef] [PubMed]
6. Dzimitrowicz, A.; Bielawska-Pohl, A.; DiCenzo, G.C.; Jamroz, P.; Macioszczyk, J.; Klimczak, A.; Pohl, P. Pulse-Modulated Radio-Frequency Alternating-Current-Driven Atmospheric-Pressure Glow Discharge for Continuous-Flow Synthesis of Silver Nanoparticles and Evaluation of Their Cytotoxicity toward Human Melanoma Cells. *Nanomaterials* **2018**, *8*, 398. [CrossRef] [PubMed]
7. Ke, C.-B.; Lu, T.-L.; Chen, J.-L. Capacitively Coupled Plasma Discharge of Ionic Liquid Solutions to Synthesize Carbon Dots as Fluorescent Sensors. *Nanomaterials* **2018**, *8*, 372. [CrossRef] [PubMed]
8. Saito, G.; Sasaki, H.; Takahashi, H.; Sakaguchi, N. Solution-Plasma-Mediated Synthesis of Si Nanoparticles for Anode Material of Lithium-Ion Batteries. *Nanomaterials* **2018**, *8*, 286. [CrossRef] [PubMed]
9. Lee, H.; Lee, W.-J.; Park, Y.-K.; Ki, S.; Kim, B.-J.; Jung, S.-C. Liquid Phase Plasma Synthesis of Iron Oxide Nanoparticles on Nitrogen-Doped Activated Carbon Resulting in Nanocomposite for Supercapacitor Applications. *Nanomaterials* **2018**, *8*, 190. [CrossRef]

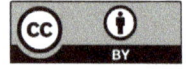

© 2019 by the author. Licensee MDPI, Basel, Switzerland. This article is an open access article distributed under the terms and conditions of the Creative Commons Attribution (CC BY) license (http://creativecommons.org/licenses/by/4.0/).

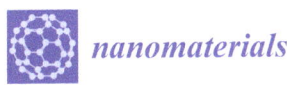

Article

Liquid Phase Plasma Synthesis of Iron Oxide Nanoparticles on Nitrogen-Doped Activated Carbon Resulting in Nanocomposite for Supercapacitor Applications

Heon Lee [1], Won-June Lee [1], Young-Kwon Park [2], Seo Jin Ki [3], Byung-Joo Kim [4] and Sang-Chul Jung [1],*

[1] Department of Environmental Engineering, Sunchon National University, Suncheon 57922, Korea; honylee@hanmail.net (H.L.); lone0486@naver.com (W.-J.L.)
[2] School of Environmental Engineering, University of Seoul, Seoul 02504, Korea; catalica@uos.ac.kr
[3] Department of Environmental Engineering, Gyeongnam National University of Science and Technology, Jinju 52725, Korea; seojinki@gmail.com
[4] R&D Division, Korea Institute of Carbon Convergence Technology, Jeonju 54853, Korea; kimbj2015@gmail.com
* Correspondence: jsc@sunchon.ac.kr; Tel.: +82-61-750-3814

Received: 3 March 2018; Accepted: 23 March 2018; Published: 25 March 2018

Abstract: Iron oxide nanoparticles supported on nitrogen-doped activated carbon powder were synthesized using an innovative plasma-in-liquid method, called the liquid phase plasma (LPP) method. Nitrogen-doped carbon (NC) was prepared by a primary LPP reaction using an ammonium chloride reactant solution, and an iron oxide/NC composite (IONCC) was prepared by a secondary LPP reaction using an iron chloride reactant solution. The nitrogen component at 3.77 at. % formed uniformly over the activated carbon (AC) surface after a 1 h LPP reaction. Iron oxide nanoparticles, 40~100 nm in size, were impregnated homogeneously over the NC surface after the LPP reaction, and were identified as Fe_3O_4 by X-ray photoelectron spectroscopy and X-ray diffraction. NC and IONCCs exhibited pseudo-capacitive characteristics, and their specific capacitance and cycling stability were superior to those of bare AC. The nitrogen content on the NC surface increased the compatibility and charge transfer rate, and the composites containing iron oxide exhibited a lower equivalent series resistance.

Keywords: liquid phase plasma; activated carbon powder; iron oxide nanoparticle; nitrogen-doped carbon; pseudo-capacitive characteristics

1. Introduction

Recently, the hybrid electric vehicles (HEV) and plug-in electric vehicles (PEV) have attracted attention and are showing rapid growth [1–3]. HEV and PEV require a low-resistance, high-voltage secondary battery and a supercapacitor [4,5]. Supercapacitors have received a great deal of interest because of their higher power densities compared to batteries and higher energy densities than conventional capacitors [6,7].

The capacitance of a supercapacitor can be changed according to the electrode material [8,9]. Therefore, there has been considerable interest in discovering ideal materials for supercapacitor electrodes with respect to different metal oxides [10,11] and carbonaceous materials [12,13]. Among the metal oxides investigated thus far, iron oxide is considered one of the most attractive because it displays high theoretical capacity, and is inexpensive [14–16]. Carbonaceous materials, particularly activated carbon (AC), are the most widely used electrode materials of electrochemical double layer capacitors

(EDLCs) because of their large specific surface area, size adjustment of pores, chemical stability, lower weight, low cost, excellent electrical conductivity, and environmental friendliness [17,18]. Many researchers have prepared carbon electrode materials with a high specific capacitance for EDLCs [19,20]. The introduction of electronic conductivity by doping the carbon matrix with nitrogen is a promising alternative to enhancing the specific surface area [21,22]. Two methods for nitrogen doping have been reported: carbonization of abundant nitrogen such as polypyrrole from nitrogen-containing precursors [23,24] and introducing nitrogen-containing reagents such as ammonia, urea, amines, and melamine to the carbon matrix [25–27]. Recently, the plasma generated from the liquid phase has been used to synthesize metal oxide nanoparticles, which were then impregnated with carbonaceous materials [28–30]. In previous studies, carbon composites impregnated with metal oxide nanoparticles were synthesized using a liquid phase plasma (LPP) method and applied to EDLCs [31–33]. In particular, the LPP method does not require the use of any additional reducing agent, and is a very simple process for producing composites in a single step [29,34].

In this study, the LPP method was used to dope nitrogen and impregnate iron oxide nanoparticles on the AC surface. The composition, shape, and chemical state of the fabricated composite produced from the LPP reaction was quantitatively and qualitatively analyzed by various instruments. Also, the effects of the amounts of nitrogen loaded and iron oxide particles impregnated on the AC surface on the electrochemical performance for the prepared composites were investigated in detail. Specifically, the main research questions of this research are (1) whether the specific capacitance of the prepared composite increased with increasing quantity of iron oxide precipitate or not, and (2) whether the composite showed resistance with the highest initial resistance slope or not.

2. Materials and Methods

2.1. Materials and Chemicals

Activated carbon powder (YP-50F, Kuraray Chemical Co. Ltd., Osaka, Japan) was used as the electrode active material. Ammonium chloride (NH_4Cl, Daejung Chemicals & Metals Co., Siheung, Republic of Korea) was used for doping the activated carbon powder with nitrogen. We specifically selected ammonium chloride that were an alkaline substance with high solubility in water, as compared to urea, glycine, nitric acid, etc., to minimize the effect of precursor type and concentration on the LPP process in terms of both conductivity and pH. However, a significant reduction of pH was still observed in the reactant solution after the LPP reaction. Nitrogen-doped activated carbon powder was subjected to the LPP reaction to impregnate iron oxide nanoparticles using iron chloride tetrahydrate ($FeCl_2 \cdot 4H_2O$, Kanto Chemical, Tokyo, Japan) as the precursor. Cetrimonium bromide (CTAB, $CH_3(CH_2)_{15}N(Br)(CH_3)_3$, Sigma-Aldrich, St. Louis, MO, USA) was added to the LPP reactant solution to disperse iron oxide nanoparticles on the surface of nitrogen doped activated carbon. All chemicals used in this study were reagent-grade chemicals and ultra-pure water (Biological industries, Beit, Israel) was used to prepare the aqueous LPP reaction solutions.

2.2. Experimental Device

The LPP system was used in the same process for the nitrogen doping on the surface of AC or impregnating iron oxide nanoparticles on nitrogen doped activated carbon. The LPP device consisted of a power generator, a reaction unit, and a cooling system. Details of the configuration and specifications of the LPP device are reported elsewhere [31,32]. In both processes, the plasma operating conditions were a frequency of 30 kHz, a pulse width of 5 µs, and an applied voltage of 250 V. The quartz LPP reactor is a double tube type with an outer diameter and height of 40 and 80 mm, respectively. The batch type reactor was filled with the reaction aqueous solution, and the outer channel was circulated with cooling water at 268 K. The cooling system played an important role in eliminating the effect of temperature, which is highly elevated during the LPP reaction due to energy released by arc plasma in the reactant solution on the generated nanoparticles. The spacing of the tungsten electrodes embedded in the ceramic insulators was maintained at 1.0 mm.

2.3. Preparation of Nitrogen Doped Carbon

Nitrogen doped carbon (NC) was synthesized through the LPP reaction. NH_4Cl, as the nitrogen precursor, was added to 200 mL of ultrapure water to make a 10 mM solution and 0.5 g of AC was then added and stirred for 30 min to prepare the LPP reaction aqueous solution. Plasma was generated in this aqueous reaction solution for 60 min to dope the AC with nitrogen. This is because both the amount of iron oxide nanoparticles generated and the efficiency of nitrogen doped carbon are increased only up to 60 min of the LPP reaction. After the LPP reaction, the NC powder was centrifuged and washed three times with ultrapure water to remove the impurities. Finally, NC was prepared by drying in a vacuum oven at 353 K for 24 h.

2.4. Preparation of IONCC

Iron oxide nanoparticles were impregnated into NC using the LPP reaction. A 0.5 g sample of NC powder prepared by the LPP reaction was added to 200 mL of ultrapure water containing CTAB and dispersed by stirring. Iron chloride (5 and 10 mM) was then added to the reactant solution, which was then dissolved by stirring for 10 min. Plasma was generated for 60 min to prepare the NC composite impregnated with iron oxide nanoparticles. The resulting iron oxide/NC composite (IONCC) powder was washed and dried using the same method for NC production.

2.5. Electrochemical Test

A half-coin cell was prepared using IONCC powders and its electrical properties as a supercapacitor electrode were assessed. The slurry for the coin cell was prepared by dissolving the active material (80%), conductive agent (acetylene black, 10%), and binder (polyvinylidene fluoride, 10%) in a N-methyl pyrrolidinone solvent. The active material:conductive agent:binder were mixed at a ratio of 80:10:10 wt. % to prepare the slurry. Here, IONCC powders, super-P (TIMCAL graphite & carbon com., Bironico, Switzerland), and polyvinylidene fluoride were used as the active material, conductive agent, and binder, respectively. The slurry was coated on Ni foil and dried for 60 min in a convection oven at 393 K. The resulting powder was then roll-pressed and dried in a vacuum oven at 373 K for 60 min to produce a half-coin cell. The electrolyte was a 6M KOH solution and the separator was 150 µm glass felt. The current-voltage (C–V) curve was measured at a scan rate of 10 mV/s, and actuation voltage from 0.1 to 0.8 V. All electrochemical properties were measured using VSP potentiostat (Bio-logic Science Instruments, Seyssinet-Pariset, France). Three coin cells were prepared under the same conditions, and the electrochemical properties reported are the mean values.

2.6. Structural Characterization

The elemental composition and dispersity of the as-prepared NC composite and IONCC were examined by field-emission scanning electron microscopy (FE-SEM, JSM-7100F, JEOL, Tokyo, Japan). The size and shape of the iron oxide nanoparticles in the IONCC were observed by high resolution field emission transmission electron microscopy (HR-FETEM, JEM-2100F, JEOL, Tokyo, Japan). The chemical structures of NC and IONCC were analyzed by X-photoelectron spectroscopy (XPS, Multilab 2000 system, Thermo Fisher Scientific, Waltham, MA, USA) and X-ray diffraction (XRD, XRD-7000, SHIMADZU Corp., Kyoto, Japan). The specific surface area and pore size distribution of the IONCC were examined using a surface area analyzer (Belsorp mini II, MicrotracBEL Corp., Osaka, Japan).

3. Results and Discussion

3.1. Characteristics of IONCC

The chemical composition and dispersibility of the IONCCs prepared by the LPP process were measured by energy dispersive spectroscopy (EDS) and element-mapping attached to the FE-SEM. Figure 1 presents the EDS spectrum, real image, and the mapping image of each chemical component of the IONCC produced by the LPP process.

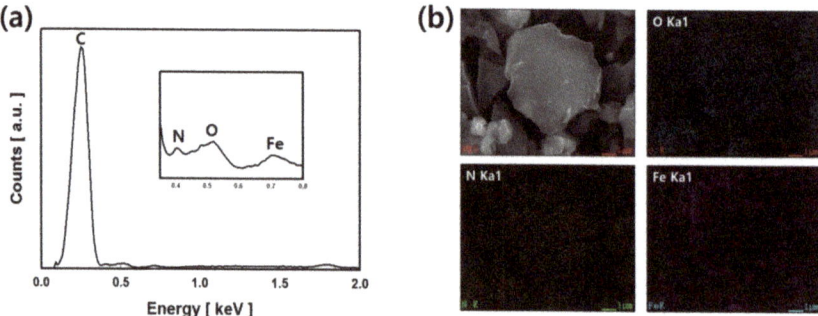

Figure 1. EDS spectrum (**a**); SEM image and element-mapping images; (**b**) of IONCC prepared by two LPP reactions.

The sample was prepared by first fabricating a NC by the LPP reaction in an aqueous ammonium chloride solution, followed by a second LPP reaction at an iron chloride concentration of 10 mM. A strong peak of carbon was observed at 0.25 keV in the EDS spectrum. Doped nitrogen (N kα) was observed at 0.39 keV after the first LPP reaction, and iron (Fe Kα) impregnated was noted at 0.77 keV after the second LPP reaction. In the mapping images, oxygen, nitrogen, and iron were marked with green dots, yellow dots, and purple dots, respectively. The mapping image revealed nitrogen and iron well dispersed over the AC surface. These results suggest that AC is doped with nitrogen by the plasma generated in the ammonium chloride solution. The iron nanoparticles adhered to the AC surface by the LPP reaction.

Table 1 lists the chemical compositions of NC and IONCCs prepared by the LPP reactions determined by EDS. The chemical composition of bare AC (YP-50F) used as an electrode active material in this study was composed of 97.06% carbon and 2.29% oxygen (at. %). Approximately 3% oxygen was detected from the oxygen-containing functional groups attached to the AC surface. Oxygen-containing functional groups are formed in the acid treatment during the production of AC. On the other hand, the nitrogen component at 3.77 at. % was detected in NC. Therefore, a nitrogen-containing functional group is formed on the AC surface when the LPP process is performed for 60 min in an aqueous ammonium chloride solution containing AC. The IONCCs were prepared by varying the initial iron chloride concentration to 5 mM (IONCC-5) and 10 mM (IONCC-10), respectively. The iron content of IONCC-5 and IONCC-10 was 0.51 and 0.89 at. %, respectively. The quantity of iron nanoparticles impregnated in the AC surface increased with increasing initial iron chloride concentration. Generating plasma in the liquid phase is usually based on a streamer discharge or spark discharge. When spark discharge occurs in the liquid phase, a large quantity of electrons, ozone and oxygen bubbles, strong ultraviolet rays, various free radicals, and over-pressure shock waves are generated [35]. Therefore, ammonium ions (NH_4^+) are reduced by the many electrons generated in the reaction solution to form nitrogen-containing functional groups on the AC surface. In addition, the iron ions are also reduced by these electrons and imprinted on the AC surface. The amount of oxygen contained in the NC was higher than that in bare AC, which means that AC was oxidized by the LPP reaction. In addition, the amount of oxygen contained in the IONCC was higher than that of NC. Therefore, NC was oxidized by the LPP reaction, in which iron nanoparticles were impregnated. When plasma is generated in the liquid phase, it can instantaneously generate a strong electric field, which produces a range of active chemical species (O_2^-, $^1O_2$, O^*, O_3, OH^*, HO_2, H_2O_2, etc.) [36,37]. The AC and NC were assumed to be oxidized by these strong oxidizing active species generated in the LPP reaction aqueous solution to increase the oxygen content. On the other hand, the oxygen content of IONCC-10 synthesized at high initial iron precursor concentrations was higher than that of IONCC-5. This was caused by the impregnation reaction of iron nanoparticles, and it was presumed that iron oxide nanoparticles are formed in the LPP reaction of this study.

Table 1. Chemical composition of bare AC and as-prepared composites using the LPP reaction with different initial iron precursor concentrations

Samples	Carbon		Oxygen		Nitrogen		Iron	
	wt. %	at. %	wt. %	at. %	wt. %	at. %	wt. %	at. %
Bare AC	96.13	97.06	3.87	2.94	0.00	0.00	0.00	0.00
NC	91.40	92.96	4.28	3.27	4.32	3.77	0.00	0.00
IONCC-5	88.94	92.21	4.83	3.76	3.96	3.52	2.27	0.51
IONCC-10	87.55	92.02	5.24	4.14	3.27	2.95	3.94	0.89

Various chemically active species can be formed in the plasma field provided to the reactant aqueous solution. In this study, the chemically active species were characterized by optical emission spectroscopy (OES, AvaSpec-3648, Avantes, Apeldoorn, the Netherlands). Figure 2 shows the spectra emitted from the ultrapure water and IONCC-10 LPP reactant aqueous solution. In ultrapure water, molecular bands of hydroxyl radicals (OH•) with the excited states of atomic H and atomic O were observed in the emission spectrum [38,39]. In the reactant solution of IONCC-10, iron peaks were newly observed in the 340 to 440 nm regions along with those chemical species observed in ultrapure water. They revealed atomic iron (Fe_I ground state electron configuration $1s^2 2s^2 2p^6 3s^2 3p^6 3d^6 4s^2$, $^5D^4$) peaks at 344.0, 358.1, 373.7, 382.0, 404.5, and 438.3 nm [40]. The LPP process can produce powerful plasma instantaneously and releases strong electric fields that generate numerous electrochemical species [35]. In addition, a very rapid reaction is followed by the active species and radicals generated under the high temperature of the LPP process cause very rapid reactions [36]. The LPP reaction applied in this study is caused by electrons and these active species. Iron oxide particles are formed by reacting charged species (i.e., ions) from iron precursor in the reactant solution with active species generated from the LPP process.

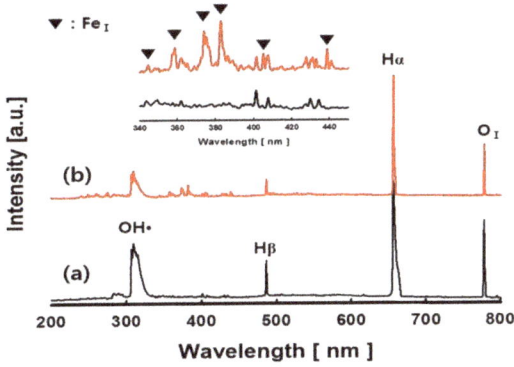

Figure 2. Spatially and temporally integrated emission spectra for the pulsed electric discharge. (a) ultrapure water, (b) IONCC-10 reactant solution.

XPS was performed to examine the chemical state and structure of nitrogen and iron particles of the IONCC synthesized by the LPP method. Figure 3 shows the high resolution narrow-range XPS spectrum of carbon, oxygen, nitrogen, and iron of IONCC-10. In the C 1s region, peaks were observed at 282.9, 284.3, 285.2, 286.6, and 288.7 eV, which were assigned to carbide carbon, graphitic carbon, C=N, C–O, and C=O bonds, respectively [41,42]. These results show that ammonium in the reactant aqueous solution reacts with AC to form a C=N bond by the LPP reaction. The observed C–O and C=O bonds can be attributed to an approximately 3% carbon content originally contained in the AC, or oxidized AC surface by the excited oxygen and hydroxyl radicals produced by the LPP process. In the O 1s region, a large Fe–O peak was observed at 530.0 eV and peaks due to C–O and C–O–C were observed at 531.4 and 533.2 eV, respectively [43]. These results show that iron doped on the NC surface by the LPP method is in the form of iron oxide nanoparticles. C–O–C and C–O bonds were observed in the C 1s region. This may also be the carbon bond that the AC had from the beginning, or it could have been formed by the LPP reaction. In the N 1s region, peaks were observed at 399.3, 400.3, and 401.6 eV, which were assigned to N-pyridinic, N-pyrrolic/pyridonic, and graphitic nitrogen, respectively [44,45]. The LPP process shows that various nitrogen-containing functional groups are generated on the AC surface. Similar peaks in the N1s region were observed between NC and IONCC, which indicated the iron oxide nanoparticles generated from the LPP reaction did not affect nitrogen loaded on the AC surface. In the Fe 2p region, peaks were observed at 710.9 and 724.6 eV, which were assigned to Fe $2p_{1/2}$ and Fe $2p_{3/2}$, respectively. The spin orbital splitting (SOS) interval of Fe $2p_{1/2}$ and Fe $2p_{3/2}$ peaks was 13.6 eV. Therefore, the iron oxide nanoparticles synthesized by the LPP method are Fe_3O_4 [46]. The peaks at 710.9 and 712.8 eV in the Fe $2p_{3/2}$ region were attributed to Fe^{2+} and Fe^{3+}, and are associated with the peaks at 724.3 and 726.7 eV in the Fe $2p_{1/2}$ region [47]. In addition, the peaks observed at 714.6 and 718.8 eV are the satellite peaks of Fe^{2+} and Fe^{3+}, respectively, which are similar to previous reports [48,49]. When the chemical state of as-prepared composites as well as their chemical composition were reviewed by XPS, the elemental composition for IONCC-5, 10, and NC was in good agreement with that of EDS in FE-SEM (see Table 1).

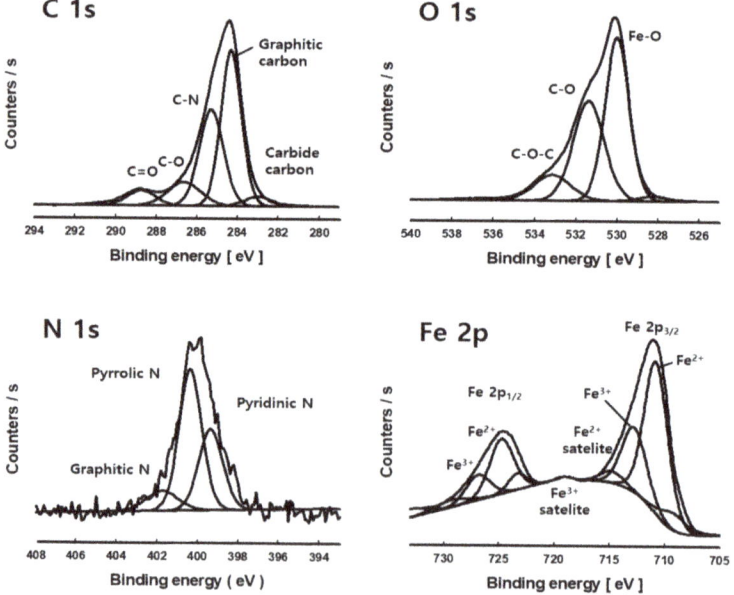

Figure 3. High resolution XPS spectra of C 1s, O 1s, N 1s, and Fe 2p region of IONCC-10 prepared by the LPP method.

Figure 4 presents XRD patterns of NC and IONCC-10 synthesized by the LPP process along with the pattern of AC. In the spectrum of bare AC, the 002 and 101 planes of carbon were observed at 24.5 and 43.9° 2θ. NC showed a similar pattern to bare AC but the peak of the 002 plane was broader, which was assigned to amorphous nitrogen doping of the AC surface by the LPP reaction [50,51]. As shown in Table 1, the content of iron oxide nanoparticles impregnated in IONCCs was less than 1 at. %, which was difficult to observe by XRD. On the other hand, in the IONCC-10 samples, the peaks for the 311 and 440 planes Fe_3O_4 were observed at 35.4 and 62.5° 2θ, respectively [52,53]. Therefore, the iron impregnated on the NC surface by the LPP reaction is iron oxide, which agrees with the EDS and XPS results.

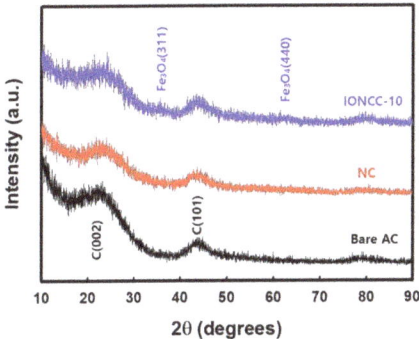

Figure 4. X-ray diffraction pattern of bare AC, NC, and IONCC-10.

Iron oxide nanoparticles on the IONCC-10 synthesized by the LPP method was observed by FE-TEM, as shown in Figure 5, along with the elemental mapping image. The iron oxide nanoparticles produced by the LPP reaction had a size ranging from 40 to 100 nm. As shown in Figure 5a, approximately 40–100 nm of iron oxide nanoparticles were clustered on the IONCC surface. In the mapping images, iron, oxygen, and nitrogen were marked with yellow, white, and red dots, respectively. The particles on the NC surface were composed of iron and oxygen components. Oxygen was also found on the IONCC surface, which is consistent with the EDS and XPS results. On the other hand, nitrogen was distributed uniformly over the IONCC surface. The LPP reaction using the ammonium chloride reactant solution resulted in nitrogen being doped uniformly over the AC surface.

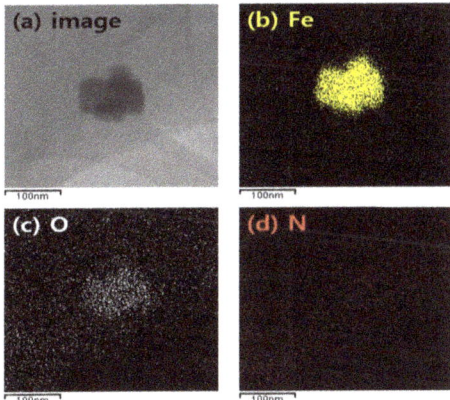

Figure 5. FE-TEM image and elemental mapped results of iron oxide nanoparticle on the IONCC-10; (**a**) TEM image; (**b**) iron; (**c**) oxygen; and (**d**) nitrogen element.

The effects of nitrogen doping and the impregnation of iron oxide nanoparticles on the surface area and pore diameter of AC were evaluated. Figure 6a shows the adsorption-desorption isotherm curves of N_2 gas at 77 K for each sample. The hysteresis zone of the mesopore was observed in all samples and the hysteresis area of NC and IONCC decreased compared to bare AC. In the case of NC, the pores were blocked by the nitrogen generated on the AC surface in the LPP reaction, and the hysteresis area of the mesopore decreased [54,55]. In the case of the IONCCs, the N_2 isotherm curves were affected by the iron oxide nanoparticles produced on the NC surface. Figure 6b presents the pore size distribution (PSD) measured by the Barrett, Joyner, and Halenda (BJH) method. Bare AC had a structure with developed mesopores, 2–5 nm in size. On the other hand, the pore size distribution of the mesopore tended to decrease in NC and IONACCs, as shown in Figure 6a, which is similar to the N_2 isotherm curve.

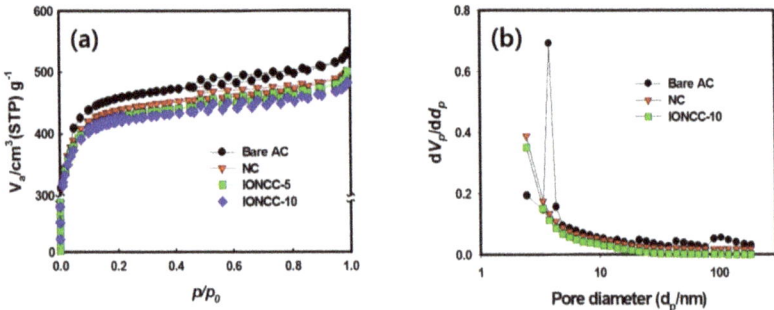

Figure 6. N_2 adsorption-desorption isotherm curve (**a**) and pore size distribution (PSD) (**b**) of bare AC and as-prepared composites.

Table 2 lists the surface area, total pore, and mean pore diameter measured using the Brunauer–Emmett–Teller (BET) method. The surface area and total pore volume of NC were smaller than those of bare AC and the mean pore size was also decreased. The micro- and mesopores are affected by the nitrogen generated on the AC surface by the LPP process and these values were reduced [42]. The surface area and total pore volume of IONCC-10 were smaller than IONCC-5 due to an increase in the amount of iron oxide nanoparticles added. This is because the proportion of iron oxide in the composite increases. In the case of the mean pore size, IONCCs were larger than NC. In addition, the mean pore size of IONCC-10 was larger than that of IONCC-5. The micro- and mesopore sizes of NC might have been blocked by the iron oxide particles produced by the LPP reaction.

Table 2. Textural properties of bare AC and as-prepared composite obtained through the LPP process with different iron precursor concentrations

Sample	BET Surface Area ($m^2 \cdot g^{-1}$)	Total Pore Volume ($cm^3 \cdot g^{-1}$)	Average Pore Size (nm)
Bare AC	1700.7	0.8189	1.9261
NC	1592.6	0.7756	1.8328
IONCC-5	1547.7	0.7691	1.8534
IONCC-10	1504.5	0.7435	1.8670

3.2. Electrochemical Measurement

The electrochemical properties of NC and IONCCs synthesized by the LPP process were measured and compared with those of bare AC. The results are shown in Figure 7. Figure 7a presents the C–V curve results measured by CV over the range of 0.1 to 0.8 V, at a rate of 10 mV/s. Bare AC showed a typical rectangular shape and the characteristics of the EDLC. On the other hand, NC and IONCCs exhibited pseudo-capacitive behavior, and the area of the C–V curve was increased compared to that of bare AC. Nitrogen bonded to the surface of the NC reduced the surface area (see Table 2), but improved the faradic interactions with 6M KOH due to the improved wettability [56]. In addition, the C–V curve area tended to increase with increasing amount of iron oxide impregnated in IONCC because of the redox reaction by iron oxide [57]. Figure 7b shows the change in capacitance measured by repeating the charge–discharge process for 300 cycles. The initial specific capacitance of bare AC was 115.12 F/g, which decreased to 99.96 F/g after 300 cycles, showing 13.16% capacitance loss. The initial specific capacitance of NC was 119.98 F/g, which decreased to 105.18 F/g after 300 cycles, showing 12.33% capacitance loss. This has higher specific capacitance and stable cycling stability than that of bare AC because the hydrophilicity and reversibility of the redox reaction by nitrogen are increased [58]. The initial specific capacitance of IONCC-5 and IONCC-10 were 122.64 and 127.11, respectively. The specific capacitance increased with increasing amount of iron oxide impregnated by the LPP reaction, which can be observed as an increase in specific capacitance due to the redox reaction. The specific capacitance after the 300th cycle was 108.50 and 114.25 F/g, respectively, which showed a corresponding 11.52% and 10.11% loss ratio, indicating stable cycling stability compared to bare AC. Figure 7c presents a voltage-time (V–t) curve measured at a charge-discharge rate of 2 mA; the bare AC showed a typical symmetrical shape. Composites (NC, IONCCs) prepared by the LPP process exhibited pseudocapacitance behavior with a slight increase in the discharging process time. Figure 7d shows the results for a composite resistor measured over the range of 0.01 to 300 kHz. The semicircle in the high frequency region indicates the charge transfer resistance between the electrolyte and electrode, which is 9.18 Ω in the bare AC, and 8.41, 7.90, and 7.22 Ω in the NC, IONCC-5, and IONCC-10, respectively. The nitrogen content on the NC surface increased the compatibility and charge transfer rate. In the case of IONCCs, the conductivity of the electrode was improved by the iron oxide in the composites [59,60]. The slope in the low frequency region represents the capacitive behavior. Compared to the bare AC, the composites containing nitrogen and iron oxide exhibited pure capacitive behavior.

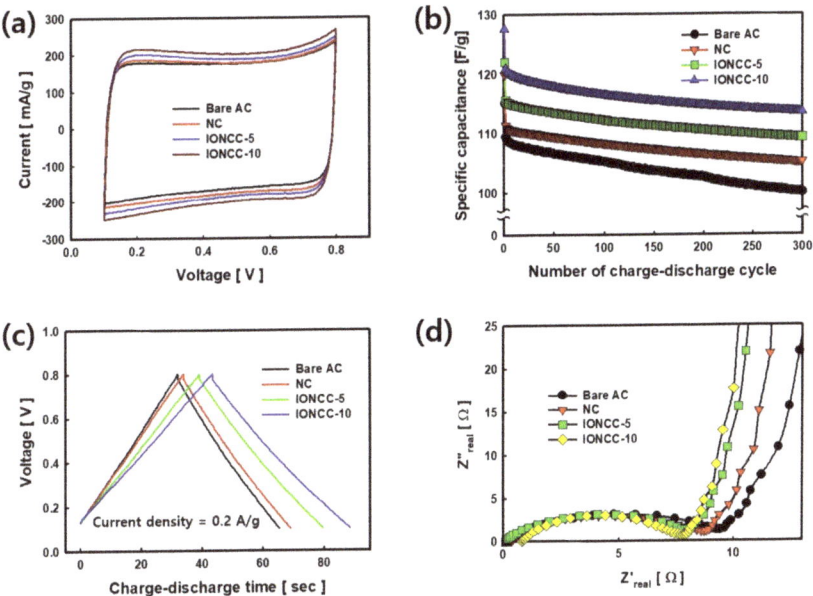

Figure 7. C–V curve (**a**); Cycling performance (**b**); V–t curve (**c**); and Nyquist plot (**d**) of bare AC and as-prepared composites using LPP method.

4. Conclusions

An electrochemical capacitor electrode was fabricated by doping with nitrogen and forming iron oxide nanoparticles on the AC surface using a LPP process. The following conclusions were obtained:

1. Nitrogen-doped carbon (NC) was prepared by a primary LPP reaction using an ammonium chloride reactant solution and nitrogen at a concentration of 3.77 at. % was formed uniformly over the AC surface.
2. Iron oxide/NC composite (IONCC) was prepared by a secondary LPP reaction using an iron chloride reactant solution. Iron oxide nanoparticles, 40–100 nm in size, were impregnated homogeneously over the NC surface, which were identified as Fe_3O_4 by XPS and XRD.
3. The amount of iron nanoparticles impregnated in the AC surface increased with increasing initial iron chloride concentration. The oxidation of AC and NC by the LPP reaction increased the oxygen content in the composites.
4. Bare AC exhibited a typical rectangular shape and the characteristic of EDLC. On the other hand, pseudo-capacitive behavior was observed in the NC and IONCCs, and the area of the C–V curve was greater than that of bare AC.
5. The nitrogen content on the NC surface increased the compatibility and charge transfer rate.
6. The impregnation of iron oxide nanoparticles on the NC by the LPP process improved the cycling stability of the EDLC and reduced the equivalent series resistance.

Acknowledgments: This work was supported by the Technology Innovation Program (10050391, Development of carbon-based electrode materials with 2000 m^2/g grade surface area for energy storage device) funded by the Ministry of Trade, industry & Energy (MI, Korea).

Author Contributions: H.L. and S.C.J. conceived and designed the experiments; H.L. and W.-J.L. performed the experiments; Y.-K.P., and B.-J.K. contributed to the analysis and the interpretation of data; H.L., S.J.K., and S.-C.J. wrote/edited/revised the paper.

Conflicts of Interest: The authors declare no conflict of interest.

References

1. Li, L.; Wang, X.; Song, J. Fuel consumption optimization for smart hybrid electric vehicle during a car-following process. *Mech. Syst. Signal Process.* **2017**, *87*, 17–29. [CrossRef]
2. He, X.; Wu, Y.; Zhang, S.; Tamor, M.A.; Wallington, T.J.; Shen, W.; Han, W.; Fu, L.; Hao, J. Individual trip chain distributions for passenger cars: Implications for market acceptance of battery electric vehicles and energy consumption by plug-in hybrid electric vehicles. *Appl. Energy* **2016**, *180*, 650–660. [CrossRef]
3. Guana, J.C.; Chena, B.C. Adaptive Power Management Strategy for a Four-Mode Hybrid Electric Vehicle. *Energy Procedia* **2017**, *105*, 2403–2408. [CrossRef]
4. Zhang, Z.; Zhang, X.; Chen, W.; Rasim, Y.; Salman, W.; Pan, H.; Yuan, Y.; Wang, C. A high-efficiency energy regenerative shock absorber using supercapacitors for renewable energy applications in range extended electric vehicle. *Appl. Energy* **2016**, *178*, 177–188. [CrossRef]
5. Capasso, C.; Veneri, O. Integration between super-capacitors and ZEBRA batteries as high performance hybrid storage system for electric vehicles. *Energy Procedia* **2017**, *105*, 2539–2544. [CrossRef]
6. Liu, Y.; Peng, X. Recent advances of supercapacitors based on two-dimensional materials. *Appl. Mater. Today* **2017**, *8*, 104–115. [CrossRef]
7. Yanik, M.O.; Yigit, E.A.; Akansu, Y.E.; Sahmetlioglu, E. Magnetic conductive polymer-graphene nanocomposites based supercapacitors for energy storage. *Energy* **2017**, *138*, 883–889. [CrossRef]
8. Tian, X.; Ma, H.; Li, Z.; Yan, S.; Ma, L.; Yu, F.; Wang, G.; Guo, X.; Ma, Y.; Wong, C. Flute type micropores activated carbon from cotton stalk for high performance supercapacitors. *J. Power Sources* **2017**, *359*, 88–96. [CrossRef]
9. Jin, E.M.; Lee, H.J.; Jun, H.B.; Jeong, S.M. Electrochemical properties of α-Co(OH)$_2$/graphene nano-flake thin film for use as a hybrid supercapacitor. *Korean J. Chem. Eng.* **2017**, *34*, 885–891. [CrossRef]

10. Gu, J.; Fan, X.; Liu, X.; Li, S.; Wang, Z.; Tang, S.; Yuan, D. Mesoporous manganese oxide with large specific surface area for high-performance asymmetric supercapacitor with enhanced cycling stability. *Chem. Eng. J.* **2017**, *324*, 35–43. [CrossRef]
11. Maheswari, N.; Muralidharan, G. Controlled synthesis of nanostructured molybdenum oxide electrodes for high performance supercapacitor devices. *Appl. Surf. Sci.* **2017**, *416*, 461–469. [CrossRef]
12. De, B.; Kuila, T.; Kim, N.H.; Lee, J.H. Carbon dot stabilized copper sulphide nanoparticles decorated graphene oxide hydrogel for high performance asymmetric supercapacitor. *Carbon* **2017**, *122*, 247–257. [CrossRef]
13. Tian, K.; Wei, L.; Zhang, X.; Jin, Y.; Guo, X. Membranes of carbon nanofibers with embedded MoO_3 nanoparticles showing superior cycling performance for all-solid-state flexible supercapacitors. *Mater. Today Energy* **2017**, *6*, 27–35. [CrossRef]
14. Yang, Q.; Bi, R.; Yung, K.; Pecht, M. Electrochemically reduced graphene oxides/nanostructured iron oxides as binder-free electrodes for supercapacitors. *Electrochim. Acta* **2017**, *231*, 125–134. [CrossRef]
15. Ghasemi, S.; Ahmadi, F. Effect of surfactant on the electrochemical performance of graphene/iron oxide electrode for supercapacitor. *J. Power Sources* **2015**, *289*, 129–137. [CrossRef]
16. Oh, I.; Kim, M.; Kim, J. Controlling hydrazine reduction to deposit iron oxides on oxidized activated carbon for supercapacitor application. *Energy* **2015**, *86*, 292–299. [CrossRef]
17. Bang, J.H.; Lee, H.M.; An, K.H.; Kim, B.J. A study on optimal pore development of modified commercial activated carbons for electrode materials of supercapacitors. *App. Surf. Sci.* **2017**, *415*, 61–66. [CrossRef]
18. Yu, M.; Han, Y.; Li, J.; Wang, L. CO_2-activated porous carbon derived from cattail biomass for removal of malachite green dye and application as supercapacitors. *Chem. Eng. J.* **2017**, *317*, 493–502. [CrossRef]
19. Zhao, C.; Ren, F.; Xue, X.; Zheng, W.; Wang, X.; Chang, L. A high-performance asymmetric supercapacitor based on $Co(OH)_2$/graphene and activated carbon electrodes. *J. Electroanal. Chem.* **2016**, *782*, 98–102. [CrossRef]
20. Ran, F.; Shen, K.; Tan, Y.; Peng, B.; Chen, S.; Zhang, W.; Niu, X.; Kong, L.; Kang, L. Activated hierarchical porous carbon as electrode membrane accommodated with triblock copolymer for supercapacitors. *J. Membr. Sci.* **2016**, *514*, 366–375. [CrossRef]
21. Ning, X.; Li, F.; Zhou, Y.; Miao, Y.; Wei, C.; Liu, T. Confined growth of uniformly dispersed $NiCo_2S_4$ nanoparticles on nitrogen-doped carbon nanofibers for high-performance asymmetric supercapacitors. *Chem. Eng. J.* **2017**, *328*, 599–608. [CrossRef]
22. Wang, C.; Wu, D.; Wang, H.; Gao, Z.; Xu, F.; Jiang, K. Nitrogen-doped two-dimensional porous carbon sheets derived from clover biomass for high performance supercapacitors. *J. Power Sources* **2017**, *363*, 375–383. [CrossRef]
23. Hulicova, D.; Yamashita, J.; Soneda, Y.; Hatori, H.; Kodama, M. Supercapacitors Prepared from Melamine-Based Carbon. *Chem. Mater.* **2005**, *17*, 1241–1247 [CrossRef]
24. Su, F.; Poh, C.K.; Chen, J.S.; Xu, G.; Wang, D.; Li, Q.; Lin, J.; Lou, X.W. Nitrogen-containing microporous carbon nanospheres with improved capacitive properties. *Energy Environ. Sci.* **2011**, *4*, 717–724. [CrossRef]
25. Hulicova-Jurcakova, D.; Kodama, M.; Shiraishi, S.; Hatori, H.; Zhu, Z.H.; Lu, G.Q. Nitrogen-Enriched Nonporous Carbon Electrodes with Extraordinary Supercapacitance. *Adv. Funct. Mater.* **2009**, *19*, 1800–1809. [CrossRef]
26. Candelaria, S.L.; Garcia, B.B.; Liu, D.; Cao, G. Nitrogen modification of highly porous carbon for improved supercapacitor performance. *J. Mater. Chem.* **2012**, *22*, 9884–9889. [CrossRef]
27. Tatsuru, S.; Yohei, N.; Taibou, Y.; Junko, H.; Nagahiro, S.; Osamu, T.; Akiharu, T.; Kazuhiro, N.; Youji, O. Functionalization of Multiwalled Carbon Nanotubes by Solution Plasma Processing in Ammonia Aqueous Solution and Preparation of Composite Material with Polyamide 6. *Jpn. J. Appl. Phys.* **2013**, *52*, 125101. [CrossRef]
28. Lee, H.; Park, Y.K.; Kim, S.J.; Kim, B.J.; An, K.H.; Kim, B.H.; Jung, S.C. Facile Synthesis of Iron Oxide/Graphene Nanocomposites Using Liquid Phase Plasma Method. *J. Nanosci. Nanotech.* **2016**, *16*, 4483–4486. [CrossRef]
29. Sun, S.H.; Jung, S.C. Facile synthesis of bimetallic Ni-Cu nanoparticles using liquid phase plasma method. *Korean J. Chem. Eng.* **2016**, *33*, 1075–1079. [CrossRef]
30. Chen, Q.; Li, J.; Li, Y. A review of plasma–liquid interactions for nanomaterial synthesis. *J. Phys. D Appl. Phys.* **2015**, *48*, 424005. [CrossRef]

31. Lee, H.; Kim, B.H.; Park, Y.K.; An, K.H.; Choi, Y.J.; Jung, S.C. Synthesis of cobalt oxide-manganese oxide on activated carbon electrodes for electrochemical capacitor application using a liquid phase plasma method. *Int. J. Hydrog. Energy* **2016**, *41*, 7582–7589. [CrossRef]
32. Lee, H.; Park, S.H.; Kim, S.J.; Park, Y.K.; Kim, B.J.; An, K.H.; Ki, S.J.; Jung, S.C. Synthesis of manganese oxide/activated carbon composites for supercapacitor application using a liquid phase plasma reduction system. *Int. J. Hydrog. Energy* **2015**, *40*, 754–759. [CrossRef]
33. Jung, S.C.; Kim, B.H.; Park, Y.K.; An, K.H.; Lee, H. Precipitation of Manganese and Nickel Nanoparticles on an Activated Carbon Powder for Electrochemical Capacitor Applications. *J. Nanosci. Nanotechnol.* **2016**, *16*, 11460–11464. [CrossRef]
34. Lee, H.; Kim, S.J.; An, K.H.; Kim, J.S.; Kim, B.H.; Jung, S.C. Application of Liquid Phase Plasma Process to the Synthesize Rutenium Oxide/activated Carbon Composite as Dielectric Naterial for Supercapacitor. *Adv. Mater. Lett.* **2016**, *7*, 98–103. [CrossRef]
35. Baroch, P.; Anita, V.; Saito, N.; Takai, O. Bipolar pulsed electrical discharge for decomposition of organic compounds in water. *J. Electrostat.* **2008**, *66*, 294–299. [CrossRef]
36. Saito, N.; Hieda, J.; Takai, O. Synthesis process of gold nanoparticles in solution plasma. *Thin Solid Films* **2009**, *518*, 912–917. [CrossRef]
37. Jamroz, P.; Greda, K.; Pohl, P.; Zyrnicki, W. Atmospheric Pressure Glow Discharges Generated in Contact with Flowing Liquid Cathode: Production of Active Species and Application in Wastewater Purification Processes. *Plasma Chem. Plasma Process.* **2014**, *34*, 25–37. [CrossRef]
38. Pootawang, P.; Saito, N.; Takai, O. Solution plasma for template removal in mesoporous silica: pH and discharge time varying characteristics. *Thin Solid Films* **2011**, *519*, 7030–7035. [CrossRef]
39. Horikoshi, S.; Serpone, N. In-liquid plasma: A novel tool in the fabrication of nanomaterials and in the treatment of wastewaters. *RSC Adv.* **2017**, *7*, 47196–47218. [CrossRef]
40. Sansonetti, J.E.; Martin, W.C. Handbook of basic spectroscopic. *Phys. J. Chem. Ref. Data* **2005**, *34*, 1559–2259. [CrossRef]
41. Puziya, A.M.; Poddubnaya, O.I.; Socha, R.P.; Gurgul, J.; Wisniewski, M. XPS and NMR studies of phosphoric acid activated carbons. *Carbon* **2008**, *46*, 2113–2123. [CrossRef]
42. Li, M.; Xue, J. Integrated Synthesis of Nitrogen-Doped Mesoporous Carbon from Melamine Resins with Superior Performance in Supercapacitors. *J. Phys. Chem. C* **2014**, *118*, 2507–2517. [CrossRef]
43. Zubir, N.A.; Yacou, C.; Motuzas, J.; Zhang, X.; Costa, J.C.D. Structural and functional investigation of graphene oxide–Fe_3O_4 nanocomposites for the heterogeneous Fenton-like reaction. *Sci. Rep.* **2014**, *4*, 4594. [CrossRef] [PubMed]
44. Yang, J.H.; Kim, B.J.; Kim, Y.H.; Lee, Y.J.; Ha, B.H.; Shin, Y.S.; Park, S.Y.; Kim, H.S.; Park, C.Y.; Yang, C.W.; et al. Nitrogen-incorporated multiwalled carbon nanotubes grown by direct current plasma-enhanced chemical vapor deposition. *J. Vac. Sci. Technol. B* **2005**, *23*, 930–933. [CrossRef]
45. Karikalan, N.; Velmurugan, M.; Chen, S.M.; Karuppiah, C.; Al-Anazi, K.M.; Ajmal Ali, M.; Lou, B.S. Flame synthesis of nitrogen doped carbon for the oxygen reduction reaction and non-enzymatic methyl parathion sensor. *RSC Adv.* **2016**, *6*, 71507–71516. [CrossRef]
46. Liu, Y.; Zhang, W.; Li, X.; Le, X.; Ma, J. Catalysis of the hydro-dechlorination of 4-chlorophenol and the reduction of 4-nitrophenol by Pd/Fe_3O_4@SiO_2@m-SiO_2. *New J. Chem.* **2015**, *39*, 6474–6481. [CrossRef]
47. Kireeti, K.V.M.K.; Chandrakanth, G.; Kadam, M.M.; Jha, N. A sodium modified reduced graphene oxide–Fe_3O_4 nanocomposite for efficient lead(II) adsorption. *RSC Adv.* **2016**, *6*, 84825–84836. [CrossRef]
48. Yang, Y.; Li, J.; Chen, D.; Zhao, J. A Facile Electrophoretic Deposition Route to the Fe_3O_4/CNTs/rGO Composite Electrode as a Binder-Free Anode for Lithium Ion Battery. *ACS Appl. Mater. Interfaces* **2016**, *8*, 26730–26739. [CrossRef] [PubMed]
49. Bhargava, G.; Gouzman, I.; Chun, C.M.; Ramanarayanan, T.A.; Bernasek, S.L. Characterization of the "native" surface thin film on pure polycrystalline iron: A high resolution XPS and TEM study. *Appl. Surf. Sci.* **2007**, *253*, 4322–4329. [CrossRef]
50. Vinayan, B.P.; Nagar, R.; Ramaprabhu, S. Solar light assisted green synthesis of palladium nanoparticle decorated nitrogen doped graphene for hydrogen storage application. *J. Mater. Chem. A* **2013**, *1*, 11192–11199. [CrossRef]

51. Wang, L.; Gao, Z.; Chang, J.; Liu, X.; Wu, D.; Xu, F.; Guo, Y.; Jiang, K. Nitrogen-Doped Porous Carbons As Electrode Materials for High-Performance Supercapacitor and Dye-Sensitized Solar Cell. *ACS Appl. Mater. Interfaces* **2015**, *7*, 20234–20244. [CrossRef] [PubMed]
52. Li, Y.; Meng, Q.; Zhu, S.; Sun, Z.; Yang, H.; Chen, Z.; Zhu, C.; Guo, Z.; Zhang, D. A Fe/Fe$_3$O$_4$/N-carbon composite with hierarchical porous structure and in situ formed N-doped graphene-like layers for high-performance lithium ion batteries. *Dalton Trans.* **2015**, *44*, 4594–4600. [CrossRef] [PubMed]
53. Qiu, P.; Cui, D.; Khim, J. Facile synthesis of uniform magnetic graphitic carbon for an efficient adsorption of pentachlorophenol. *RSC Adv.* **2017**, *7*, 35012–35015. [CrossRef]
54. Le, H.N.T.; Jeong, H.K. Synthesis and Characterization of Nitrogen-doped Activated Carbon by Using Melamine. *New Phys.* **2015**, *65*, 86–89. [CrossRef]
55. Liu, Y.; Li, K.; Liu, Y.; Pu, L.; Chen, Z.; Deng, S. The high-performance and mechanism of P-doped activated carbon as a catalyst for air-cathode microbial fuel cells. *J. Mater. Chem. A* **2015**, *3*, 21149–21158. [CrossRef]
56. Shen, W.; Fan, W. Nitrogen-containing porous carbons: Synthesis and application. *J. Mater. Chem. A* **2013**, *1*, 999–1013. [CrossRef]
57. Kim, D.W.; Kim, K.S.; Park, S.J. Synthesis and Electrochemical Performance of Polypyrrole Coated Iron Oxide/Carbon Nanotube Composites. *Carbon Lett.* **2012**, *13*, 157–160. [CrossRef]
58. Hsieh, C.T.; Teng, H.; Chen, W.Y.; Cheng, Y.S. Synthesis, characterization, and electrochemical capacitance of amino-functionalized carbon nanotube/carbon paper electrodes. *Carbon* **2010**, *48*, 4219–4229. [CrossRef]
59. Khiew, P.; Ho, M.; Tan, T.; Chiu, W.; Shamsudin, R.; Abd-Hamid, M.A. Synthesis and Electrochemical Characterization of Iron Oxide/Activated Carbon Composite Electrode for Symmetrical Supercapacitor. *World Acad. Sci. Eng. Technol. Int. J. Chem. Mole. Nuc. Mater. Metal. Eng.* **2013**, *7*, 615–619.
60. Lim, Y.S.; Lai, C.W.; Hamid, S.B.A. Porous 3D carbon decorated Fe$_3$O$_4$ nanocomposite electrode for highly symmetrical supercapacitor performance. *RSC Adv.* **2017**, *7*, 23030–23040. [CrossRef]

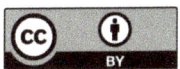

© 2018 by the authors. Licensee MDPI, Basel, Switzerland. This article is an open access article distributed under the terms and conditions of the Creative Commons Attribution (CC BY) license (http://creativecommons.org/licenses/by/4.0/).

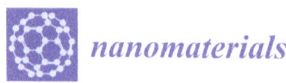

Article

Solution-Plasma-Mediated Synthesis of Si Nanoparticles for Anode Material of Lithium-Ion Batteries

Genki Saito [1,*], Hitoshi Sasaki [2], Heishichiro Takahashi [1,2] and Norihito Sakaguchi [1]

1. Faculty of Engineering, Hokkaido University, Kita 13 Nishi 8, Kitaku, Sapporo 060-8628, Japan; takahash@ufml.caret.hokudai.ac.jp (H.T.); sakaguchi@eng.hokudai.ac.jp (N.S.)
2. Kankyou-Engineering Co., Ltd. Kita 19 Higashi 1, Higashiku, Sapporo 065-0019, Japan; ht-sasaki@kankyou-eng.co.jp
* Correspondence: genki@eng.hokudai.ac.jp; Tel.: +81-11-706-6345

Received: 8 April 2018; Accepted: 25 April 2018; Published: 27 April 2018

Abstract: Silicon anodes have attracted considerable attention for their use in lithium-ion batteries because of their extremely high theoretical capacity; however, they are prone to extensive volume expansion during lithiation, which causes disintegration and poor cycling stability. In this article, we use two approaches to address this issue, by reducing the size of the Si particles to nanoscale and incorporating them into a carbon composite to help modulate the volume expansion problems. We improve our previous work on the solution-plasma-mediated synthesis of Si nanoparticles (NPs) by adjusting the electrolyte medium to mild buffer solutions rather than strong acids, successfully generating Si-NPs with <10 nm diameters. We then combined these Si-NPs with carbon using MgO-template-assisted sol-gel combustion synthesis, which afforded porous carbon composite materials. Among the preparations, the composite material obtained from the LiCl 0.2 M + H_3BO_3 0.15 M solution-based Si-NPs exhibited a high reversible capacity of 537 mAh/g after 30 discharge/charge cycles at a current rate of 0.5 A/g. We attribute this increased reversible capacity to the decreased particle size of the Si-NPs. These results clearly show the applicability of this facile and environmentally friendly solution-plasma technique for producing Si-NPs as an anode material for lithium-ion batteries.

Keywords: solution plasma; nanoparticles; batteries; silicon; anode materials

1. Introduction

Rechargeable lithium-ion batteries (LIBs) have been widely used as energy-storage devices for applications such as portable electronic devices and electric vehicles. Among the newer anode materials with higher capacities, silicon anodes have attracted considerable attention because of their high theoretical capacity of 4200 mAh·g^{-1}, which exceeds that of commercialized graphite anodes [1–4]. During the lithium insertion-extraction process, however, a large volume change (>280%) inevitably occurs, which leads to pulverization of the silicon anode and loss of electrical contact with the current collector, resulting in poor cycling performance [2,5]. To mitigate this volume-change issue, several strategies have been proposed, including reducing the particle size to nanoscale [6,7], fabricating Si nanostructures such as nanowires and nanoporous materials [8–11], utilizing hollow core-shell structures [12], and dispersing nano-Si in a conductive carbon matrix to form Si-carbon composites [13–19]. Liu et al. clarified that the critical particle diameter for a Si anode should be less than 150 nm to avoid surface cracking and subsequent fracturing during lithiation [5]. In addition, dispersing silicon nanoparticles (Si-NPs) into a carbon matrix is a technique that has been well developed; here, the carbonaceous material acts to buffer the volume expansion and improves the electrical conductivity of the Si active materials [13].

As an effective synthetic route for Si-NPs, this study proposes the solution-plasma-mediated synthesis [20–30]. In this process, Si-NPs are directly synthesized from a Si bar electrode via a solution-plasma treatment. Our previous study revealed that the use of a strong acid electrolyte solution was effective for producing Si-NPs without oxidation [31]. In general, the solution plasma technique offers many advantages, such as (1) simple experimental setup, (2) use of readily available precursors, and (3) applicability to mass production. Unfortunately, with respect to the last point, strong acid solution is not applicable on large scale. Furthermore, the performance of LIBs based on Si-NPs synthesized from solution plasma is still unclear. Therefore, in this study, we have optimized the Si-NPs synthesis conditions using mild buffer solutions.

In addition to the Si-NPs synthesis, the fabrication of a composite material consisting of the Si-NPs and porous carbon is also important for overcoming the volume-change issue. This study applied a sol-gel solution-combustion synthesis (SCS) approach, which is a highly exothermic and self-sustaining process involving heating a homogeneous solution of aqueous metal salts and fuels such as urea, citric acid, glycine acid, or glycine [32–37]. This method has been applied to synthesize a Sn-NP-embedded porous carbon structure, using nanosized MgO as the template upon which to construct the porous structure; this material displayed good cycle performance as an LIB anode [38]. Based on this result, a Si-C composite material was synthesized via MgO template-assisted SCS, in which the starting material was a gel containing the Si-NPs, glycine ($C_2H_5O_2N$) as the carbon source, and $Mg(NO_3)_2 \cdot 6H_2O$ as the template. After the combustion reaction, the generated MgO was removed from the carbon, leaving the Si-NPs dispersed throughout the porous carbon structure after calcination in N_2. The obtained materials were characterized by X-ray diffractometry (XRD) and transmission electron microscopy (TEM). Finally, the electrochemical properties of the product as an LIB anode material were investigated.

2. Materials and Methods

Figure 1 shows the experimental setup for producing the Si particles and a schematic diagram for the solution-combustion synthesis of the Si-C composite. A B-doped p-type Si bar with a square cross-sectional width of 5.0 mm (Shin-Etsu Chemical Co., Ltd., Tokyo, Japan) and electrical resistance of 0.00494–0.00478 Ω cm was used as the cathode. The upper part of the Si bar was shielded by a quartz glass tube to generate a plasma at the bottom tip of the electrode. A counter electrode was the Pt mesh. A voltage was applied using a direct current power supply. To study the effect of the electrolyte on the generation of the Si-NPs, solutions of $KCl + H_3BO_3$, $KH_2PO_4 + K_2HPO_4$, and $LiCl + H_3BO_3$ were used. The electrolyte concentrations and applied voltages are summarized in Table 1. After the synthesis, the products were collected by filtration and then washed several times with deionized water.

Table 1. Summary of experimental conditions and changes in pH and electrical conductivity for each electrolyte.

Electrolyte	Voltage (V)	Current (A)	Before			After		
			pH (-)	Electrical Conductivity (mS/m)	Electrolyte Temperature (°C)	pH (-)	Electrical Conductivity (mS/m)	Electrolyte Temperature (°C)
KCl 0.125 M + H_3BO_3 0.125 M	195	2.01	4.84	1509	93.4	-	-	94.8
KH_2PO_4 0.249 M + K_2HPO_4 0.001 M	189	2.46	4.54	1879	92.3	4.59	1848	95.6
LiCl 0.2 M + H_3BO_3 0.15 M	180	1.56	5.11	1716	94.7	7.52	1670	98.7

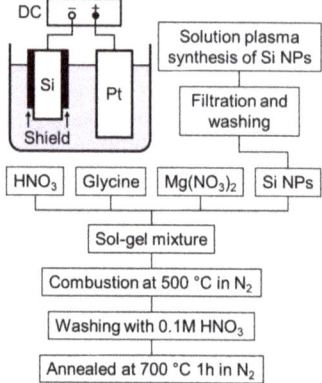

Figure 1. (Color online) Experimental setup for producing Si particles and schematic diagram for the solution combustion synthesis of Si-C the composite.

To synthesize the Si-C composite, commercially available $Mg(NO_3)_2 \cdot 6H_2O$ (1.282 g, 0.005 M) and $C_2H_5O_2N$ (2.252 g, 0.03 M) were added to 20% HNO_3 solution (20 mL). After agitation, the Si-NPs (30 mg) synthesized as described above were added to the HNO_3 solution and then dispersed with a thin-film spin system high-speed mixer (Filmix Model 30-L, PRIMIX Corp., Osaka, Japan) at 5000 rpm for 15 min. The resulting solution was then dried on a hot plate at 90 °C. The prepared gel was transferred to a furnace for combustion synthesis. The furnace was evacuated to below 100 Pa and then nitrogen was introduced at 2 L/min. The annealing temperature was set at 500 °C. Upon reaching 200–300 °C, the gel quickly combusted, releasing a large amount of gases. After SCS, the obtained particles were washed sequentially with 0.1 M HNO_3 solution and deionized water to remove the MgO phase. After drying, the sample was calcined at 700 °C for 1 h under N_2 atmosphere.

The particles obtained at the end of each step were analyzed via XRD (Miniflex600, Rigaku, Tokyo, Japan), employing Cu Kα radiation (λ = 1.5418 Å). The microstructure of the samples was observed using a field-emission scanning electron microscope (SEM; JSM–7001FA, JEOL, Tokyo, Japan), in which the inner structure of the porous particle was observed by the ion-milling technique using a cross-sectional polisher (CP, IB-19510CP, JEOL, Tokyo, Japan). TEM imaging (JEOL JEM-2010F, Tokyo, Japan) was also performed. Raman spectra of the porous carbon were acquired from a LabRam 1B Raman spectrometer (HORIBA, Kyoto, Japan).

Electrochemical characterization was performed in two-electrode Swagelok-type cells. The working electrode consisted of the active material, conductive carbon (acetylene black), and a polymer binder of sodium carboxymethyl cellulose (CMC) and poly(acrylic acid) (PAA) in a weight ratio of 75:15:5:5. The well-blended solution-based slurry was spread onto copper foil and dried at 60 °C for 3 h under vacuum. The dried electrode was punched into a 14-mm-diameter disc with a mass loading of 2–3 mg. A metallic lithium disc (15-mm diameter) was used as the counter and reference electrodes. The cells were assembled in an Ar-filled glove box (UNICO), using a solution of 1 M $LiPF_6$ dissolved in ethylene carbonate (EC)/dimethyl carbonate (DMC) (1:1 v/v) as the electrolyte and a polypropylene membrane as the separator. The cells were galvanostatically cycled from 0.01 to 2.0 V versus Li/Li^+ at 0.5 A/g in the constant current mode using a battery charge/discharge system (MSTAT4, Arbin Instruments, College station, TX, USA) at a constant temperature of 25 °C.

3. Results and Discussion

The Si-NPs were synthesized using solution plasma generated by contact glow discharge electrolysis (CGDE). Two electrodes consisting of a Si bar and Pt mesh were placed in a glass cell and a direct-current voltage was applied. When the voltage was increased above 1.3 V, the current increased linearly in accordance with Ohm's law, corresponding to the occurrence of water electrolysis. Since the electrode surface of Si is smaller than the Pt mesh, the thermal loss concentrates at the Si anode-solution interface. When a higher voltage is applied, the increased current heats the solution near the Si electrode, and finally, the solution temperature surrounding Si electrode exceeds the boiling point and a gas layer consisting of steam is generated. Once the gas layer is generated, the cathode and solution are no longer in contact and the current is decreased. When the voltage is sufficiently high (>150 V) [39,40], a discharge with intense light emission begins in the gas layer. The surface of the electrode partially melts to produce nanoparticles, owing to the concentration of the current caused by the electrothermal instability [41,42]. Control parameters for size of Si-NPs are applied voltage and plasma mode. When the plasma mode is kept as a partial plasma region, the particle size decreases with an increase of applied voltage [43,44]. However, the higher applied voltage induces the transition from partial plasma to full plasma region, in which coarse particles are formed under the high excitation temperature. Thus, we have selected the appropriate voltage for each electrolyte, as shown in Table 1.

In our previous study, K_2CO_3, KNO_3, KCl, HNO_3, and HCl electrolytes were used for Si-NPs synthesis; among these, the acid solutions were effective for producing Si-NPs without oxidation [31]. When the electrolyte was either a strong acid or strong base, the pH remained constant. The pH of KNO_3 and KCl increased during electrolysis because of the consumption of negative ions and formation of OH^- ions. In principle, the electrolysis of an acidic solution can be described as follows:

$$2H_2O = 4H^+ + O_2(g) + 2e^- \tag{1}$$

However, the reduction of Cl^- ions is favored over the decomposition of H_2O:

$$2Cl^- = Cl_2(g) + 2e^- \tag{2}$$

Therefore, the pH in the neutral solution increases during electrolysis due to the generation of Cl_2 gas, and oxidized Si particles are then formed to react with the OH^- ions, which produce Cl^- ions instead. At certain hot spots on the electrode surface during the plasma electrolysis, the Si^{2+} ions were generated, and they combined with OH^- to form SiO_2: $Si^{2+} + 2OH^- \rightarrow Si(OH)_2 \rightarrow SiO_2 + H_2O$. Etching of Si in KOH and NaOH was also reported by other research groups [45,46]. Thus, the pH value of the electrolyte might have affected the product phase. In the case of KNO_3 solution as the electrolyte, the reduction of NO_3^- to NO_2^- may occur at the cathode electrode [47].

$$NO_3^- + 2e^- + H_2O = NO_2^- + 2OH^- \tag{3}$$

Previously, we found that the pH values of 0.1 M KCl and KNO_3 solutions were increased from 6.13 and 6.87 to 8.71 and 9.88, respectively, during the solution-plasma synthesis of Si-NPs [44]. When the electrolyte solution becomes too alkaline, the synthesized Si-NPs tend to be oxidized. In contrast, strong acids such as HCl and HNO_3 are effective for Si-NPs synthesis, but such strong acids are harmful and corrosive. Thus, the use of neutral solutions is attractive because of their safety and non-corrosive natures. This study investigates the non-volatile buffer solutions, KCl 0.125 M + H_3BO_3 0.125 M, KH_2PO_4 0.249 M + K_2HPO_4 0.001 M, and LiCl 0.2 M + H_3BO_3 0.15 M. In the experiments, solution plasma is successfully generated in each electrolyte. As shown in Table 1, the changes in pH are smaller compared to the cases of neutral single-electrolyte solutions, suggesting the effectiveness of the buffered systems. The initial solution temperature was over 92 °C because the pre-warming of the electrolysis was effective for initiate the plasma generation [48]. During Si-NPs production, solution temperature was controlled in the range of 94~99 °C.

The produced Si-NPs were collected and characterized by XRD, SEM, and TEM. Figure 2 shows the XRD patterns of the synthesized crystalline Si-NPs. generated in the three buffer solutions. Figure 3a–c shows the SEM images of the synthesized Si-NPs. The synthesized particles are almost spherical, and some particles have an oval sphere shape. During melting and solidification process, the generated particles forms sphere due to a surface tension. The particle size was measured using low magnification TEM as shown in Figure 4, in which the particle size with over 50 nm were analyzed using low magnification TEM. In the case of the KCl + H_3BO_3 solution, the particle size of Si particles widely distributed from 50 nm to over 1 μm. Although the KH_2PO_4 + K_2HPO_4 solution produces smaller particles, the LiCl + H_3BO_3 solution is the most effective for producing small Si-NPs. Although the detailed mechanism is still unclear, ions such as K^+, Na^+, and Li^+ are excited in the light-emitting plasma layer [49], and these excited species might affect the generated plasma and local current concentration, resulting in the change in product size. Figure 5 shows high-resolution TEM images of the Si-NPs synthesized in the LiCl + H_3BO_3 solution, in which Si-NPs with diameters of less than 10 nm can also be observed. From the high-resolution TEM image shown in Figure 4b, small Si-NPs have a single-crystalline structure, in which the obtained d spacing matched to the {111} plane of cubic diamond-structured Si.

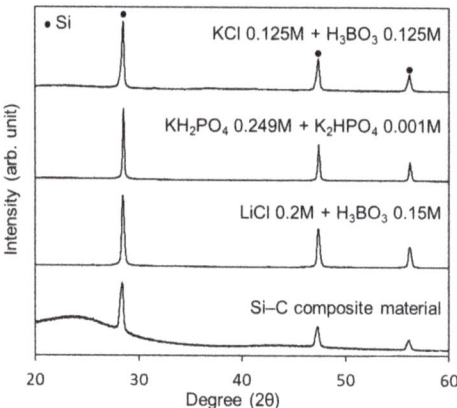

Figure 2. XRD patterns of the synthesized Si-NPs, as well as the Si-C composite prepared from Si-NPs generated in LiCl + H_3BO_3 solution.

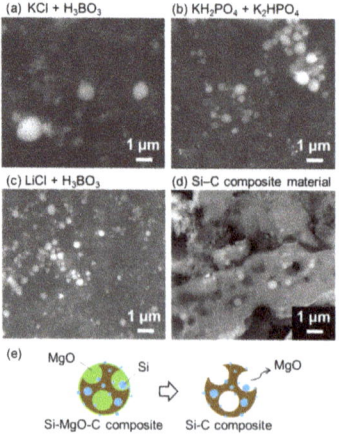

Figure 3. (a–c) SEM images of Si-NPs synthesized in different buffers; and (d) cross-sectional SEM image of Si-C composite (LiCl + H_3BO_3 solution); (e) Illustration of porous Si-C composite material.

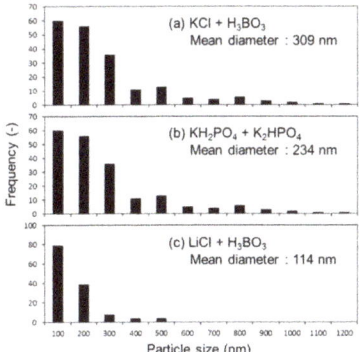

Figure 4. The particle size distribution of Si-NPs, in which the particle sizes with over 50 nm were analyzed using a low magnification TEM.

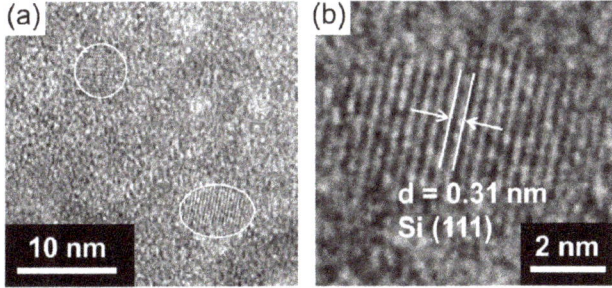

Figure 5. (a) High-resolution TEM image of Si-NPs synthesized using LiCl + H_3BO_3 solution. The white circle indicates the Si-NPs; (b) Enlarged image of Si-NPs. The obtained d spacing matched to the {111} plane of cubic diamond-structured Si.

For the LIB measurements, composite materials of porous carbon and Si-NPs were synthesized via MgO template-assisted SCS to accommodate the huge volume expansion of Si-NPs during the lithiation reaction. As indicated in Figure 1, the starting material is a gel containing the Si-NPs, glycine as the carbon source, and $Mg(NO_3)_2 \cdot 6H_2O$ as the template. After the combustion reaction, the generated MgO is removed from the carbon, and the Si-NPs remain dispersed throughout the porous carbon structure after calcination under N_2, as shown in the schematic illustration in Figure 3e. This process has been applied to fabricate a composite material of Sn-NPs and carbon, which successfully improved battery properties [37]. Figure 2 shows the XRD pattern of the synthesized Si-C composite. After combustion synthesis, the crystal structure of the Si is unchanged and a broad peak originating from the carbon structure has appeared. Figure 6 shows the Raman spectrum of the Si-C composite. The peak at around 500 cm^{-1} corresponds to a silicon band [50,51]. Two strong peaks at around 1350 and 1570 cm^{-1} are D-band and G-band of carbon, indicating the disordered carbon and ordered graphitic carbon, respectively. The ratios of the intensities of the D-band to G-band, I_D/I_G, are higher than 1 for Si-C composite. This indicates that the synthesized porous carbon has disordered carbon structure, rather than highly graphitic structure. It is reported that the generated carbon contains nitrogen after SCS using glycine and nitrate [38,52]. The existence of nitrogen might affect to the crystallinity of the generated carbon.

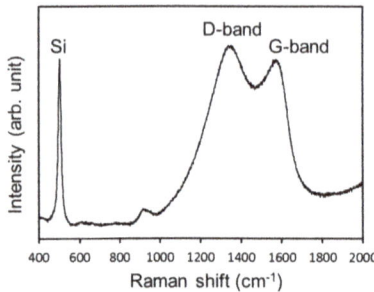

Figure 6. Raman spectrum of the Si-C composite prepared from Si-NPs generated in LiCl + H$_3$BO$_3$ solution.

The electrochemical properties of the synthesized composites were investigated using a Li disk as the reference and counter electrodes at a current density of 0.5 A/g. Figure 7 shows the cyclic performance of the materials synthesized in the different electrolytes. The Si-C composite containing the LiCl + H$_3$BO$_3$ solution-based Si-NPs shows a higher initial discharge capacity (over 1300 mAh/g) compared to the other electrolyte-derived composites, and the capacity gradually decreases with increasing cycle number. This same composite material (using Si-NPs from prepared in LiCl + H$_3$BO$_3$ solution) exhibits a higher reversible capacity (537 mAh/g) after 30 discharge/charge cycles at a current rate of 0.5 A/g, compared to the 283 mAh/g observed for the composite prepared with KCl + H$_3$BO$_3$ solution-based Si-NPs. Because the theoretical capacity of graphite is 360 mAh/g, these results reveal that the synthesized Si-NPs can function as anode materials. The difference in capacity is mainly due to the particle size of the Si-NPs. When the particle size of the Si-NPs is less than 150 nm [5], their fracture during cycling can be avoided. Thus, the small Si-NPs produced in the LiCl + H$_3$BO$_3$ solution are effective for increasing the capacity. However, the discharge capacity continuously decreases. Because the volume expansion of the Si-NPs during lithiation exceeds 400%, the synthesized porous structure might be insufficient to accommodate this expansion, resulting in the fracture of the carbon electrode. In the case of the Sn-C composite synthesized by the solution-combustion method [38], the synthesized SnO$_2$ nanoparticles are reduced by the surrounding carbon to form a Sn melt during calcination. This Sn melt moves to the surface of the porous carbon, resulting in the "attachment" of the Sn nanoparticles to the carbon structure to afford excellent battery performance. In the case of the Si-NPs, the solid Si-NPs are "embedded" in the carbon structure, as shown in Figure 3d, which might have induced the pulverization of the composite. A smaller particle size, use of a polymer, and a well-organized porous structure should increase the cycle stability.

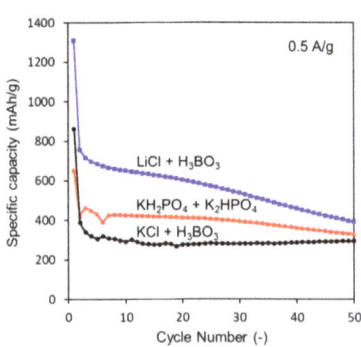

Figure 7. Cycling performance of Si-C composite anode materials at 0.5 A/g ranging from 0.01 to 2.00 V.

4. Conclusions

In this study, Si nanoparticles (Si-NPs) were synthesized via a facile solution-plasma-mediated synthesis, and composites consisting of Si-NPs and porous carbon were fabricated as the anode materials for lithium-ion batteries. Among several mild buffer solutions investigated, the LiCl 0.2 M + H_3BO_3 0.15 M solution effectively produced smaller Si-NPs. These Si-NPs were formed from a solid Si bar via local current concentration during the solution-plasma treatment. High-resolution TEM imaging confirmed the synthesis of Si-NPs with diameters of less than 10 nm. The Si-C composite material was synthesized via MgO template-assisted solution-combustion synthesis. The composite material obtained from the LiCl 0.2 M + H_3BO_3 0.15 M solution exhibited a reversible capacity of 537 mAh/g after 30 discharge/charge cycles at a current rate of 0.5 A/g, as compared to the 283 mAh/g observed for the KCl 0.125 M + H_3BO_3 0.125 M solution. The increased reversible capacity is mainly due to the decreased particle size of the Si-NPs. These results clearly show the applicability of this facile and environmentally friendly solution-plasma technique for producing Si-NPs as an anode material for LIBs.

Author Contributions: Genki Saito measured the electrochemical performance and wrote the manuscript. Hitoshi Sasaki synthesized the Si nanoparticles. Heishichiro Takahashi and Norihito Sakaguchi contributed to the analysis by electron microscopy. All authors approved the final version of the manuscript.

Acknowledgments: A part of this work was conducted at "Joint-Use Facilities: Laboratory of Nano-Micro Material Analysis" at Hokkaido University, supported by the "Material Analysis and Structure Analysis Open Unit (MASAOU)" and "Nanotechnology Platform" Program of the Ministry of Education, Culture, Sports, Science and Technology (MEXT), Japan. This work was supported by the Iketani Science and Technology Foundation.

Conflicts of Interest: The authors declare no conflict of interest.

References

1. Obrovac, M.N.; Christensen, L. Structural Changes in Silicon Anodes during Lithium Insertion/Extraction. *Electrochem. Solid-State Lett.* **2004**, *7*, A93–A96. [CrossRef]
2. Kasavajjula, U.; Wang, C.; Appleby, A.J. Nano- and bulk-silicon-based insertion anodes for lithium-ion secondary cells. *J. Power Sources* **2007**, *163*, 1003–1039. [CrossRef]
3. Zhang, W.-J. A review of the electrochemical performance of alloy anodes for lithium-ion batteries. *J. Power Sources* **2011**, *196*, 13–24. [CrossRef]
4. Ozanam, F.; Rosso, M. Silicon as anode material for Li-ion batteries. *Mater. Sci. Eng. B* **2016**, *213*, 2–11. [CrossRef]
5. Liu, X.H.; Zhong, L.; Huang, S.; Mao, S.X.; Zhu, T.; Huang, J.Y. Size-Dependent Fracture of Silicon Nanoparticles During Lithiation. *ACS Nano* **2012**, *6*, 1522–1531. [CrossRef] [PubMed]
6. Xun, S.; Song, X.; Grass, M.E.; Roseguo, D.K.; Liu, Z.; Battaglia, V.S.; Liu, G. Improved Initial Performance of Si Nanoparticles by Surface Oxide Reduction for Lithium-Ion Battery Application. *Electrochem. Solid-State Lett.* **2011**, *14*, A61–A63. [CrossRef]
7. Wu, H.; Zheng, G.; Liu, N.; Carney, T.J.; Yang, Y.; Cui, Y. Engineering Empty Space between Si Nanoparticles for Lithium-Ion Battery Anodes. *Nano Lett.* **2012**, *12*, 904–909. [CrossRef] [PubMed]
8. Zuo, X.; Zhu, J.; Müller-Buschbaum, P.; Cheng, Y.-J. Silicon based lithium-ion battery anodes: A chronicle perspective review. *Nano Energy* **2017**, *31*, 113–143. [CrossRef]
9. Ikonen, T.; Nissinen, T.; Pohjalainen, E.; Sorsa, O.; Kallio, T.; Lehto, V.P. Electrochemically anodized porous silicon: Towards simple and affordable anode material for Li-ion batteries. *Sci. Rep.* **2017**, *7*, 7880. [CrossRef] [PubMed]
10. Gao, P.; Tang, H.; Xing, A.; Bao, Z. Porous silicon from the magnesiothermic reaction as a high-performance anode material for lithium ion battery applications. *Electrochim. Acta* **2017**, *228*, 545–552. [CrossRef]
11. Cho, J. Porous Si anode materials for lithium rechargeable batteries. *J. Mater. Chem.* **2010**, *20*, 4009–4014. [CrossRef]
12. Chen, Y.; Hu, Y.; Shen, Z.; Chen, R.; He, X.; Zhang, X.; Li, Y.; Wu, K. Hollow core–shell structured silicon@carbon nanoparticles embed in carbon nanofibers as binder-free anodes for lithium-ion batteries. *J. Power Sources* **2017**, *342*, 467–475. [CrossRef]

13. Zhou, M.; Cai, T.; Pu, F.; Chen, H.; Wang, Z.; Zhang, H.; Guan, S. Graphene/Carbon-Coated Si Nanoparticle Hybrids as High-Performance Anode Materials for Li-Ion Batteries. *ACS Appl. Mater. Interfaces* **2013**, *5*, 3449–3455. [CrossRef] [PubMed]
14. Gomez-Camer, J.L.; Morales, J.; Sanchez, L. Anchoring Si nanoparticles to carbon nanofibers: An efficient procedure for improving Si performance in Li batteries. *J. Mater. Chem.* **2011**, *21*, 811–818. [CrossRef]
15. Tao, H.-C.; Fan, L.-Z.; Mei, Y.; Qu, X. Self-supporting Si/Reduced Graphene Oxide nanocomposite films as anode for lithium ion batteries. *Electrochem. Commun.* **2011**, *13*, 1332–1335. [CrossRef]
16. Zhou, M.; Pu, F.; Wang, Z.; Cai, T.; Chen, H.; Zhang, H.; Guan, S. Facile synthesis of novel Si nanoparticles-graphene composites as high-performance anode materials for Li-ion batteries. *Phys. Chem. Chem. Phys.* **2013**, *15*, 11394–11401. [CrossRef] [PubMed]
17. Luo, Z.; Xiao, Q.; Lei, G.; Li, Z.; Tang, C. Si nanoparticles/graphene composite membrane for high performance silicon anode in lithium ion batteries. *Carbon* **2016**, *98* (Suppl. C), 373–380. [CrossRef]
18. Zhou, X.; Yin, Y.-X.; Wan, L.-J.; Guo, Y.-G. Facile synthesis of silicon nanoparticles inserted into graphene sheets as improved anode materials for lithium-ion batteries. *Chem. Commun.* **2012**, *48*, 2198–2200. [CrossRef] [PubMed]
19. Zhang, T.; Gao, J.; Fu, L.J.; Yang, L.C.; Wu, Y.P.; Wu, H.Q. Natural graphite coated by Si nanoparticles as anode materials for lithium ion batteries. *J. Mater. Chem.* **2007**, *17*, 1321–1325. [CrossRef]
20. Saito, G.; Akiyama, T. Nanomaterial synthesis using plasma generation in liquid. *J. Nanomater.* **2015**, *16*, 299. [CrossRef]
21. Yatsu, S.; Takahashi, H.; Sasaki, H.; Sakaguchi, N.; Ohkubo, K.; Muramoto, T.; Watanabe, S. Fabrication of Nanoparticles by Electric Discharge Plasma in Liquid. *Arch. Metall. Mater.* **2013**, *58*, 425. [CrossRef]
22. Saito, G.; Hosokai, S.; Tsubota, M.; Akiyama, T. Synthesis of copper/copper oxide nanoparticles by solution plasma. *J. Appl. Phys.* **2011**, *110*, 023302. [CrossRef]
23. Jiang, B.; Zheng, J.; Qiu, S.; Wu, M.; Zhang, Q.; Yan, Z.; Xue, Q. Review on electrical discharge plasma technology for wastewater remediation. *Chem. Eng. J.* **2014**, *236*, 348–368. [CrossRef]
24. Chen, Q.; Li, J.; Li, Y.; Zhang, X.; Yang, S. Plasma-Liquid Interaction: A New Way to Synthesize Nanomaterials. *arXiv* **2014**, arXiv:1404.2515.
25. Švrček, V.; Mariotti, D.; Kondo, M. Microplasma-induced surface engineering of silicon nanocrystals in colloidal dispersion. *Appl. Phys. Lett.* **2010**, *97*. [CrossRef]
26. Liu, S.-M.; Kobayashi, M.; Sato, S.; Kimura, K. Synthesis of silicon nanowires and nanoparticles by arc-discharge in water. *Chem. Commun.* **2005**, 4690–4692. [CrossRef] [PubMed]
27. Tokushige, M.; Tsujimura, H.; Nishikiori, T.; Ito, Y. Formation of metallic Si and SiC nanoparticles from SiO_2 particles by plasma-induced cathodic discharge electrolysis in chloride melt. *Electrochim. Acta* **2013**, *100*, 300–303. [CrossRef]
28. Tokushige, M.; Nishikiori, T.; Ito, Y. Plasma-induced cathodic discharge electrolysis to form various metal/alloy nanoparticles. *Russ. J. Electrochem.* **2010**, *46*, 619–626. [CrossRef]
29. Lee, H.; Lee, W.-J.; Park, Y.-K.; Ki, S.; Kim, B.-J.; Jung, S.-C. Liquid Phase Plasma Synthesis of Iron Oxide Nanoparticles on Nitrogen-Doped Activated Carbon Resulting in Nanocomposite for Supercapacitor Applications. *Nanomaterials* **2018**, *8*, 190. [CrossRef] [PubMed]
30. Show, Y.; Ueno, Y. Formation of Platinum Catalyst on Carbon Black Using an In-Liquid Plasma Method for Fuel Cells. *Nanomaterials* **2017**, *7*, 31. [CrossRef] [PubMed]
31. Saito, G.; Sakaguchi, N. Solution plasma synthesis of Si nanoparticles. *Nanotechnology* **2015**, *26*, 23560. [CrossRef] [PubMed]
32. Da Conceição, L.; Ribeiro, N.F.P.; Furtado, J.G.M.; Souza, M.M.V.M. Effect of propellant on the combustion synthesized Sr-doped $LaMnO_3$ powders. *Ceram. Int.* **2009**, *35*, 1683–1687. [CrossRef]
33. Blennow, P.; Hansen, K.K.; Wallenberg, L.R.; Mogensen, M. Synthesis of Nb-doped $SrTiO_3$ by a modified glycine-nitrate process. *J. Eur. Ceram. Soc.* **2007**, *27*, 3609–3612. [CrossRef]
34. Nomura, T.; Zhu, C.; Sheng, N.; Murai, R.; Akiyama, T. Solution combustion synthesis of Brownmillerite-type Ca_2AlMnO_5 as an oxygen storage material. *J. Alloys Compd.* **2015**, *646*, 900–905. [CrossRef]
35. Zhu, C.; Saito, G.; Akiyama, T. A facile solution combustion synthesis of nanosized amorphous iron oxide incorporated in a carbon matrix for use as a high-performance lithium ion battery anode material. *J. Alloys Compd.* **2015**, *633*, 424–429. [CrossRef]

36. Zhu, C.; Saito, G.; Akiyama, T. A new CaCO$_3$-template method to synthesize nanoporous manganese oxide hollow structures and their transformation to high-performance LiMn$_2$O$_4$ cathodes for lithium-ion batteries. *J. Mater. Chem. A* **2013**, *1*, 7077–7082. [CrossRef]
37. Saito, G.; Nakasugi, Y.; Sakaguchi, N.; Zhu, C.; Akiyama, T. Glycine-nitrate-based solution-combustion synthesis of SrTiO$_3$. *J. Alloys Compd.* **2015**, *652*, 496–502. [CrossRef]
38. Saito, G.; Zhu, C.; Han, C.-G.; Sakaguchi, N.; Akiyama, T. Solution combustion synthesis of porous Sn-C composite as anode material for lithium ion batteries. *Adv. Powder Technol.* **2016**, *27*, 1730–1737. [CrossRef]
39. Sengupta, S.K.; Singh, R.; Srivastava, A.K. A Study on the Origin of Nonfaradaic Behavior of Anodic Contact Glow Discharge Electrolysis. *J. Electrochem. Soc.* **1998**, *145*, 2209–2213. [CrossRef]
40. Yerokhin, A.L.; Nie, X.; Leyland, A.; Matthews, A.; Dowey, S.J. Plasma electrolysis for surface engineering. *Surf. Coat. Technol.* **1999**, *122*, 73–93. [CrossRef]
41. Okazaki, K.; Mori, Y.; Hijikata, K.; Ohtake, K. Electrothermal instability in the seeded combustion gas boundary layer near cold electrodes. *AIAA J.* **1978**, *16*, 334–339. [CrossRef]
42. Uncles, R.; Nelson, A. Dynamic stabilization of the electrothermal instability. *Plasma Phys.* **1970**, *12*, 917. [CrossRef]
43. Saito, G.; Hosokai, S.; Akiyama, T.; Yoshida, S.; Yatsu, S.; Watanabe, S. Size-Controlled Ni Nanoparticles Formation by Solution Glow Discharge. *J. Phys. Soc. Jpn.* **2010**, *79*, 083501. [CrossRef]
44. Saito, G.; Hosokai, S.; Tsubota, M.; Akiyama, T. Nickel nanoparticles formation from solution plasma using edge-shielded electrode. *Plasma Chem. Plasma Process.* **2011**, *31*, 719–728. [CrossRef]
45. Seidel, H.; Csepregi, L.; Heuberger, A.; Baumgärtel, H. Anisotropic Etching of Crystalline Silicon in Alkaline Solutions: I. Orientation Dependence and Behavior of Passivation Layers. *J. Electrochem. Soc.* **1990**, *137*, 3612–3626. [CrossRef]
46. Glembocki, O.J.; Stahlbush, R.E.; Tomkiewicz, M. Bias-Dependent Etching of Silicon in Aqueous KOH. *J. Electrochem. Soc.* **1985**, *132*, 145–151. [CrossRef]
47. Polatides, C.; Dortsiou, M.; Kyriacou, G. Electrochemical removal of nitrate ion from aqueous solution by pulsing potential electrolysis. *Electrochim. Acta* **2005**, *50*, 5237–5241. [CrossRef]
48. Saito, G.; Nakasugi, Y.; Akiyama, T. Generation of solution plasma over a large electrode surface area. *J. Appl. Phys.* **2015**, *118*, 023303. [CrossRef]
49. Saito, G.; Nakasugi, Y.; Akiyama, T. Excitation temperature of a solution plasma during nanoparticle synthesis. *J. Appl. Phys.* **2014**, *116*. [CrossRef]
50. Reichert, F.; Pérez-Mas, A.M.; Barreda, D.; Blanco, C.; Santamaria, R.; Kuttner, C.; Fery, A.; Langhof, N.; Krenkel, W. Influence of the carbonization temperature on the mechanical properties of thermoplastic polymer derived C/C-SiC composites. *J. Eur. Ceram. Soc.* **2017**, *37*, 523–529. [CrossRef]
51. Nanda, J.; Datta, M.K.; Remillard, J.T.; O'Neill, A.; Kumta, P.N. In situ Raman microscopy during discharge of a high capacity silicon–carbon composite Li-ion battery negative electrode. *Electrochem. Commun.* **2009**, *11*, 235–237. [CrossRef]
52. Zhu, C.; Han, C.-G.; Saito, G.; Akiyama, T. MnO nanocrystals incorporated in a N-containing carbon matrix for Li ion battery anodes. *RSC Adv.* **2016**, *6*, 30445–30453. [CrossRef]

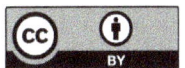

© 2018 by the authors. Licensee MDPI, Basel, Switzerland. This article is an open access article distributed under the terms and conditions of the Creative Commons Attribution (CC BY) license (http://creativecommons.org/licenses/by/4.0/).

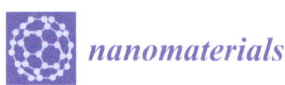

Article

Capacitively Coupled Plasma Discharge of Ionic Liquid Solutions to Synthesize Carbon Dots as Fluorescent Sensors

Ching-Bin Ke [1], Te-Ling Lu [2] and Jian-Lian Chen [2],*

1. Department of Beauty and Health Care, Min-Hwei Junior College of Health Care Management, No. 1116, Sec. 2, Zhongshan E. Rd., Tainan 73658, Taiwan; cbke@mail.mhchcm.edu.tw
2. School of Pharmacy, China Medical University, No. 91 Hsueh-Shih Road, Taichung 40402, Taiwan; lutl@mail.cmu.edu.tw
* Correspondance: cjl@mail.cmu.edu.tw; Tel.: +886-4-22-053-366

Received: 25 April 2018; Accepted: 23 May 2018; Published: 26 May 2018

Abstract: Oxygen and nitrogen capacitively coupled plasma (CCP) was used to irradiate mixtures of aliphatic acids in high boiling point solvents to synthesize fluorescent carbon dots (C-dots). With a high fluorescence intensity, the C-dots obtained from the O_2/CCP radiation of a 1-ethyl-3-methylimidazolium dicyanamide ionic liquid solution of citric acid were characterized with an average diameter of 8.6 nm (σ = 1.1 nm), nitrogen and oxygen bonding functionalities, excitation-independent emissions, and upconversion fluorescence. Through dialysis of the CCP-treated C-dots, two emissive surface states corresponding to their respective functionalities and emissions were identified. The fluorescence spectrum of the CCP-treated C-dots was different from that of the microwave irradiation and possessed higher intensity than that of hydrothermal pyrolysis. By evaluation of the fluorescence quenching effect on flavonoids and metal ions, the CCP-treated C-dots showed a high selectivity for quercetin and sensitivity to Hg^{2+}. Based on the Perrin model, a calibration curve (R^2 = 0.9992) was established for quercetin ranging from 2.4 μM to 119 μM with an LOD (limit of detection) = 0.5 μM. The quercetin in the ethanol extract of the sun-dried peel of *Citrus reticulata* cv. Chachiensis was determined by a standard addition method to be 4.20 ± 0.15 mg/g with a matrix effect of 8.16%.

Keywords: capacitively coupled plasma; carbon dots; ionic liquid; mercury ion; quercetin; upconversion

---

1. Introduction

Carbon dots (C-dots) have readily acquired predominance over commercial dyes and conventional semiconductor quantum dots in a wide variety of analytical and biomedical applications, including (bio)chemical sensing, photocatalysis, electrochemiluminescence, photoelectrochemical sensing, bioimaging, and drug delivery, because of their tunable photoluminescence, fine resistance to photobleaching, excellent water solubility, good biocompatibility, and ease of synthesis [1–4]. Based on the chosen carbonaceous precursors, the approaches to synthesize C-dots are divided into top-down and bottom-up routes [3–6]. The former involves cleaving or breaking down relatively macroscopic carbonaceous materials, such as carbon nanotubes, graphite columns, and graphene powder, via acidic and electrochemical oxidation, arc-discharge, and laser ablation. The latter is realized through carbonization of small organic molecules via solvothermal and hydrothermal pyrolysis, microwave and ultrasonic irradiation, and plasma treatment. The low requirement for carbon molecules in the bottom-up route is advantageous for obtaining C-dots with desirable morphological, functional, and spectral properties.

Due to equipment availability, plasma treatment is less reported than other approaches, especially compared to the mainly utilized microwave and hydrothermal syntheses. However, the ability to control the nanoscale localization of energy and matter delivered from bulk plasmas to form nano-solids is capable of unique self-organized processes [7]. In 2010, C-dots were first generated by the reaction of benzene with atmosphere helium cavitation gas in a submerged-arc plasma reactor [8]. Another plasma–liquid system used argon atmospheric-pressure microplasma as gaseous electrodes to purge an aqueous solution containing citric acid and ethylenediamine to produce C-dots [9]. Without the need for a well-designed reactor, the plasma-gas system can use gaseous and solid organic precursors. Methane, hydrogen, and nitrogen were used as the reactive gases in a plasma-enhanced hot filament chemical vapor deposition of carbon nanofilms and nanodots [10]. Ethylene gas was introduced continuously along with the thermal argon plasma jet at sound velocity to produce graphene quantum dots [11,12]. Also, solid egg white, yolk, acrylamide, and ashes of plant leaves were irradiated by air atmospheric-pressure dielectric barrier discharge plasmas to generate C-dots [13–15]. No liquid precursors have been irradiated in a plasma-gas system to obtain C-dots.

In this study, aliphatic acids dispersed in viscous media, ionic liquids and high b.p. solvents, were irradiated with capacitively coupled plasma (CCP) between regular plate electrodes in a low-pressure chamber, in presence of oxygen; to obtain C-dots. Due to its high fluorescence intensity, the C-dots synthesized via O_2/CCP treatment of 1-ethyl-3-methylimidazolium dicyanamide solution of citric acid were further characterized to determine the physical dimensions, crystallinity, functionality, and spectral properties of the C-dots. A possible fluorescence mechanism was proposed. After comparison with hydrothermal and microwave treatments, the O_2/CCP-treated C-dots were applied to detect metal ions and flavonoids.

2. Materials and Methods

2.1. Materials and Chemicals

Citric acid was purchased from Acros (Thermo Fisher Scientific, Geel, Belgium). Malic acid, ethylene glycol, 1,4-butanediol, and poly(ethylene imide) (PEI, branched, Mn = 600, Mw = 800) were from Aldrich (Milwaukee, WI, USA). Poly(ethylene glycol) (PEG, Mn = 1000) was purchased from Alfa Aesar (Ward Hill, MA, USA). Adipic acid, succinic acid, and glycerol were from Showa (Tokyo, Japan). Ionic liquids were purchased from Aldrich (1-ethyl-3-methylimidazolium dicyanamide, [EMIM]N(CN)$_2$; 1-ethyl-3-methylimidazolium tetrachloroaluminate, [EMIM]AlCl$_4$; 1-methyl-3-octylimidazolium chloride, [MOIM]Cl); and trihexyltetradecylphosphonium dicyanamide, [P6,6,6,14]N(CN)$_2$) and Alfa Aesar (1-butyl-3-methylimidazolium tetrafluoroborate, [BMIM]BF$_4$; 1-butyl-3-methylimidazolium chloride, [BMIM]Cl; and 1-butyl-3-methylimidazolium bromide, [BMIM]Br). Nine flavonoids (5-methoxyflavone (Met), hesperidin (Hpd), naringin (Nag), catechin (Cat), epicatechin (Epi), hesperetin (Hpt), daidzein (Dai), naringenin (Nar), and quercetin (Que)) were from Aldrich. All metal and phosphate salts were of analytical grade and were obtained from Aldrich and Acros. Purified water (18 MΩ·cm) from a Milli-Q water purification system (Millipore, Bedford, MA, USA) was used to prepare the standard salt and buffer solutions. All standard solutions were protected from light and kept at 4 °C in a refrigerator.

2.2. Synthesis and Characterization of C-Dots

For the capacitively coupled plasma (CCP) treatment, a crucible containing a mixture of an aliphatic acid (100 mg) and a viscous solvent (500 µL) was placed on a flat aluminum tray adapted for a cylindrical, stainless-steel, low pressure chamber (diameter of 10 cm and depth of 27.8 cm), which was evacuated by a rotary vane pump (3.0 $m^3 \cdot h^{-1}$) in a modular plasma system (Femto SRS, Diener electronic GmbH + Co. KG, Ebhausen, Germany). The system was initiated by an RF generator (13.56 MHz, 0~100 W) to discharge the inlet gas (O_2 or N_2) between an aluminum planar electrode and the flat tray under a working pressure of 0.285 torr. The gas flow was manually adjusted by a needle valve (0~50 sccm), and the chamber pressure was measured by a Pirani sensor (10^{-2}~10 mbar). The small-footprint, table-top system was semi-automatically processed through evacuation pumping, gas inlet, plasma ignition, and ventilation. For comparison, the crucible was placed in a domestic microwave oven (0~1150 Watt, 2450 MHz) or in a Teflon-lined vessel, sealed in a stainless-steel autoclave (50 mL) and calcined at a constant temperature (200 °C) for a specified period of time.

After treatment, the crucible was rinsed with 1.0 mL of H_2O to collect the synthesized C-dot products. The 1.0 mL C-dot solutions were diluted at different ratios with water for characterization or with phosphate buffers (50 mM, pH 7.0) to build a calibration curve. The diluted aqueous solutions were characterized by a ultraviolet-visible (UV-Vis) spectrometer (Lambda 35, Perkin Elmer, Cambridge, MA, USA), spectrofluorometer (LS55, Perkin Elmer, Cambridge, MA, USA), Fourier transform infrared (FTIR) spectrometer (Prestige-21, Shimadzu, Japan) equipped with a single reflection horizontal ATR accessory (MIRacle, PIKE Technologies, Fitchburg, WI, USA), high-resolution transmission electron microscopy (JEM-2100, JEOL, Tokyo, Japan) operated at an accelerating voltage of 200 kV, and laboratory-built electrophoresis apparatus consisting of a ± 30 kV high-voltage power supply (TriSep TM-2100, Unimicro Technologies, Pleasanton, CA, USA) and a UV-Vis detector (LCD 2083.2 CE, ECOM, Prague, Czech). Some product solutions were dried to evaporate the water at 70 °C in a vacuum oven for 24 h to prepare solid samples for high-resolution X-ray diffraction (D8 Discover, Bruker, MA, USA) and X-ray photoelectron spectroscopy (ULVAC-PHI PHI 5000 VersaProbe, Physical Electronics, Eden Prairie, MN, USA). Some product solutions (1.0 mL) were dialyzed against ultra-pure water through a molecular weight cutoff membrane (500–1000 Dalton, Float-A-Lyzer G2, 1 mL capacity, Spectrum Laboratories Inc., Savannah, GA, USA) to study the effect of the dialysis on the separation of the C-dot products.

2.3. Fluorescence Measurement of Samples with the CCP-Treated C-Dots

The CCP treatment of the mixture of citric acid (100 mg) and the ionic liquid (500 µL) [EMIM]N(CN)$_2$ was performed with 10 sccm O_2 inlet, 90 Watt RF power, and a 30 min duration. The as-prepared 1.0 mL C-dot solution possessed high fluorescence intensity and was capable of sensing samples. A small volume (0.2 µL) of the C-dot solution was added to each sample containing metal ions (33.3 µM) or flavonoids (8.33 µg/mL) in 3.0 mL of phosphate buffer (50 mM, pH 7.0) to measure the fluorescence intensities (I) at 430 nm (excitation at 330 nm) and 480 nm (excitation at 390 nm). These I values were compared with those (I_0) observed in the blank samples to evaluate the quenching effect (I/I_0) on the samples and to further establish the calibration curves for quercetin, a flavonoid.

A flavonoid-rich traditional Chinese medicine (TCM), called "Guang-Chen-Pi" in Chinese, was purchased from a TCM store in Taichung, Taiwan, and the amount of quercetin in the medicine was determined. After cleaning with deionized water, 5.0 g of dried Guang-Chen-Pi was triturated and refluxed in 50 mL ethanol for two hours. After filtering through a glass microfiber disc (GF/A, Whatman, England), 25 mL of the filtrate was concentrated to dryness on a rotary evaporator. The remaining residue was dissolved with 7.2 mL ethanol and became the sample solution. Five 3.0 mL vials were each spiked with 6.0 µL of the sample solution, and four of the five vials were further spiked with 1.0, 2.0, 3.0, and 4.0 µL of the quercetin standard solution (7.24×10^{-3} M). The quercetin in the ethanol extract of the Guang-Chen-Pi was calculated from the standard addition curve established by the I values of the five vials.

3. Results and Discussion

3.1. Choice of Short Aliphatic Acids and Solvents

Four short aliphatic acids, including citric acid (CA), succinic acid, adipic acid, and malic acid (MA), were separately dispersed in high b.p. solvents, including glycerol, PEG 1000, PEI 600, and seven ionic liquids, which are listed in Section 2.1. Then, the mixtures were treated with the oxygen-gas (10 sccm), RF-discharge (90 Watt) plasma produced between the capacitive-coupling, parallel-plate electrodes. If lower b.p. solvents, such as ethylene glycol (b.p. 197 °C) and 1,4-butanediol (b.p. 235 °C), were substituted for the high b.p. solvents, a large amount of vaporized solvent was rapidly produced just after the plasma initiation, and the vacuum pumping and RF power were quickly stopped. If only the acids were treated by the capacitively coupled plasma (CCP) without the addition of solvents, the white powder products looked like the native, untreated acids and showed no fluorescence. After dispersion in the high b.p. solvents and a 30 min treatment with O_2/CCP, dark brown products were obtained, re-dispersed in water, and measured by UV-Vis and fluorescence spectroscopies. The observed spectra are shown in Table S1 in the Electronic supplementary information (ESI). Except for glycerol and PEG 1000, for which the CCP products did not show any fluorescence, most of the solvents had excitation-dependent emissions. Glycerol and PEG do not contain any nitrogen atoms in their chemical structures, but the other solvents do. The nitrogen involvement in O_2/CCP carbonization of the acids is crucial for obtaining fluorescent C-dots. Although some fluorescent C-dots were obtained from non-nitrogen-containing materials by solvothermal [16], pyrolysis [17], hydrothermal [18], and microwave heating [19], nitrogen gas in air can enter the heating apparatuses and encounter the reactants to introduce nitrogen atoms into the C-dot structures. Even heating glycerol or PEG solvents alone in a domestic microwave oven resulted in fluorescent C-dots [20,21]. In this study, the nitrogen in air could not enter the CCP vacuum chamber. The only nitrogen source was the high b.p. solvents. Currently, most fluorescent C-dots are synthesized from nitrogen-containing carbon sources, solvents, or additives. In these cases, nitrogen-containing solvents act both as a dispersant and a passivant.

As shown in Table S1, the highest photoluminescence (PL) intensity (I_{max}) observed at the corresponding emission ($\lambda_{em,max}$) and excitation ($\lambda_{ex,max}$) wavelengths varied with the acid and nitrogen-containing solvent used. Some of the solvents, including PEI 600, [BMIM]AlCl$_4$, [BMIM]BF$_4$, and [MOIM]Cl, possessed similar $\lambda_{em,max}$ and $\lambda_{ex,max}$ values for all the acids, but other solvents did not. Most of the CCP products possessed an obvious dependence of λ_{em} on λ_{ex}, but a few of them did not. Interestingly, the C-dots obtained from the O_2/CCP treatment of CA and MA in [EMIM]N(CN)$_2$ possessed the first and second highest photoluminescence (PL) intensities among the CCP products in Table S1, but their dependence of λ_{em} on λ_{ex} was obscure. As shown in Figure 1a and Table S1, the emission redshifts were only 11 nm and 26 nm as an increase of 80 nm in λ_{ex} was applied to the CA-based C-dots (350 nm to 430 nm) and MA-based C-dots (300 nm to 380 nm), respectively. In contrast, as shown in Figure 1(b), an obvious 58 nm redshift emission (λ_{ex} = 350~430 nm) was observed for the O_2/CCP of [EMIM]N(CN)$_2$ alone. Moreover, the $\lambda_{em,max}$ position and the smaller PL intensity in Figure 1b were different from those of the CA- and MA-based C-dots. There should be a synergistic effect of [EMIM]N(CN)$_2$ and the acids, CA and MA, on the formation of fluorescent C-dots in the O_2/CCP carbonization. Further discussion about the independence of λ_{ex} for the CA-based C-dots is addressed in Section 3.2.

Instead of O_2/CCP, the N_2/CCP treatment of CA in glycerol under the same CCP conditions converted non-fluorescent C-dots to fluorescent ones, as shown in Figure 1c, and they present a $\lambda_{em,max}$ of 400 nm with a $\lambda_{ex,max}$ of 330 nm and a 19 nm redshift emission with an excitation from 290 nm to 370 nm. The definite difference in the fluorescence and UV-Vis spectra between Figure 1a,c implies the different routes of C-dot formation. Although the N_2/CCP treatment aided the use of non-nitrogen-containing glycerol, its PL intensity was much lower than that of the product from the O_2/CCP treatment of CA in [EMIM]N(CN)$_2$ at the same dilution factor. Because a fluorophore with a high PL intensity is advantageous for analytical uses, CA dispersed in [EMIM]N(CN)$_2$ was selected to be the carbon source for the O_2/CCP carbonization in the following discussion.

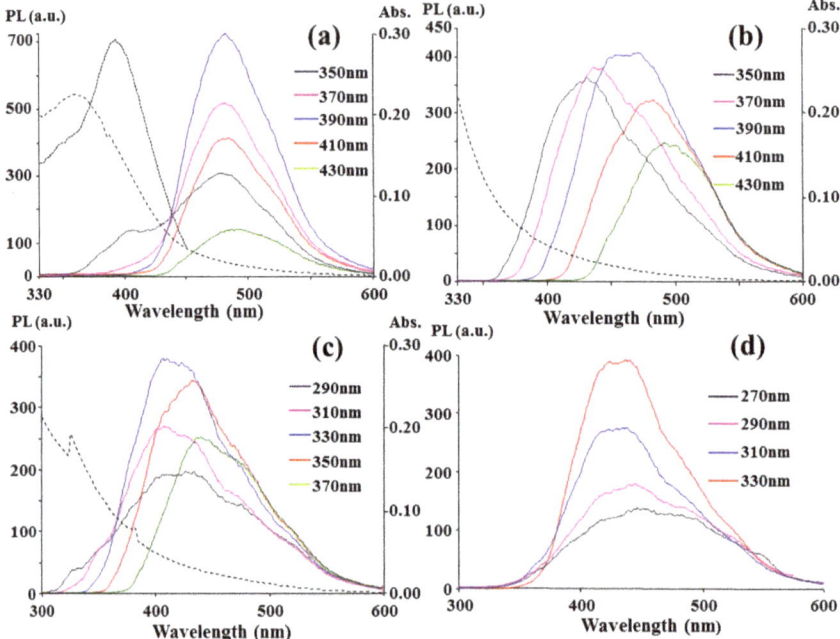

Figure 1. Fluorescence spectra of (**a,d**) CA + [EMIM]N(CN)$_2$; (**b**) [EMIM]N(CN)$_2$; and (**c**) CA + glycerol treated by O$_2$/CCP (**a,b,d**) and N$_2$/CCP (**c**). The mixtures of CA (100 mg) and solvents (500 µL) were treated by CCP (10 sccm of gas flow, RF power 90 W, 30 min). After the addition of 1.0 mL of H$_2$O to the treated products, different volumes of the product solutions (0.2 µL for (**a,d**) and 20 µL for (**b,c**)) were separately transferred to cuvettes filled with 3.0 mL of H$_2$O for spectrometric measurements. (—) and (····) curves denote UV-Vis absorption and PL (emission at 480 nm) spectra, respectively.

3.2. Characterization of CCP-Treated C-Dots

The high-resolution TEM (HRTEM) image of the C-dots obtained in the conditions of Figure 1a is shown in Figure S1, and the average size of the 55 particles analyzed by the ImageJ freeware was 8.6 nm (σ = 1.1 nm). Most of the C-dots did not have any clear lattice fringes in the HRTEM image, but a few indicated spaces between the graphene layers, as shown in Figure 2a and Figure S1. This was further supported by the X-ray diffraction (XRD) pattern in Figure 2b, which displayed a broad diffraction peak due to the amorphous nature of the sample and a distinct peak centered at 2θ = 27.3° for the (002) facet of graphite. The prepared C-dots would be classified as carbon quantum dots rather than carbon nanodots according to the classification in a recent paper [22]. Capillary zone electrophoresis was used to analyze the changes in the surface charge of the C-dots via the electrophoretic mobility (μ_{ep}) at the pH of the running buffers. As shown in Figure 2c, the μ_{ep} values, which were determined by subtracting the electroosmotic mobilities (μ_{eof}) from the apparent mobilities (μ_{app}) and inferred net charge on the C-dot surface, were positive below pH 5.0 and negative above pH 8.9. The dissociation of carboxylic acid and protonated amine or 1.3-diketones would occur on the C-dot surface as their pKa values are near to 5.0 and 8.9, respectively. The full scan of the XPS spectrum presents the main peaks of C 1s, N 1s, and O 1s in Figure 2d. The carbon content (49.5%) in the O$_2$/CCP product was reasonable and in the range between the reactants CA (C: 37.5%) and [EMIM]N(CN)$_2$ (C: 58.9%). However, a large decrease in the oxygen percentage from 58.3% in CA to 13.2% in the product was distinct from the slight increase in the nitrogen percentage from 34.4% in [EMIM]N(CN)$_2$ to 37.4% in the product. This indicates that the oxygen atoms in CA were more easily subtracted by the oxygen plasma than the nitrogen atoms bound in the imidazole ring in [EMIM]N(CN)$_2$. The deconvolution of the main peaks is shown in Figure S2. In detail, four peaks related to the C–C (284.3 eV), C–N (284.9 eV), C–O (285.9 eV), and C=O/C=N (287.6 eV) functional groups were deconvoluted from the C 1s spectrum. The N 1s spectrum contained three nitrogen bonding groups, including C–N–C (399.5 eV), N–(C)$_3$ (400.2 eV), and N–H (401.9 eV). The O 1s spectrum contained two characteristic peaks corresponding to the C=O (530.7 ev) and C–OH/C–O–C (532.3 eV) groups. Although the peaks of C=N and N–(C)$_3$ may support the existence of the imidazole group, the peaks for C–N, C–N–C, and N–H imply that parts of the imidazole rings were pyrolyzed. Further evidence of the decomposition of imidazole rings was given by the FTIR spectra in Figure 2e, which show that the characteristic absorption bands of the aromatic CN heterocycles observed at 1465 to 1600 cm^{-1} in [EMIM]N(CN)$_2$ disappeared after the O$_2$/CCP treatment. Even the dicyanamide anion decomposed, and its C≡N group absorption at 2145 cm^{-1} also vanished after the plasma action. The other typical peaks of the plasma product were recognized as specific chemical bonding in Figure 2e.

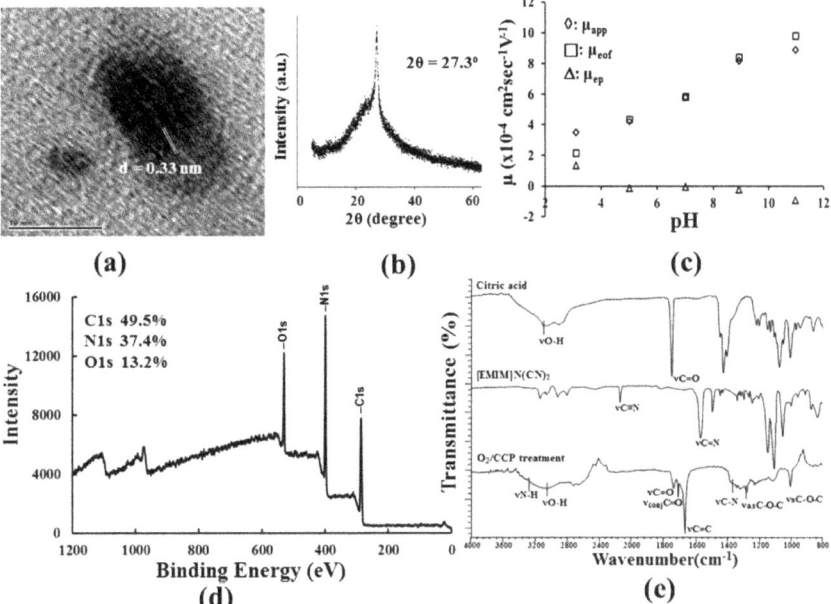

Figure 2. Characterization of the C-dots prepared in the conditions of Figure 1a. (a) HRTEM image; (b) XRD spectrum; (c) the plot of mobility with the pH of the running buffers; (d) XPS spectrum, and (e) FTIR spectrum.

The PL, PLE (PL excitation), and UV-Vis absorption spectra of the as-prepared C-dots are shown in Figure 1a, and an excitation-independent PL and an absorption peak at 360 nm, which was different from $\lambda_{ex,max}$ = 390 nm, were observed. The emission at approximately 480 nm is independent of the excited light beam from 350 nm to 430 nm. At $\lambda_{ex,max}$ = 390 nm, the quantum yield of the C-dots was 12.4% based on a calibration against the reference quinine sulfate in 0.5 M H$_2$SO$_4$, as shown in Figure S3. The same phenomenon occurred in Figure 1d, and the excited light beam from 270 to 330 nm produced another independent emission at approximately 430 nm for the C-dots. At $\lambda_{ex,max}$ = 330 nm, the quantum yield was calculated to be 7.2% with reference to 2-aminopyridine in 0.5 M H$_2$SO$_4$, as shown in Figure S3. The two λ_{ex}-independent emissions at 430 nm and 480 nm indicate two emissive states for each uniform energy distribution on the C-dots. Neither of the two emissions could be categorized as an intrinsic emission ($\pi^* \rightarrow \pi$) from the carbon core because the quantum confinement effect determines that 8.6 nm in diameter C-dots would have a longer-wavelength emission than near infrared but not visible emissions [23]. The molecule states, which are determined solely by the fluorescent molecules connected on the surface or interior of the C-dots, may be emissive states because λ_{ex} independence is a characteristic of a molecule state [24–27]. However, the possibility of forming molecule states on the C-dots was excluded because no reasonable route to form a fluorophore molecule via the reaction of CA and [EMIM]N(CN)$_2$ could be inferred, whereas fluorophores were reasonably formed by the reaction of CA and a primary amine, such as ethanolamine and ethylene diamine [24,27]. Therefore, the two emissions should come from the surface states, which consisted of hybridization of the carbon backbone and the connected chemical groups because the π^* and molecule states were excluded as the emissive states [28].

A dialysis membrane (cellulose ester, 500–1000 Da molecular weight cut-off) was used as an ultrafilter for the as-prepared C-dots to separate the two surface states. As shown in Figure 3a, the 430 nm emission of the dialyzed C-dots that collected outside the membrane grew stronger after the first 2 h dialysis, but the 480 nm emission was weaker than that inside the membrane. Moreover, the UV absorption peak at approximately 360 nm for the dialyzed C-dots vanished, and this could be related to the weakness of the 480 nm emission. The fluorescence spectra of the C-dots dialyzed at various times are assembled in Figure S4, and the changes in the ratio of the PL intensity at 430 nm to that at 480 nm with the dialysis time are plotted in Figure 3b. The plot shows that the C-dot particles with higher ratio values penetrate through membrane faster than those with lower ratios, and each as-prepared C-dot particle did not have a uniform surface composition with an identical PL intensity ratio. The faster penetration was apparently not due to the smaller particle size because the average diameter (3.1 nm, σ = 1.0 nm) of the C-dots dialyzed for the first two hours was close to that (3.6 nm, σ = 1.1 nm) for those dialyzed for 8 h, as shown in Figure S5. The main reason for different penetration rate is that some of the functional groups or surface states leading to the 430 nm emission favored penetration, but other surface states that lead to the 480 nm emission did not favor penetration. These two groups simultaneously collected on a C-dot particle, but the buildup of the groups on the particles was in different mole ratios. Figure 3c shows a possible energy level diagram for a C-dot particle. For the two emissions, the excitation radiation beams actuated the valence π electrons in the core of the C-dot particle to the π^* conduction band. Then, the excited electrons transitioned to the emissive surface states via radiationless relaxation between the lower π^* levels and/or their hybrid states, which were hybridized with core carbon and heteroatoms, such as nitrogen and oxygen atoms, during the nucleation step in the carbonation.

The upconversion emission at $\lambda_{em,max}$ = 480 nm was observed for the C-dots with 710–790 nm excitation ($\lambda_{ex,max}$ = 790 nm), as shown in Figure S6. The emission intensity increased with the excitation wavelength. A longer-wavelength light than 800 nm was not available due to the limitations of the fluorospectrophotometer used in this study, but a longer wavelength source, such as a near-IR laser, might induce a higher PL intensity. A 790 nm light stimulated the 480 nm up-conversion emission, and a 390 nm light also stimulated the 480 nm emission, as shown in Figure 1a. This was expected because 790 nm is nearly double 390 nm and is suitable for the sequential absorption of two long wavelength photons. However, a 430 nm up-conversion emission was not observed in the excitation range from 430 to 790 nm. The π^* transit states (2λ = 660 nm) that correlated with the 430 nm emission at $\lambda_{ex,max}$ = 330 nm, as shown in Figure 1d, would be less stable for the sequential absorption than those (2λ = 780 nm) that correlated with the 480 nm and underwent radiationless relaxation.

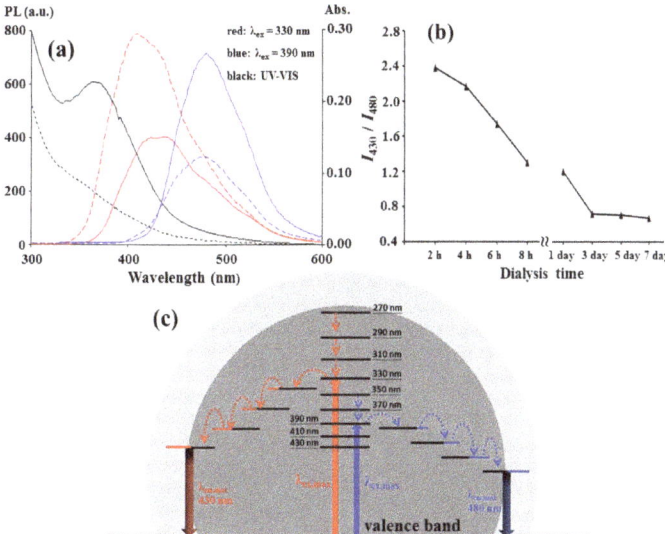

Figure 3. (a) Fluorescence and UV-Vis absorption spectra of the C-dots prepared in the conditions of Figure 1a before (solid lines) and after (dashed lines) dialysis in H$_2$O by a 500–1000 Da cut-off membrane for two hours; (b) The plot of the PL intensity ratios of 430 nm PL intensity to 480 nm PL intensity with the dialysis duration; (c) The proposed PL mechanism.

3.3. Comparison between CCP, Microwave, and Hydrothermal Carbonation

For a comparison, CA and [EMIM]N(CN)$_2$ were mixed in a crucible and heated in a domestic microwave oven at 90 Watt. The heating was stopped after 4.5 min because a severe burning flame appeared on the crucible during the microwave irradiation. As shown in Figure 4a, the microwave-treated product emission at 430 nm is stronger than its emission at 480 nm. Therefore, the number of surface states corresponding to the 430 nm emission should be larger than the number corresponding to the 480 nm emission. Furthermore, the chemical composition corresponding to the two surface states caused by microwave radiation with a sufficient oxygen supply should be different from that caused by the CCP ion bombardment under a limited oxygen supply. The stronger 430 nm emission obtained with a sufficient oxygen supply implied that the formation of the 430 nm emissive surface states involved oxygen atoms. Figure 4a shows the $\lambda_{ex,max}$ was 370 nm or 390 nm for the maximum emission at $\lambda_{em,max}$ = 430 nm, and the $\lambda_{ex,max}$ was 430 nm for that at $\lambda_{em,max}$ = 480 nm. The two $\lambda_{ex,max}$ values are larger (approximately 40 nm) than those in Figure 1d ($\lambda_{ex,max}$ = 330 nm) and Figure 1a ($\lambda_{ex,max}$ = 390 nm), respectively. In addition to the changes in the surface composition, the severe carbonation in a microwave oven might extend the domain of the double bond and shrink the energy gap between π and π^* to cause the 40 nm redshift compared with that for the CCP treatment. Without the addition of CA, heating [EMIM]N(CN)$_2$ alone in a microwave could not provide the considerable 480 nm emission and only resulted in a strong 430 nm emission ($\lambda_{em,max}$ = 400 nm) at a shorter λ_{ex} (290~350 nm), as shown in Figure 4b. In comparison with Figure 4a, the participation of CA in the carbonation could mainly contribute the 480 nm emissive states and the extension of the conjugated double bonds to the C-dot structure.

The mixture of CA and [EMIM]N(CN)$_2$ was also placed in a Teflon-lined autoclave and heated in a hot-air oven at 200 °C for 30 min. The PL and UV-Vis absorption spectra of the hydrothermal products are plotted in Figure 4c and are similar to those in Figure 1a, which were obtained from O$_2$/CCP at 10 sccm, except the PL intensity was smaller than that in Figure 1a. Furthermore, the spectrum of the [EMIM]N(CN)$_2$ alone sample treated by a hydrothermal method was similar to that from the CCP method, i.e., comparison of Figure 4d with Figure 1b. It is believed that fine tuning the temperature and duration of the hydrothermal reaction in an autoclave could enhance the similarity of the reaction to the CCP carbonation in a vacuum chamber with a low O_2 supply, i.e., 10 sccm in our system. Figure 4d shows the results from 5.0 h of heating [EMIM]N(CN)$_2$ alone in an autoclave. Only 30 min of heating by the hydrothermal method could not obtain a PL spectrum, but Figure 1b spectrum by the O_2/CCP method was obtained.

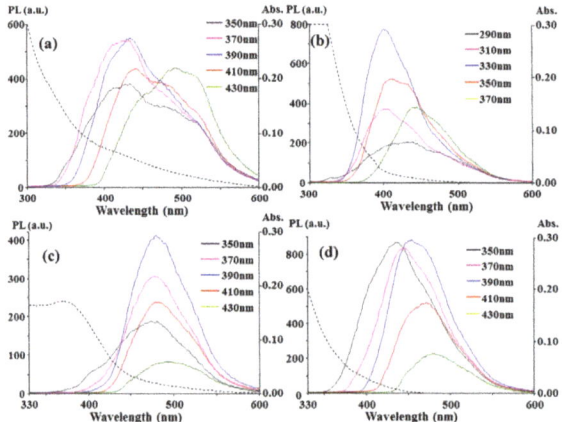

Figure 4. Fluorescence and UV-Vis absorption spectra for the CA + [EMIM]N(CN)$_2$ (**a**,**c**) and [EMIM]N(CN)$_2$ alone (**b**,**d**) samples heated in a 90 W microwave oven for 4.5 min (**a**,**b**) and in an autoclave at 200 °C for 30 min (**c**) and 5.0 h (**d**). After the addition of 1.0 mL of H$_2$O to the heated products, the product solutions of 0.2 µL for (**a**); 0.3 µL for (**b**); 2.0 µL for (**c**); and 15 µL for (**d**) were diluted with 3.0 mL of H$_2$O to measure the spectra.

3.4. Fluorescent Sensing by the O$_2$/CCP-Treated C-Dots

The fluorescent C-dots prepared by O_2/CCP of a mixture of CA and [EMIM]N(CN)$_2$ in the conditions shown in the legend of Figure 1a were used to separately probe fifteen metal ions and nine flavonoids. At first, the λ_{ex}-independent emissions at 430 nm ($\lambda_{ex,max}$ = 330 nm) and 480 nm ($\lambda_{ex,max}$ = 390 nm) of the C-dots were used to evaluate their responses to the analytes. The 480 nm emission was quenched by Cu^{2+}, Ag^+, and Hg^{2+}, while the 430 nm emission was further quenched by Fe^{3+} in addition to those ions, as shown in Figure 5a, where I and I_0 are the emission intensities in the absence and presence of the sample, respectively. The ions, Fe^{3+}, Cu^{2+}, and Ag^+, quenched 10~15% of each emission, and nearly 30% of the 430 nm emission and 65% of the 480 nm emission could be heavily quenched by Hg^{2+}. The quenching was sensitive to Hg^{2+}, especially the 480 nm emission, but the coexistence of the Fe^{3+}, Cu^{2+}, and Ag^+ ions in a real sample would interfere with the detection of Hg^{2+}. However, the synthetic C-dots are good starting fluorescent materials for further ligand attachment on them to improve a sensor's specificity for Hg^{2+} in the presence of interfering ions.

For the flavonoid samples, quercetin, hesperetin, and naringenin could quench nearly half of the 430 nm emission, but daidzein and 5-methoxyflavone passivated some unknown surface traps and enhanced the 430 nm PL intensity, as shown in Figure 5b. In contrast to the 430 nm emission, the 480 nm emission was only selectively quenched by quercetin, and the other flavonoids did not affect the 480 nm emission. Therefore, the C-dots would directly sense quercetin in a flavonoid-rich sample, such as *Citrus reticulata* cv. Chachiensis, which is a sun-dried peel used as a traditional Chinese medicine, called "Guang-Chen-Pi" in Chinese. For quantification, the 480 nm PL intensities were measured (Figure 5c) after equilibrium with quercetin standards in a phosphate buffer, pH 7.0, 50 mM, and they were plotted against the quercetin concentrations ranging from 2.4 µM to 119 µM in Figure 5d.

As shown in Figure 5d, the Stern–Volmer plot, I_0/I v.s. [quercetin], is not linear. The deviation from linearity is frequently attributed to a combination of dynamic and static quenching and can be corrected using a modified Stern–Volmer plot, i.e., the Perrin model:

$$\ln (I_0/I) = N_A V \text{[Quencher]}$$

where $\alpha = N_A V$, where N_A is Avogadro's number and V is the volume of the active sphere of quenching. Based on the good linearity ($R^2 = 0.9992$) and high slope (1.96×10^4 M^{-1}) of the Perrin relationship, the radius of the effective quenching sphere was calculated to be 19.8 nm, which is 2.3 times the C-dot radius (8.6 nm) and allowed an efficient, photoinduced electron-transfer process of the encounter pair between the C-dot (as an electron donor) and quercetin (as an electron acceptor) without coupling reagents. The relative standard deviation for seven replicate measurements of 12.1 µM quercetin solutions was 3.3%. Based on the 3σ of the blank response ($\sigma = 3.1\%$, $n = 10$), the detection limit was calculated to be 0.5 µM. As shown in the inset of Figure 5d, the quercetin in the ethanol extract of Guang-Chen-Pi was determined by a standard addition method to be 4.20 ± 0.15 mg/g, which was nearly nine times higher than 0.47 mg/g found in the air-dried peel of *Citrus reticulate* Blanco [29]. Some factors, such as the citrus species used, growth environment, and method of drying the peel, accounted for the difference. The matrix effect was evaluated by the ratio defined as $(S_1 - S_2) \times 100\%/S_2$, where S_1 and S_2 are the slopes of the calibration curves obtained by standard addition ($S_1 = 2.12 \times 10^4$ M^{-1}, $R^2 = 0.9990$) and external standard ($S_2 = 1.96 \times 10^4$ M^{-1}) methods, respectively [30]. The calculated ratio, 8.16%, was lower than 10%, which suggested that the matrix effect could be ignored by the standard addition method. The selectivity of the 480 nm emission from the C-dots for quercetin helped reduce the matrix effect.

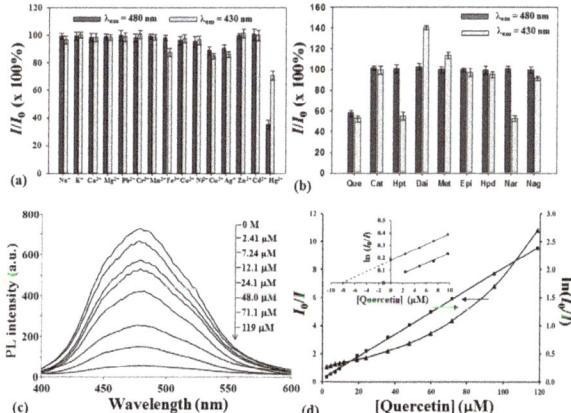

Figure 5. Effect of different metal ions (33.3 µM) (**a**) and flavonoids (8.33 µg/mL) (**b**) on the relative PL intensity (I/I_0) of the C-dots prepared in the conditions of Figure 1a; (**c**): Emission spectra of the prepared C-dots before and after the addition of various concentrations of quercetin; (**d**): The respective emission intensities are plotted versus the quercetin concentrations according to the Stern–Volmer (▲) and Perrin (■) models. The curve of the standard addition calibration (♦) for the determination of quercetin in the ethanol extract of Guang-Chen-Pi is inserted in (**d**). I and I_0 are the PL intensities observed in the presence (I) and absence (I_0), respectively, of the samples in a 50 mM phosphate buffer at pH 7.0.

4. Conclusions

The use of O_2/CCP in the carbonation of mixtures of aliphatic acids and nitrogen-containing viscous liquids, such as ionic liquids and PEI, was successful in forming fluorescent molecules.

The dispersion of citric acid in [EMIM]N(CN)$_2$ possessed the highest fluorescence intensity among the mixtures, and the characteristics of the carbon quantum dots with C–N, C–O, O–H, and N–H functionalities were two excitation-independent emissions emerging from two surface states and upconversion of the fluorescence. In a comparison of the fluorescence spectra, the CCP-treated C-dots were similar to the hydrothermally synthesized ones because they were operated in an oxygen-limited environment, but they were different from the MW-irradiated ones in an open environment. With specificity for quercetin among nine flavonoids, the CCP-treated C-dots were applied to determine the quercetin content in Guang-Chen-Pi, 4.20 ± 0.15 mg/g. Among fifteen metal ions, mercury ions most effectively quenched the fluorescence of the CCP-treated C-dots. Instead of O$_2$/CCP, the N$_2$/CCP treatment of citric acid in glycerol under the same CCP conditions converted non-fluorescent C-dots to fluorescent ones. This CCP-gas system can, not only provide carbonization of carbonaceous materials but doping of heteroatoms or afterwards.

Supplementary Materials: The following are available online at http://www.mdpi.com/2079-4991/8/6/372/s1, Figure S1: TEM images of the as-prepared C-dots; Figure S2: The deconvolution of the C 1s, N 1s, and O 1s XPS peaks from the O$_2$/CCP of the mixture of CA and [EMIM]N(CN)$_2$; Figure S3: Plot of the normalized PL intensity against the UV-Vis absorbance for the determination of the quantum yield; Figure S4: The fluorescence spectra of the C-dots collected after different dialysis times; Figure S5: TEM images of the C-dots dialyzed for two hours and their size distribution; Figure S6: Up-conversion emissions of the prepared C-dots under different wavelength excitations; Table S1: The UV-Vis and fluorescence spectra of the products obtained by CCP treatments.

Author Contributions: J.-L.C. supervised the experiments and assured the high quality of the scientific content. C.-B.K. and T.-L.L. conducted experiments and wrote the paper. All authors read and approved the final manuscript.

Acknowledgments: Support for this work by the Ministry of Science and Technology of Taiwan under Grant no. MOST–106-2113-M-039-006 and the China Medical University under Grant no. CMU106-S-17 is gratefully acknowledged.

Conflicts of Interest: The authors declare no conflict of interest.

References

1. Qi, B.-P.; Bao, L.; Zhang, Z.-L.; Pang, D.-W. Electrochemical methods to study photoluminescent carbon nanodots: Preparation, photoluminescence mechanism and sensing. *ACS Appl. Mater. Interfaces* **2016**, *8*, 28372–28382. [CrossRef] [PubMed]
2. Du, Y.; Guo, S. Chemically doped fluorescent carbon and graphene quantum dots for bioimaging, sensor, catalytic and photoelectronic applications. *Nanoscale* **2016**, *8*, 2532–2543. [CrossRef] [PubMed]
3. Gao, X.; Du, C.; Zhuang, Z.; Chen, W. Carbon quantum dot-based nanoprobes for metal ion detection. *J. Mater. Chem. C* **2016**, *4*, 6927–6945. [CrossRef]
4. Namdari, P.; Negahdari, B.; Eatemadi, A. Synthesis, properties and biomedical applications of carbon-based quantum dots: An updated review. *Biomed. Pharmacother.* **2017**, *87*, 209–222. [CrossRef] [PubMed]
5. Miao, P.; Han, K.; Tang, Y.; Wang, B.; Lin, T.; Cheng, W. Recent advances in carbon nanodots: Synthesis, properties and biomedical applications. *Nanoscale* **2015**, *7*, 1586–1595. [CrossRef] [PubMed]
6. Zheng, X.T.; Ananthanarayanan, A.; Luo, K.Q.; Chen, P. Glowing graphene quantum dots and carbon dots: Properties, syntheses, and biological applications. *Small* **2015**, *11*, 1620–1636. [CrossRef] [PubMed]
7. Ostrikov, K.; Neyts, E.C.; Meyyappan, M. Plasma nanoscience: From nano-solids in plasmas to nano-plasmas in solids. *Adv. Phys.* **2013**, *62*, 113–224. [CrossRef]
8. Jiang, H.; Chen, F.; Lagally, M.G.; Denes, F.S. New strategy for synthesis and functionalization of carbon nanoparticles. *Langmuir* **2010**, *26*, 1991–1995. [CrossRef] [PubMed]
9. Wang, Z.; Lu, Y.; Yuan, H.; Ren, Z.; Xu, C.; Chen, J. Microplasma-assisted rapid synthesis of luminescent nitrogen-doped carbon dots and their application in pH sensing and uranium detection. *Nanoscale* **2015**, *7*, 20743–20748. [CrossRef] [PubMed]
10. Wang, B.B.; Chen, C.C.; Zheng, K.; Cheng, Q.J.; Wang, L.; Wang, R.Z. Comparative study of the carbon nanofilm and nanodots grown by plasma-enhanced hot filament chemical vapor deposition. *Mater. Sci. Semicond. Process.* **2014**, *21*, 146–153. [CrossRef]

11. Kim, J.; Suh, J.S. Size-controllable and low-cost fabrication of graphene quantum dots using thermal plasma jet. *ACS Nano* **2014**, *8*, 4190–4196. [CrossRef] [PubMed]
12. Lee, M.W.; Kim, J.; Suh, J.S. Characteristics of graphene quantum dots determined by edge structures: Three kinds of dots fabricated using thermal plasma jet. *RSC Adv.* **2015**, *5*, 67669–67675. [CrossRef]
13. Wang, J.; Wang, C.-F.; Chen, S. Amphiphilic egg-derived carbon dots: Rapid plasma fabrication, pyrolysis process, and multicolor printing patterns. *Angew. Chem. Int. Ed.* **2015**, *51*, 9297–9301. [CrossRef] [PubMed]
14. Li, C.-X.; Yu, C.; Wang, C.-F.; Chen, S. Facile plasma-induced fabrication of fluorescent carbon dots toward high-performance white LEDs. *J. Mater. Sci.* **2013**, *48*, 6307–6311. [CrossRef]
15. Zhu, L.; Yin, Y.; Wang, C.-F.; Chen, S. Plant leaf-derived fluorescent carbon dots for sensing, patterning and coding. *J. Mater. Chem. C* **2013**, *1*, 4925–4932. [CrossRef]
16. Jia, X.; Wang, E. One-pot green synthesis of optically pH-sensitive carbon dots with upconversion luminescence. *Nanoscale* **2012**, *4*, 5572–5575. [CrossRef] [PubMed]
17. Lai, C.-W.; Hsiao, Y.-H.; Peng, Y.-K.; Chou, P.-T. Facile synthesis of highly emissive carbon dots from pyrolysis of glycerol; gram scale production of carbon dots/mSiO$_2$ for cell imaging and drug release. *J. Mater. Chem.* **2012**, *22*, 14403–14409. [CrossRef]
18. Yang, Z.-C.; Wang, M.; Yong, A.M.; Wong, S.Y.; Zhang, X.-H.; Tan, H.; Chang, A.Y.; Li, X.; Wang, J. Intrinsically fluorescent carbon dots with tunable emission derived from hydrothermal treatment of glucose in the presence of monopotassium phosphate. *Chem. Commun.* **2011**, *47*, 11615–11617. [CrossRef] [PubMed]
19. Zhu, H.; Wang, X.; Li, Y.; Wang, Z.; Yang, F.; Yang, X. Microwave synthesis of fluorescent carbon nanoparticles with electrochemiluminescence properties. *Chem. Commun.* **2009**, 5118–5120. [CrossRef] [PubMed]
20. Wang, X.; Qu, K.; Xu, B.; Ren, J.; Qu, X. Microwave assisted one-step green synthesis of cell-permeable multicolor photoluminescent carbon dots without surface passivation reagents. *J. Mater. Chem.* **2011**, *21*, 2445–2450. [CrossRef]
21. Jaiswal, A.; Ghosh, S.S.; Chattopadhyay, A. One step synthesis of C-dots by microwave mediated caramelization of poly(ethylene glycol). *Chem. Commun.* **2012**, *48*, 407–409. [CrossRef] [PubMed]
22. Cayuela, A.; Soriano, M.L.; Carrillo-Carrión, C.; Valcárcel, M. Semiconductor and carbon-based fluorescent nanodots: The need for consistency. *Chem. Commun.* **2016**, *52*, 1311–1326. [CrossRef] [PubMed]
23. Li, H.; He, X.; Kang, Z.; Huang, H.; Liu, Y.; Liu, J.; Lian, S.; Tsang, C.H.A.; Yang, X.; Lee, S.-T. Water-soluble fluorescent carbon quantum dots and photocatalyst design. *Angew. Chem. Int. Ed.* **2010**, *49*, 4430–4434. [CrossRef] [PubMed]
24. Krysmann, M.J.; Kelarakis, A.; Dallas, P.; Giannelis, E.P. Formation mechanism of carbogenic nanoparticles with dual photoluminescence emission. *J. Am. Chem. Soc.* **2012**, *134*, 747–750. [CrossRef] [PubMed]
25. Zhu, S.; Meng, Q.; Wang, L.; Zhang, J.; Song, Y.; Jin, H.; Zhang, K.; Sun, H.; Wang, H.; Yang, B. Highly photoluminescent carbon dots for multicolor patterning, sensors, and bioimaging. *Angew. Chem. Int. Ed.* **2013**, *52*, 3953–3957. [CrossRef] [PubMed]
26. Song, Y.; Zhu, S.; Xiang, S.; Zhao, X.; Zhang, J.; Zhang, H.; Fu, Y.; Yang, B. Investigation into the fluorescence quenching behaviors and applications of carbon dots. *Nanoscale* **2014**, *6*, 4676–4682. [CrossRef] [PubMed]
27. Song, Y.; Zhu, S.; Zhang, S.; Fu, Y.; Wang, L.; Zhao, X.; Yang, B. Investigation from chemical structure to photoluminescent mechanism: A type of carbon dots from the pyrolysis of citric acid and an amine. *J. Mater. Chem. C* **2015**, *3*, 5976–5984. [CrossRef]
28. Zhu, S.; Song, Y.; Zhao, X.; Shao, J.; Zhang, J.; Yang, B. The photoluminescence mechanism in carbon dots (graphene quantum dots, carbon nanodots, and polymer dots): Current state and future perspective. *Nano Res.* **2015**, *8*, 355–381. [CrossRef]
29. Wang, Y.-C.; Chuang, Y.-C.; Hsu, H.-W. The flavonoid, carotenoid and pectin content in peels of citrus cultivated in Taiwan. *Food Chem.* **2008**, *106*, 277–284. [CrossRef]
30. Fernández, P.; González, M.; Regenjo, M.; Ares, A.M.; Fernández, A.M.; Lorenzo, R.A.; Carro, A.M. Analysis of drugs of abuse in human plasma using microextraction by packed sorbents and ultra-high-performance liquid chromatography. *J. Chromato. A* **2017**, *1485*, 8–19. [CrossRef] [PubMed]

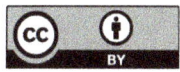

© 2018 by the authors. Licensee MDPI, Basel, Switzerland. This article is an open access article distributed under the terms and conditions of the Creative Commons Attribution (CC BY) license (http://creativecommons.org/licenses/by/4.0/).

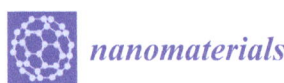

Article

Pulse-Modulated Radio-Frequency Alternating-Current-Driven Atmospheric-Pressure Glow Discharge for Continuous-Flow Synthesis of Silver Nanoparticles and Evaluation of Their Cytotoxicity toward Human Melanoma Cells

Anna Dzimitrowicz [1], Aleksandra Bielawska-Pohl [2], George C. diCenzo [3], Piotr Jamroz [1], Jan Macioszczyk [4], Aleksandra Klimczak [2] and Pawel Pohl [1,*]

[1] Department of Analytical Chemistry and Chemical Metallurgy, Faculty of Chemistry, Wroclaw University of Science and Technology, Wybrzeze St. Wyspianskiego 27, 50-370 Wroclaw, Poland; anna.dzimitrowicz@pwr.edu.pl (A.D.); piotr.jamroz@pwr.edu.pl (P.J.)

[2] Laboratory of Biology of Stem and Neoplastic Cells, Hirszfeld Institute of Immunology and Experimental Therapy Polish Academy of Science, R. Weigla 12, 53-114 Wroclaw, Poland; aleksandra.bielawska@iitd.pan.wroc.pl (A.B.-P.); klimczak@iitd.pan.wroc.pl (A.K.)

[3] Department of Biology, University of Florence, via Madonna del Piano 6, 50017 Sesto Fiorentino, Italy; georgecolin.dicenzo@unifi.it

[4] Faculty of Microsystem Electronics and Photonics, Wroclaw University of Science and Technology, Wybrzeze St. Wyspianskiego 27, 50-370 Wroclaw, Poland; jan.macioszczyk@pwr.edu.pl

* Correspondence: pawel.pohl@pwr.edu.pl; Tel.: +48-71-320-24-94

Received: 14 May 2018; Accepted: 30 May 2018; Published: 2 June 2018

Abstract: An innovative and environmentally friendly method for the synthesis of size-controlled silver nanoparticles (AgNPs) is presented. Pectin-stabilized AgNPs were synthesized in a plasma-reaction system in which pulse-modulated radio-frequency atmospheric-pressure glow discharge (pm-rf-APGD) was operated in contact with a flowing liquid electrode. The use of pm-rf-APGD allows for better control of the size of AgNPs and their stability and monodispersity. AgNPs synthesized under defined operating conditions exhibited average sizes of 41.62 ± 12.08 nm and 10.38 ± 4.56 nm, as determined by dynamic light scattering and transmission electron microscopy (TEM), respectively. Energy-dispersive X-ray spectroscopy (EDS) confirmed that the nanoparticles were composed of metallic Ag. Furthermore, the ξ-potential of the AgNPs was shown to be -43.11 ± 0.96 mV, which will facilitate their application in biological systems. Between 70% and 90% of the cancerous cells of the human melanoma Hs 294T cell line underwent necrosis following treatment with the synthesized AgNPs. Furthermore, optical emission spectrometry (OES) identified reactive species, such as NO, NH, N_2, O, and H, as pm-rf-APGD produced compounds that may be involved in the reduction of the Ag(I) ions.

Keywords: cold atmospheric-pressure plasma; nanostructures; necrosis

1. Introduction

Since ancient times, the many special properties of metallic silver have been well known and widely utilized because of its antibacterial [1], conductive [2], and optical [3] applications. Special attention has been given to silver nanoparticles (AgNPs), as their high surface-area-to-volume ratio [4] increases their number of possible applications. Most commonly, AgNPs are utilized in surface-enhanced Raman spectroscopy [5] and metal-enhanced fluorescence [6]. Furthermore, because of the excellent antibacterial activities of AgNPs, they are included in antibacterial clothing [7].

One promising utilization of AgNPs, and nanoparticles in general, is their application in medicine, for example, serving as drug delivery vectors [8,9]. The antiproliferating and antitumor activities of AgNPs have been the focus of much scientific effort, having been reviewed by Banti et al. and Zhang et al. among others [10,11]. In particular, AgNPs have gained interest in the field of nanomedicine because of their unique properties and their therapeutic potential in the treatment of at least some human cancers, with a particular focus on breast cancer [12,13]. Notably, a significant difference in the effects of AgNPs on tumor and non-tumor cell lines has been observed [14], supporting their potential as a cancer therapy agent. The effects of AgNPs on cancer cells are dependent on the concentration [13] and size [15] of the AgNPs. For example, smaller AgNPs at a lower concentration induced apoptosis and necrosis in a human pancreatic ductal adenocarcinoma cell line, while larger AgNPs at higher concentrations induced autophagy in this cell line [15].

The cytotoxic and genotoxic effects of AgNPs against mammalian cells [16,17], as well as their antimicrobial properties [18], has led to increased demand for methods for the reproducible production of AgNPs with defined characteristics, such as size and shape. An intriguing technique for AgNP synthesis is the use of cold atmospheric-pressure plasmas (CAPPs) in direct interaction with $AgNO_3$ solutions. The synthesis of AgNPs using CAPPs is a promising alternative to conventional "wet" chemical methods. It allows for the production of biocompatible AgNPs with higher monodispersity [19], without the use of potentially toxic reducing agents [20,21]. It additionally allows for the control of the optical and granulometric properties of the resulting nanomaterial, while minimizing the number of required steps and manipulations.

Among the different CAAPs applied for the production of Ag nanostructures directly in solutions, high-voltage direct-current-driven atmospheric-pressure glow discharge (dc-APGD) is the most widely used; however, the number of studies devoted to this topic is limited [22–33]. Considering experimental setups, stable dc-APGDs generated in contact with non-flowing solutions have been sustained with the aid of Ar [23,29,31–33] or He [24,26–28,30] jets. Gases were introduced through Cu [29] or stainless steel [23–28,30–33] tubes or capillaries attached to the negative polarity outputs of high voltage direct current (HV-dc) power supplies. Solutions were positively biased by immersing graphite rods [24], Pt rods [29], or Pt foils [23,28,30–33] into them, to which the ground earth outputs of the supplies were attached, or through the use of another gaseous jet [27]. Generally, these systems use a stationary $AgNO_3$ solution [20,23–27,30–34], and the reactors usually run for up to 30 min [31,32], resulting in the production of limited amounts of nanomaterials. However, a few continuous-flow systems have also been developed that significantly improve the production rate [19,22].

In the systems described above, the plasma generated in the gaps between gas-supporting capillaries and $AgNO_3$ solutions is a rich source of high-energy electrons (e_g^-) that bombard the solution surface. After thermalization (energy loss through multibody interactions with water molecules) of the e_g^- from the gas phase, solvated electrons (e_{aq}^-) are formed in the liquid phase. Redox reactions mediated by the e_{aq}^- and other reactive species, such as hydrogen radicals (H), hydrogen peroxide (H_2O_2), singlet oxygen (O), nitrogen oxide (NO), and hydroxyls (OH), result in particle nucleation and the growth of AgNPs in the solution [22–30]. This process can lead to electrostatically stabilized AgNPs without the need for additional capping agents [22,30,33]. However, various stabilizers, such as pectin [19], dextran [29], fructose [30–32], sucrose [24], polyvinyl alcohol [23], polyacrylic acid [25], and sodium dodecyl sulfate [19,26,27], are often included to prevent undesirable agglomeration and precipitation of the Ag nanostructures.

We are unaware of any studies making use of pulse-modulated radio-frequency alternating-current-driven atmospheric-pressure glow discharge (pm-rf-APGD) for the synthesis of nanomaterials. However, pm-rf-APGD presents many characteristics that make it an appealing alternative to dc-APGD for the synthesis of AgNPs. In pm-rf-APGD, there is a constant switching in the polarity of the electrodes, resulting in alternating injections of electrons (positive charge of the flowing liquid electrode) and positive ions (negative charge of the flowing liquid electrode). Both the electrons and positive ions contribute to the production of reactive oxygen and nitrogen species (RONS) responsible for the reduction of Ag(I) ions in the liquid phase. This characteristic may allow for the generation of AgNPs with improved monodispersity and long-term stability. By alternating between conditions convenient for reduction of the precursor of AgNPs (when the flowing liquid electrode of pm-rf-APGD has positive polarity) and conditions permissive for AgNPs etching due to acidification of the liquid (when the flowing liquid electrode of pm-rf-APGD has negative polarity), pm-rf-APGD may allow for better control of the shape and size of the AgNPs [34]. Moreover, the use of pm-rf-APGD is expected to reduce the power consumption of the AgNPs synthesis procedure relative to the use of dc-APGD; when 30% or 70% duty cycles are used, the plasma is off for 70% or 30% of the time, respectively [34].

Here, the properties of pm-rf-APGD-mediated AgNPs are explored. The effects of five parameters of this novel plasma-reaction system on the wavelength of the maximum (λ_{max}) of the localized surface plasmon resonance (LSPR) absorption band of the resultant AgNPs were examined using a response surface design. On the basis of the full quadratic response surface regression model, optimal conditions for the production of AgNPs of the largest and smallest sizes were selected, and the model was validated. Next, AgNPs produced under the conditions for the largest size were further characterized with respect to their optical and morphological properties and their cytotoxic activity toward human melanoma Hs 294T cells. Furthermore, the processes in the gas phase of the pm-rf-APGD were examined by optimal emission spectrometry (OES) in order to identify the reactive species possibly responsible for the synthesis of the Ag nanostructures.

2. Materials and Methods

2.1. Reagents and Solutions

To obtain a 1000 mg·L^{-1} stock solution of Ag(I) ions, 0.3937 g of solid silver nitrate (AgNO$_3$; Avantor Performance Materials, Gliwice, Poland) was dissolved in 250 mL of de-ionized water. The prepared stock solution was diluted 5, 2.86, or 2 times with de-ionized water, yielding final Ag(I) ion concentrations of 200, 350, and 500 mg·L^{-1}, respectively. Next, pectin (Agdia-Biofords, Evry Cedex, France), which is a biocompatible stabilizer, was added to aliquots of the working solutions to final concentrations of 0%, 0.25%, or 0.50% (*m*/*v*). This non-toxic biopolymer was included with the aim to stabilize the synthesized Ag nanostructures as well as to prevent their aggregation and sedimentation. All of the reagents were of analytical grade or higher purity. De-ionized water was used in all experiments.

2.2. Plasma-Reaction System for the Continuous Synthesis of AgNPs

Ag nanostructures were continuously produced in an innovative plasma-reaction system (Figure 1), in which APGD was generated between the surface of the flowing liquid electrode and a pin-type tungsten electrode (outer diameter of 4.00 mm). The APGD was generated using the rf (50 kHz) voltage wave modulated at frequencies within 500–1500 Hz with duty cycles of 30–70%. The distance between the surface of the flowing liquid electrode and the pin-type tungsten electrode was 4.00 mm. The rf voltage waveform was generated using a rf generator (Dora Electronics Equipment, Wroclaw, Poland). To charge the working solutions, a platinum wire was connected to the quartz-graphite capillary. Current and voltage measurements were made using a Rogowski coil and a voltage probe. The measured root-mean-square current was ~15 mA, while the root-mean-square voltage was 5 kV. The working solutions of the flowing liquid electrode were introduced to the developed pm-rf-APGD plasma-reaction system by a four-channel peristaltic pump (Masterflex L\S, Cole-Parme, Vernon Hill, IL, USA), at flow rates of 3.0–6.0 mL·min^{-1} *via* a quartz-graphite capillary (outer diameter of 6.00 mm). In the flowing liquid electrode working solutions, the concentration of Ag(I) ions was between 200 and 500 mg·L^{-1}, and the pectin concentration was within 0.00–0.50% (*m*/*v*). Flowing liquid electrode solutions containing Ag(I) ions of defined concentrations (with or without pectin) were continuously introduced to the plasma-reaction system and treated by pm-rf-APGD. Plasma-treated solutions containing AgNPs were collected and subjected to analysis by UV/Vis absorption spectrophotometry to acquire the λ_{max} value of the LSPR absorption band, characteristically in the range of 400–750 nm for spherical AgNPs [19,35].

2.3. Response Surface Model and Optimization of AgNP Synthesis

To examine the effects of the operating parameters of the pm-rf-APGD plasma-reaction system on the location of λ_{max} of the LSPR absorption band of the produced AgNPs, as well as to optimize this system so as to fabricate Ag nanostructures of a given size, the response surface methodology (RSM) was used to plan the experimental treatments and analyze the response surface. In this case, the Box–Behnken experimental design (BBD) was used, and the following five operating parameters were considered: the flow rate of the flowing liquid electrode solution (A) (mL·min^{-1}), the precursor concentration in the flowing liquid electrode solution (B) (mg·L^{-1}), the stabilizer concentration (C) (% (m/v)), the frequency of pulse modulation of the rf current (D) (Hz), and the duty cycle (E) (%). The response surface design included 43 randomized experimental treatments at three different levels (-1, 0, and $+1$) of the operating parameters, counting three center points. The levels of parameters were arbitrarily selected and limited to the range in which stable operation of the pm-rf-APGD plasma-reaction system was obtained, that is, 3.0–6.0 mL·min^{-1} (A), 200–500 mg·L^{-1} of Ag(I) ions as AgNO$_3$ (B), 0.00–0.50% (m/v) of pectin (C), 500–1500 Hz (D), and 30–70% (E). All experimental treatments were executed in one block within the response surface design matrix (with actual and coded values of the operating parameters) that is given in Table 1.

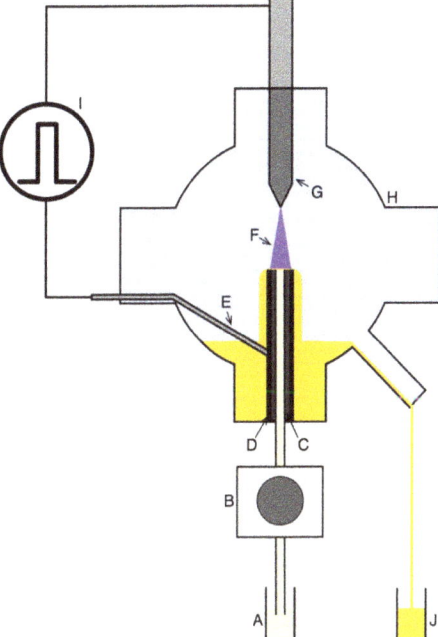

Figure 1. The scheme of the pulse-modulated radio-frequency atmospheric-pressure glow discharge (pm-rf-APGD)-based plasma-reaction system for the continuous production of silver nanoparticles (AgNPs). (A) Solution containing the AgNP precursor with or without pectin; (B) peristaltic pump; (C) quartz capillary; (D) graphite tube; (E) platinum wire; (F) pm-rf-APGD; (G) pin-type electrode; (H) quartz chamber; (I) radio-frequency (rf) voltage; (J) solution after pm-rf-APGD treatment containing AgNPs.

Table 1. The Box–Behnken response surface design with actual and coded values of operating parameters of the pulse-modulated radio-frequency atmospheric-pressure glow discharge (pm-rf-APGD) plasma-reaction system for synthesis of silver nanoparticles (AgNPs), along with the randomized run order and the response, i.e., λ_{max} of the localized surface plasmon resonance (LSPR) absorption band of AgNPs: (A) the flow rate of the flowing liquid electrode solution, (B) the precursor concentration, (C) the pectin concentration, (D) the frequency of pulse modulation of rf current, and (E) the duty cycle.

Run Order	Actual (Coded) Levels of Operating Parameters					Response
	A (mL·min^{-1})	B (mg·L^{-1})	C (%(m/v))	D (Hz)	E (%)	λ_{max} (nm)
1	6.0 (+1)	350 (0)	0.25 (0)	1500 (+1)	50 (0)	401.9
2	4.5 (0)	350 (0)	0.25 (0)	500 (−1)	70 (+1)	404.0
3	3.0 (−1)	350 (0)	0.25 (0)	1500 (+1)	50 (0)	404.0
4	3.0 (−1)	350 (0)	0.25 (0)	500 (−1)	50 (0)	404.0
5	6.0 (+1)	350 (0)	0.00 (−1)	1000 (0)	50 (0)	406.1
6 [a]	4.5 (0)	350 (0)	0.25 (0)	1000 (0)	50 (0)	405.1
7	4.5 (0)	500 (+1)	0.00 (−1)	1000 (0)	50 (0)	402.5
8	4.5 (0)	200 (−1)	0.25 (0)	1500 (+1)	50 (0)	400.3
9	4.5 (0)	500 (+1)	0.25 (0)	500 (−1)	50 (0)	415.4
10	4.5 (0)	500 (+1)	0.50 (+1)	1000 (0)	50 (0)	411.8
11	4.5 (0)	350 (0)	0.50 (+1)	1500 (+1)	50 (0)	399.7
12	4.5 (0)	200 (−1)	0.25 (0)	500 (−1)	50 (0)	397.2
13	4.5 (0)	350 (0)	0.50 (+1)	1000 (0)	30 (−1)	394.7
14	4.5 (0)	350 (0)	0.00 (−1)	1000 (0)	30 (−1)	399.3
15	3.0 (−1)	350 (0)	0.50 (+1)	1000 (0)	50 (0)	409.0
16	6.0 (+1)	350 (0)	0.50 (+1)	1000 (0)	50 (0)	394.2
17	4.5 (0)	350 (0)	0.00 (−1)	1500 (+1)	50 (0)	400.8
18	3.0 (−1)	500 (+1)	0.25 (0)	1000 (0)	50 (0)	412.4
19	3.0 (−1)	350 (0)	0.25 (0)	1000 (0)	30 (−1)	404.0
20	4.5 (0)	350 (0)	0.50 (+1)	500 (−1)	50 (0)	401.0
21	4.5 (0)	350 (0)	0.00 (−1)	1000 (0)	70 (+1)	406.3
22	4.5 (0)	500 (+1)	0.25 (0)	1000 (0)	70 (+1)	415.9
23	6.0 (+1)	350 (0)	0.25 (0)	1000 (0)	70 (+1)	397.0
24	3.0 (−1)	350 (0)	0.25 (0)	1000 (0)	70 (+1)	403.1
25	4.5 (0)	200 (−1)	0.50 (+1)	1000 (0)	50 (0)	421.5
26	6.0 (+1)	350 (0)	0.25 (0)	500 (−1)	50 (0)	394.6
27	4.5 (0)	350 (0)	0.00 (−1)	500 (−1)	50 (0)	415.1
28	6.0 (+1)	500 (+1)	0.25 (0)	1000 (0)	50 (0)	411.4
29	4.5 (0)	350 (0)	0.25 (0)	1500 (+1)	30 (−1)	426.2
30	4.5 (0)	500 (+1)	0.25 (0)	1000 (0)	30 (−1)	407.7
31	6.0 (+1)	350 (0)	0.25 (0)	1000 (0)	30 (−1)	405.9
32	4.5 (0)	200 (−1)	0.25 (0)	1000 (0)	30 (−1)	384.3
33	3.0 (−1)	350 (0)	0.00 (−1)	1000 (0)	50 (0)	419.8
34 [a]	4.5 (0)	350 (0)	0.25 (0)	1000 (0)	50 (0)	397.5
35	4.5 (0)	350 (0)	0.25 (0)	500 (−1)	30 (−1)	392.5
36	4.5 (0)	200 (−1)	0.25 (0)	1000 (0)	70 (+1)	390.1
37	6.0 (+1)	200 (−1)	0.25 (0)	1000 (0)	50 (−1)	399.7
38 [a]	4.5 (0)	350 (0)	0.25 (0)	1000 (0)	50 (0)	395.3
39	4.5 (0)	350 (0)	0.50 (+1)	1000 (0)	70 (+1)	403.1
40	4.5 (0)	200 (−1)	0.00 (−1)	1000 (0)	50 (0)	403.5
41	4.5 (0)	500 (+1)	0.25 (0)	1500 (+1)	50 (0)	411.0
42	4.5 (0)	350 (0)	0.25 (0)	1500 (+1)	70 (+1)	406.2
43	3.0 (−1)	200 (−1)	0.25 (0)	1000 (0)	50 (0)	410.6

[a] Center point.

To provide a good assessment of the curvature in the system, the acquired λ_{max} values were modeled using a complete quadratic function, including the main and quadratic effects, and the two-way interactions. To lower the dimensionality of the model for easier interpretation, insignificant terms were eliminated using a forward-selection-of-terms algorithm. The suitability of the model was evaluated using an analysis of variance (ANOVA) test, on the basis of the p-values for each of the terms in the model as well as the values of the residual standard deviation (S) and the coefficient of determination (R^2). The model was also tested for lack-of-fit, which provided evidence of the adequacy and efficacy of the full quadratic regression model for approximation of the response surface. In such a case, the respective *p*-value for the lack-of-fit test should ideally be high. Finally, the quality of the model and the reliability of its assumptions were checked by examining the residuals. To do this, scatter plots of the frequency distribution of the standardized residuals, as well as the standardized residuals *versus* fitted values, were used for identifying outliers and/or non-contact variance. This provided a good way to look for severe non-normality or heteroscedasticity (unequal variation) in residuals in the model to ensure informed decisions about acceptance or rejection of the model. The response surface design was planned and analyzed using the Minitab 17 statistical software package (Minitab Ltd., Coventry, UK) for Windows 7 (32 bit).

2.4. Characterization of the AgNPs Synthesized under Defined Operating Conditions

The optical properties of the Ag nanostructures were assessed using UV/Vis absorption spectrophotometry. The UV/Vis absorption spectra were acquired in the range from 260 to 1100 nm with a step of 0.1 nm, using a Specord 210 Plus (Analityk Jena, Jena, Germany) double-beam spectrophotometer. The UV/Vis absorption spectra were registered 1440 min after the pm-rf-APGD treatment. De-ionized water was used to zero the instrument. As the recorded UV/Vis absorption spectra were composed of more than a single band, the spectra were deconvoluted to resolve λ_{max} of the LSPR absorption band. The acquired UV/Vis absorption spectra were resolved using OriginPro 8 software (OriginLab Corp., Northampton, MA, USA) and were fitted by Gaussian functions, as was done by Calabrese et al. [36].

The size distribution by number and the polydispersity index of the synthesized Ag nanostructures (in reference to the mean hydrodynamic diameter) were estimated using a ZetaSizer Nano-ZS instrument (Malvern Instrument, Malvern, UK) with a detection angle of 173°. The measurements were performed at 25 °C in optically homogenous polystyrene cuvettes. To reveal the surface charge of the AgNPs, the ξ-potential was measured with this instrument as well. To assess the results for the particle size distribution, polydispersity index, and ξ-potential, which represent the average of three measurements, Malvern Dispersion Technology Software (version 7.11) for ZetaSizer was applied.

Next, the size and shape distributions, as well as the elemental composition and crystallographic structure, of the AgNPs produced under the optimal operating conditions were estimated *via* Tecnai G^2 20 X-TWIN transmission electron microscopy (TEM) (FEI Co., Hillsboro, OR, USA) supported by energy-dispersive X-ray spectroscopy (EDS)(FEI Co., Hillsboro, OR, USA) and selected-area electron diffraction (SAED; AztecEnergy, Oxford Instrument, Abingdon, UK). One drop of proper solution was put onto a Cu grid (CF 400-Cu-UL, Electron Microscopy Sciences, Hatfield, PA, USA) and evaporated to dry under infrared (IR) irradiation (95E, Philips Lighting, Pila, Poland). The size and shape distributions were assessed on the basis of the diameter of 60 single nanoparticles using FEI software (version 3.2, SP6 build 421, FEI Co., Hillsboro, OR, USA).

2.5. Optical Emission Spectrometry

To identify reactive species generated in the gas phase of the pm-rf-APGD, OES measurements were performed. A Shamrock SR-500i (Andor, Belfast, UK) spectrometer with a Newton DU-920P-OE CCD camera (Andor, Belfast, UK) was used to resolve the radiation emitted by the pm-rf-APGD collimated onto the entrance slit (10 µm).

2.6. Purification of AgNPs

Dialysis was applied in order to purify the AgNPs from the pm-rf-APGD-treated reaction mixture, which also contained unreacted Ag(I) ions. The plasma-treated solution was transferred into a dialysis tube (molecular weight cut-off = 14,000 Da; Sigma-Aldrich, Poznan, Poland) and placed into 500 mL of de-ionized water. The dialysis was conducted for 24 h with magnetic stirring (WIGO, Pruszkow, Poland), as was done previously [19].

2.7. Determining the Efficiency of AgNP Synthesis

The yield of AgNPs following the pm-rf-APGD treatment was measured before and after dialysis. The yield was estimated by flame atomic absorption spectrometry (FAAS) using a PerkinElmer 1100 B (Waltham, MA, USA), which is a single-beam flame atomic absorption spectrometer. The FAAS measurements were carried out after the digestion of the AgNPs in a 65% (m/m) HNO_3 solution (Avantor Performance Materials, Gliwice, Poland) at 100 °C for 30 min.

2.8. Cell Culture Conditions

Hs 294T melanoma cells are of a continuous cell line established from metastatic melanoma isolated from a human lymph node. These cells were obtained from the American Type Culture Collection (ATCC HTB-140). The cell line was cultured as monolayers in high-glucose Dulbecco's modified eagle medium (DMEM) culture medium supplemented with GlutaMAX-I, 10% heat-inactivated fetal bovine serum (BioMin Biotechnologia, Getzersdorf, Austria), 100 $\mu g \cdot mL^{-1}$ penicillin, and 100 $\mu g \cdot mL^{-1}$ streptomycin and was maintained in a cell culture incubator at 37 °C in 5% CO_2.

2.9. Experimental Groups and Exposure Conditions

In order to evaluate the effect of AgNPs on necrosis of the Hs 294T cell line, cells were treated with different concentrations of the reaction mixture compounds (for groups 2 and 3) or with the purified and non-purified Ag nanostructures (1, 5, 10, 50, and 100 $\mu g \cdot mL^{-1}$) for 24 h. As a control, culture medium was used for 24 h (group 1). The details of the experimental protocol are given in Table 2.

Table 2. Experimental groups used in the in vitro tests.

Serial No.	Treatment/Compound
Group 1 (Gr1)	Cells treated with medium alone
Group 2 (Gr2)	Cells incubated with pectin at a concentration of 2500 $mg \cdot L^{-1}$
Group 3 (Gr3)	Cells incubated with pulse-modulated radio-frequency atmospheric-pressure glow discharge (pm-rf-APGD) activated water
Group 4 (Gr4)	Purified silver nanoparticles (AgNPs) solution
Group 5 (Gr5)	Solutions of Ag(I) ions and pectin before pm-rf-APGD treatment
Group 6 (Gr6)	Solutions of Ag(I) ions before pm-rf-APGD treatment
Group 7 (Gr7)	Non-purified AgNPs solution, containing unreacted Ag(I) ions

2.10. Necrotic Assay

Necrosis was measured by flow cytometry to assess the number of human cells incorporating propidium iodide compared to control cells treated only with culture medium alone. Briefly, cells were cultured in medium containing fetal calf serum in 48-well plates and used in the experiments after reaching 80–90% confluence. A defined concentration of AgNPs was added to each well, and the cells were incubated for a further 24 h. A propidium iodide solution (1 $\mu g \cdot mL^{-1}$) was then added to each sample, and the dead cells were detected using flow cytometry in a FL3 mode, i.e., red channel, λ_{em} = 620 nm. Data were analyzed using a FACSCalibur flow cytometer (Becton Dickinson, Franklin Lakes, NJ, USA). The percentage of necrotic target cells was calculated using the Flowing Software 2 program. All values are presented as the mean ± standard error of the mean of three independent experiments, each consisting of technical triplicates. The results were analyzed through Student's t-tests using GraphPad Prism 5 software. The p-values for all investigated groups were calculated compared to the control group 1 (cells treated with medium alone).

3. Results and Discussion

3.1. Response Surface Regression Model

Nanostructures of different metals and sizes are able to absorb and reflect light of unique wavelengths, resulting in a LSPR absorption band centered around distinct wavelengths known as

λ_{max} [19]. In the case of spherical AgNPs, the LSPR absorption band typically occurs within the 400 to 750 nm range [14,19], with larger-sized AgNPs resulting in a red shift in the position of the λ_{max} values. Therefore, to evaluate the effects of the operating parameters on the size of the synthesized AgNPs, 43 independent runs of AgNPs synthesis were performed with varying experimental conditions, and the position of λ_{max} of the LSPR absorption band for each sample was recorded (Table 1).

To evaluate the quality of the data, two scatter plots were prepared: (i) the range of the values of λ_{max} measured under a given condition *versus* the mean of the λ_{max} values, and (ii) the mean value of the λ_{max} values *versus* the randomized run order. It was visually noted that the variability in the mean response between experimental treatments of the BBD was higher than the variability in the response within each treatment (for repeated measurements). Neither correlations nor trends in the scatter plots were observed. Thus, it was concluded that the variability in the results was associated with changes in the experimental conditions and that there was no need to stabilize the variance in the response through mathematical transformation [37,38]. To obtain the response surface, the values of λ_{max} for the LSPR absorption band of the 43 AgNP solutions were approximated with a full quadratic polynomial model. The response surface regression model, developed with the aid of the forward-selection-of-terms algorithm, for the λ_{max} values over the studied range of operating parameters was as follows (given in uncoded units): $\lambda_{max} = 341.8 - 2.34A + 3.37 \times 10^{-2}B + 4.27 \times 10^{-2}D + 1.54E - 7.16 \times 10^{-3}E^2 - 7.87 \times 10^{-4}DE$. The accuracy of this regression model was tested by ANOVA and the lack-of-fit test. The results of these analyses at $\alpha = 0.25$ are given in Table 3.

Table 3. Outputs of analysis of variance (ANOVA) and the lack-of-fit test for the response surface regression model established using the forward-selection-of-terms algorithm (α to enter = 0.25) for the pulse-modulated radio-frequency atmospheric-pressure glow discharge (pm-rf-APGD) plasma-reaction system used for synthesis of silver nanoparticles (AgNPs) [a].

Source of Data	DF	Adjusted SS	Adjusted MS	F-Value [b]	p-Value
Model	6	988.09	164.68	2.84	0.023
Linear	4	657.69	164.42	2.84	0.038
A	1	196.70	196.70	3.39	0.074
B	1	410.06	410.06	7.08	0.012
D	1	43.23	43.23	0.75	0.393
E	1	7.70	7.70	0.13	0.718
Square	1	82.33	82.33	1.42	0.241
E^2	1	82.33	82.33	1.42	0.241
Two-way interactions	1	248.06	248.06	4.28	0.046
DE	1	248.06	248.06	4.28	0.046
Error	36	2086.15	57.95	-	-
Lack-of-fit	34	2033.27	59.80	2.26	0.354
Pure error	2	52.88	26.44	-	-
Total	42	3074.24	-	-	-

[a] DF: Degrees of freedom. SS: Sum of squares. MS: Mean of squares. A: The flow rate of the flowing liquid electrode solution. B: The precursor concentration. D: The frequency of pulse modulation of radio-frequency (rf) current. E: The duty cycle. [b] The value of the F-test for comparing model variance with residual (error) variance.

By using an α value of 0.25, it was possible to learn more about the effects of each of the entered factors on the response and on the terms already in the model [39,40]. The terms A ($p = 0.074$), B ($p = 0.012$), E^2 ($p = 0.241$) and DE ($p = 0.046$) were statistically significant in the model. Considering the hierarchy of the terms, the statistically insignificant terms D and E ($p > 0.25$) were also included in the model. The concentration of pectin in the flowing liquid electrode solution, that is, term C, appeared to have no statistically significant effect on the position of the λ_{max} value of the LSPR absorption band of the synthesized AgNPs. The R^2 value was 32.1%, which was relatively low but acceptable, as it is a measure of how close the data fit the model and not a measure of the adequacy of the regression model. The p-value for the lack-of-fit test was higher than 0.25 ($p = 0.354$) and was therefore statistically insignificant. The S-value was also relatively low, at 7.61. Therefore, on the basis of the mentioned statistics summarizing the regression model, it was concluded that there was no reason to reject the model nor evidence that it did not fit the data. To finally check the goodness-of-fit of the regression model, the residuals were examined by plotting the following: (i) the frequency distribution of the standardized residuals (Figure 2A), and (ii) the standardized residuals *versus* the fitted values (Figure 2B). The distribution of the standardized residuals largely resembled a normal distribution with a mean of 0.015 and a standard deviation of 1.032 ($n = 43$). A random pattern of the residuals on both sides of zero was observed in the scatter plot of the standardized residuals *versus* the fitted values, indicating that a correct polynomial function was used to model the response surface of the system. Except for two outliers (points 25 and 29), no unusual structures or patterns were observed in this scatter plot. These observations confirmed the correctness of the model and the goodness-of-fit of the empirical data with those established by the regression.

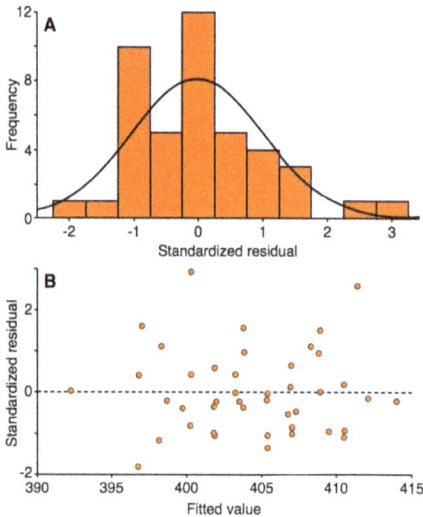

Figure 2. Frequency distribution graph of the standardized residuals (**A**) and a scatter plot of the standardized residuals *versus* the fitted values (**B**).

3.2. The Effects of Operating Parameters

The effects of the operating parameters included in the response surface regression model (i.e., A: the flow rate of the flowing liquid electrode solution; B: the precursor concentration in the flowing liquid electrode solution; D: the frequency of pulse modulation of the rf current; and E: the duty cycle) on the position of λ_{max} for the LSPR absorption band of the synthesized AgNPs is shown in Figure 3. There was an inversely linear relationship between the flow rate of the flowing liquid electrode solution and the position of the λ_{max} values; that is, a higher flow rate was associated with smaller AgNPs. As the flow rate increased, each milliliter of solution was exposed to the pm-rf-APGD for less time. Consequently, a smaller number of solvated electrons (e_{aq}^-) was likely available for reduction of the Ag(I) ions in the plasma-treated solution; that is, $Ag^+ + e_{aq}^- = Ag^0$ [22–26,34]. Considering the effect of the precursor concentration in the flowing liquid electrode solution, the lowest concentration of Ag(I) ions seemed to be preferable for obtaining small-sized AgNPs, that is, those with the lowest λ_{max} value of their LSPR absorption band. This could be explained by the Finke–Watzky two-step mechanism of nucleation and growth of AgNPs [41]. Accordingly, at higher concentrations of Ag(I) ions, faster growth and further aggregation of AgNPs can take place as a result of the reduction of these ions on the surface of the AgNPs. This would make existing AgNPs larger rather then produce new particles in the solution. In addition, at higher Ag(I) concentrations, the ionic strength of the solution could destabilize the synthesized AgNPs [41]. Finally, increasing either the frequency of pulse modulation of the rf current or its duty cycle led to a gradual increase in the position of the λ_{max} value of the LSPR absorption band. Hence, AgNPs of a greater particle size would be produced under these conditions. Both of these parameters directly affected the width of the pulses modulating the rf current in the on-and-off cycles and the duration of the interchanges of polarity set to the flowing liquid electrode solution. At the lowest settings of these parameters (i.e., D: 500 Hz; E: 30%), the pulse width at a given modulation frequency will be the shortest, while the time spent in the off state of the cycle will be the longest. Considering that the solution was continuously replenished in the flow-through system used, the above-mentioned conditions would have been responsible for the lowest production yield and the smallest size of the AgNPs. Particularly, the negative polarity of the flowing liquid electrode solution and the bombardments of the solution surface with positive ions, for example, $H_2O^+_{(g)}$, could provide convenient conditions for the etching of AgNPs. This is because H_2O molecules are ionized under these conditions ($H_2O^+_{(g)} + H_2O = 2H_2O^+_{(aq)} + e_{aq}^-$), while the resultant $H_2O^+_{(aq)}$ ions recombine with water molecules, leading to the formation of $H_3O^+(aq)$ ions and the acidification of the solution ($H_2O^+_{(aq)} + H_2O = H_3O^+_{(aq)} + OH^\bullet_{(aq)}$) [37,38]. This would be a process competitive to the formation of AgNPs through the reduction of the Ag(I) ions; however, it appeared that the longest off time in the cycle was convenient for rearrangement of synthesized nanostructures, leading to improved control over their size. The effect of the stabilizer concentration (C) was established to be statistically insignificant. This could be due to electrostatic stabilization of AgNPs, that is, negative charging of the surface of the AgNPs by electrons "injected" from the discharge through the plasma–liquid interface. This explanation was also suggested by Patel et al. [42], who reported surfactant-free synthesis of AuNPs facilitated by dc-APGD operated between a He jet (acting as a cathode) and a non-flowing solution of $AuCl_4^-$ ions (acting as an anode).

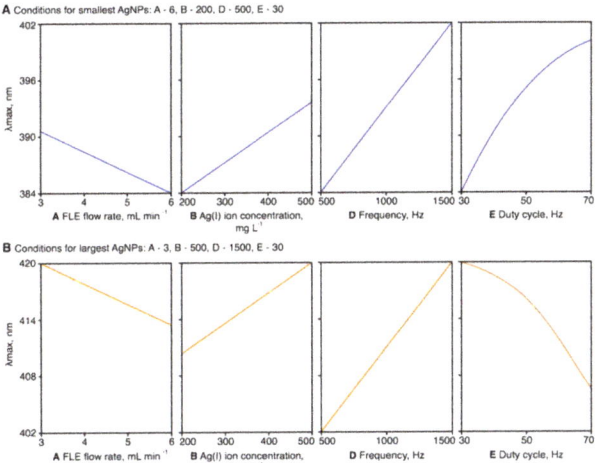

Figure 3. Graphical representation of the effects of the statistically significant parameters included in the response surface regression model on the wavelength at maximum (λ_{max}) of the localized surface plasmon resonance (LSPR) absorption band of the synthesized silver nanoparticles (AgNPs). Graphs demonstrate the effects of modifying variables when the operating conditions were otherwise optimal for the production of spherical AgNPs with the lowest (**A**) and highest (**B**) λ_{max}. A: the flow rate of the flowing liquid electrode (FLE) solution (mL·min^{-1}); B: the precursor concentration in the FLE solution (mg·L^{-1}); D: the frequency of pulse modulation of radio-frequency (rf) current (Hz); E: the duty cycle (%).

3.3. Validation of the Response Surface Regression Model

Graphical illustrations of the response surface regression model for the position of the λ_{max} value for the LSPR absorption band of the synthesized AgNPs are given in Figure 4. These are given as contour plots of the λ_{max} value for the following pairs of parameters at specific hold values: A–B, A–D, A–E, B–D, B–E, and D–E. To validate the developed regression model, two opposite sets of operating parameters were selected: condition 1, which led to the production of the smallest-size AgNPs (A: 6.0 mL·min^{-1}; B: 200 mg·L^{-1}; D: 500 Hz; E: 30%), and condition 2, which led to the production of the largest-size AgNPs (A: 3.0 mL·min^{-1}; B: 500 mg·L^{-1}; D: 1500 Hz; E: 30%). In both cases, pectin was included as a stabilizer in the flowing liquid electrode solutions at a concentration of 0.25%.

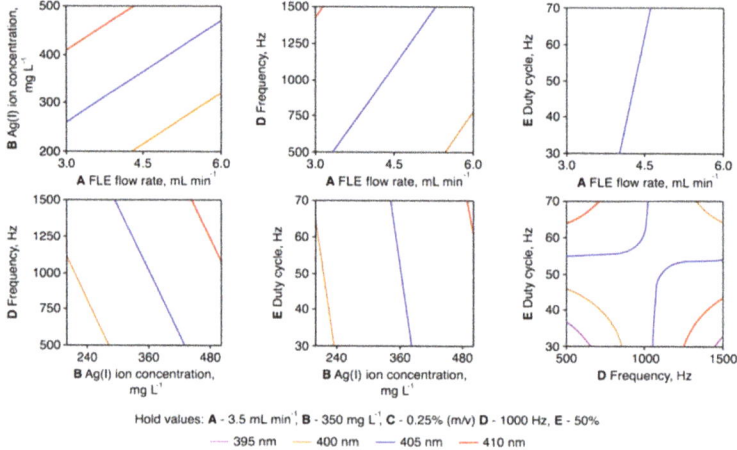

Figure 4. Counter plots of the wavelength at maximum (λ_{max}) of the localized surface plasmon resonance (LSPR) band of silver nanoparticles (AgNPs) synthesized using the pulse-modulated radio-frequency atmospheric-pressure glow discharge (pm-rf-APGD) system for pairs of statistically significant parameters in the developed response surface regression model (A–B, A–D, A–E, B–D, B–E, and D–E) at defined hold values. A: the flow rate of the flowing liquid electrode (FLE) solution (mL·min^{-1}); B: the precursor concentration in the FLE solution (mg·L^{-1}); D: the frequency of pulse modulation of rf current (Hz); E: the duty cycle (%).

According to the established regression model, the predicted value of λ_{max} of the LSPR absorption band for condition 1 was 383.7 nm, with a standard error of fit of 5.7 nm and a 95% confidence interval of 372.2–395.3 nm. The pm-rf-APGD plasma-reaction system was run with the parameter settings of condition 1, the plasma-treated solutions were collected, and the positions of the λ_{max} value of the LSPR absorption bands were determined (Figure 5). The mean value ($n = 4$) of the λ_{max} values of the LSPR band was 374.6 ± 3.4 nm with a 95% confidence interval of 371.1–378.0 nm. This corresponded well with the value predicted from the response surface regression model; the absolute error was 9.1 nm, which was lower than two standard errors of fit. Considering condition 2, the fitted value of λ_{max} of the LSPR absorption band was 419.9 nm, with a standard error of fit of 5.7 nm and a 95% confidence interval of 408.3–431.5 nm. The plasma-reaction system was run with the parameters of condition 2, and the positions of the λ_{max} values for the LSPR absorption band of the synthesized AgNPs were determined (Figure 5). The mean ($n = 4$) λ_{max} of the LSPR band was 415.8 ± 5.4 nm with a 95% confidence interval of 410.4–421.2 nm. The absolute error between the predicted and empirical values of λ_{max} was just 4.1 nm, which was lower than a single standard error of fit. These tests thus confirmed the usefulness of the developed response surface regression model for the control of the continuous-flow, one-step production process of spherical AgNPs of a given size.

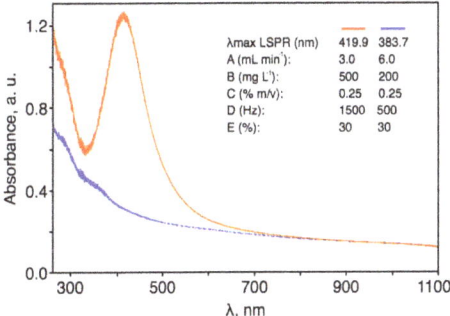

Figure 5. UV/Vis absorption spectra of silver nanoparticles (AgNPs) synthesized with the aid of the pulse-modulated radio-frequency atmospheric-pressure glow discharge (pm-rf-APGD) plasma-reaction under experimental conditions providing the smallest (condition 1) and the largest (condition 2) AgNPs according to the developed response surface regression model.

As was done in previous work [42–44], the absorbance at λ_{max} of the LSPR bands and their full width at half maximum (FWHM) values were recorded as measures of production yield and particle size distribution, respectively, of the AgNPs synthesized using conditions 1 and 2. Under condition 1, which was optimal for obtaining the smallest nanostructures, the absorbance was relatively low (0.21 ± 0.02), which was suggestive of a rather low production yield. The FWHM of the LSPR absorption band of these AgNPs was 106.8 ± 8.0 nm. Additionally, these AgNPs were stable for only 1 week, after which the color intensity of the solutions gradually decreased until they were colorless after 2 weeks. In the case of condition 2, which was optimal for the largest nanostructures, the measured absorbance was fairly high (1.16 ± 0.18), which was indicative of a much higher production yield than that using condition 1. Interestingly, the FWHM of the LSPR absorption bands for AgNPs produced under condition 2 (103.4 ± 6.2 nm) was very similar to that observed for AgNPs produced with condition 1. This suggested that a similar particle size distribution was achieved under both conditions, likely as a result of the electrostatic stabilization provided by the discharge as well as the presence of pectin. The solutions of AgNPs produced using condition 2 remained stable even 6 weeks following plasma treatment, as the shape and absorbance of the LSPR absorption band did not change within this time period. Considering the production yields and the stabilities of the AgNPs synthesized under conditions 1 and 2, only the AgNPs produced under condition 2, optimal for production of the largest nanostructures, were further characterized. According to Mie's scattering theory [45], a single intense LSPR absorption band, as was observed under condition 2, is expected in the UV/Vis absorption spectrum of monodisperse, spherical AgNPs.

To finally prove that different reactive species are formed in the gas phase of the pm-rf-APGD (as a result of alternating bombardments of the surface of the flowing liquid electrode with electrons and positive ions) and may contribute to the reduction of Ag(I) to AgNPs in the liquid phase as well as the formation of other species according to the reactions presented in the Section 3.2., OES was used to acquire the emission spectra of this unique discharge system operating under condition 2. This spectrum is provided in Figure 6 and was recorded in the spectral range from 200 to 400 nm, in the near-liquid electrode zone. It was found that the UV region of the plasma-reaction system was dominated by the emission bands of N_2 molecules (290–380 nm), which belong to the numerous transitions of the second positive system ($C^3\Pi_u$-$B^3\Pi_g$). Furthermore, bands of the NO γ-system ($A^2\Sigma^+$-$X^2\Pi$) were observed in the 200–280 nm UV region. In addition, strong bands of OH molecules at 282.9 nm (the transition 1–1) and at 308.9 nm (the transition 0–0), which belong to the $A^2\Sigma^+$-$X^2\Pi$ system, were excited. NH molecules, belonging to the $A^3\Pi$-$X^3\Sigma$ system, were also present in the spectrum, as determined by the presence of the band heads at 336.0 (the transition 0–0) and at 337.0

(the transition 1–1). Moreover, strong atomic Ag lines at 328.07 and 338.29 nm were identified, likely as a result of the formation of AgNPs in the liquid–plasma interfacial zone [46]. The NO and NH molecules were presumably produced as a result of the reaction of active nitrogen (N_2 and N) with O and H radicals, respectively [47]. On the other hand, the main source of the OH radicals observed in the emission spectrum were likely dissociative processes of water (H_2O) and its ions (e.g., H_2O^+ and H_3O^+), as was figured out on the basis of [37,38]. All reactive species, that is, NO, N_2, OH, O, NH, N_2^+, and H, identified in the gas phase of pm-rf-APGD may certainly give rise to the formation of important active species in the liquid phase of the discharge that can be directly involved in the reduction of the Ag(I) ions to AgNPs.

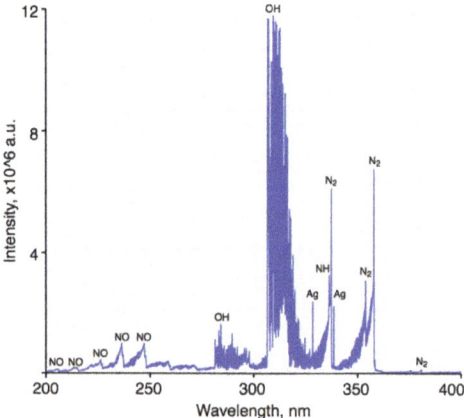

Figure 6. The optical emission spectrometry (OES) spectrum of pulse-modulated radio-frequency atmospheric-pressure glow discharge (pm-rf-APGD) generated under optimal operating conditions in the spectral range from 200 to 400 nm.

3.4. Characterization of Synthesized AgNPs under Optimal Operating Conditions

An aliquot of the AgNPs synthesized under condition 2 were purified by dialysis, and the purified and non-purified AgNPs were characterized by dynamic light scattering (DLS) to determine their average size by number, polydispersity index, and ξ-potential. The average sizes by number of the AgNPs were 32.78 ± 17.55 and 41.62 ± 12.08 nm, for the purified and non-purified AgNPs, respectively (Figure 6A,B). The similarity in sizes suggested that the purification process did not significantly influence the AgNPs population.

The polydispersities of the purified and non-purified AgNPs were determined to be 0.393 ± 0.093 and 0.490 ± 0.050, respectively. The polydispersity index [48] is a measure of the width of the size distribution. When the polydispersity index value of a colloidal suspension is higher than 0.1, the dispersion exhibits polydispersity [49]. A polydispersity index value below 0.3 is favored for pharmaceutical AgNPs. Thus, the AgNPs synthesized by pm-rf-APGD exhibited moderate polydispersity. The higher polydispersity value of the non-purified AgNPs was associated with the presence of pectin, which can impact the Brownian motions and result in a higher polydispersity value being detected. The ξ-potential of the colloidal solutions was estimated in order to predict their stability, as it has been suggested that nanoparticles with negative or positive surface charges can overcome the van der Waals forces and avoid aggregation. The ξ-potentials of the purified and non-purified AgNPs were −37.8 ± 1.85 and −43.11 ± 0.96 mV, respectively. These results are supportive of these AgNPs being highly stable, consistent with the optical results reported above. Additionally, it is significant that the AgNPs were negatively charged, as this can increase their ability to access tumor cells after injection into the circulatory system [50].

The size and morphology of the non-purified AgNPs were further characterized using TEM. It was observed that the AgNPs produced using condition 2 were approximately spherical in shape and non-aggregated (Figure 7C,D). On the basis of the TEM measurements (Figure 7C,D), the average size of the AgNPs was 10.38 ± 4.56 nm. It was noted that on the basis of the TEM measurements, the AgNPs appeared to be uniform in size. The differences in the sizes of the AgNPs as measured by DLS and TEM were expected and could be explained by the principals of these techniques [51]. In the case of DLS, the average size is based on the metallic core of the nanoparticles as well as on any compounds connected to the core, such as a stabilizer [51], which in this case was pectin. In contrast, size estimation as performed by TEM only considers the metallic structures [51].

SAED analysis was performed in order to determine whether the structure of the synthesized AgNPs was crystalline or amorphous. On the basis of the SAED pattern (Figure 7E), the following d-spacings were calculated: 2.334, 2.083, 1.452, and 1.350 Å. These d-spacing values correspond to (110), (200), (220), and (311) Miller indices [52]. Thus, it was determined that the synthesized AgNPs had a face-centered-cubic (fcc) crystalline structure.

EDS analysis was conducted to reveal the elemental composition of the synthesized Ag nanostructures (Figure 7F). Peaks corresponding to metallic Ag were detected in the EDS spectrum, confirming the formation of AgNPs. The presence of O and C was also detected, presumably because of the presence of pectin, an organic compound that was included in the reaction mixture. The peaks located at 8000 and 8900 keV were associated with the Cu sample grid onto which the sample was coated.

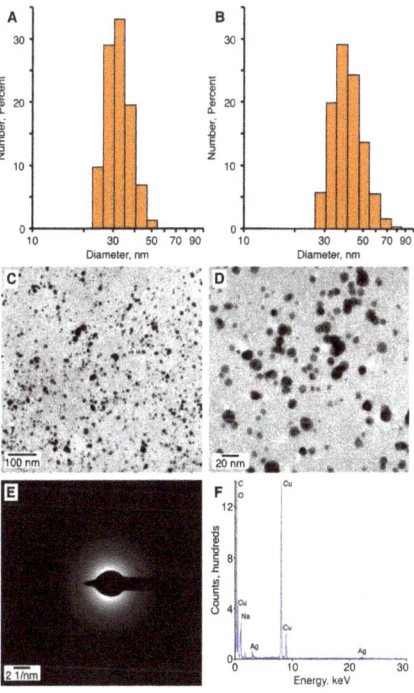

Figure 7. The morphology of silver nanoparticles (AgNPs) produced under optimal conditions. The histograms of size distribution by number of (**A**) purified AgNPs, and (**B**) non-purified AgNPs. (**C,D**) Representative transmission electron microscopy (TEM) micrographs of non-purified AgNPs, (**E**) the selected-area electron diffraction (SAED) pattern, and (**F**) the energy-dispersive X-ray spectroscopy (EDS) spectrum with prominent peaks labeled.

3.5. Influence of the Synthesized AgNPs on Necrosis of Cancer Cells

According to the American Cancer Society, cancer of the skin is the most common type of all cancers [53]. Melanoma skin cancer is responsible for the large majority of deaths related to skin cancer, with approximately 10,000 people expected to die from melanoma every year in the United States [53]. One of the most common treatments of melanoma cancer involves cell transfer therapies, based on antitumor lymphocytes and cytotoxic agents [54,55]. The cytotoxic agents might cause, for example, anemia and generation of cellular resistance [55]. A remedy to these drawbacks may be the use of AgNPs in the treatment of cancer. Previous studies have shown that nanoparticles in the range of 10–100 nm in size can have anticancer properties [56]. It is true that in vivo there are different types of cells within a tumor mass; however, all of them are activated and proliferated under a low O_2 level as well as acidic pH conditions (hypoxic conditions and tumor microenvironment) [14,15]. Certainly, it is critical to incorporate the microenvironmental characteristics into the development of physiologically relevant in vitro models, which could provide reliable, quick, and low-cost methods for toxicity studies of the synthesized nanoparticles. The use of cell lines in the testing of the cytotoxicity of AgNPs is a common practice in the field. Therefore, the activity of the AgNPs synthesized in this study using condition 2 against the human melanoma tumor cell line Hs 294T was tested (Table 2).

As shown in Figure 8, necrosis of 70–100% of the tumor cell populations was detected following treatment with 5, 10, 50, and 100 $\mu g \cdot mL^{-1}$ purified or non-purified AgNPs compared to the control cell population treated only with culture medium (p < 0.0001). The majority of the tumor cells underwent necrosis within 24 h, with the first symptoms of tumor cell death were observable as early as 6 h after the AgNPs' application (data not shown). No necrosis was detected when a concentration of 1 $\mu g \cdot mL^{-1}$ of purified or non-purified AgNPs was used (Figure 8). Similar results were observed when the tumor cells were treated with free Ag(I) ions as when treated with AgNPs (Figure 8). In contrast, treatment of the tumor cells with pectin alone or with pm-rf-APGD-treated water alone had no effect on the rate of necrosis compared to the control sample, which had a rate of necrosis of ~10% of the cell population (Figure 8). It was reported that AgNPs had a higher inhibition efficacy in tumor lines than in normal lines, which is due to the higher endocytic activity of tumor cells as compared to normal cells [14]. Therefore, additional experiments were performed, in which the antitumor activity of AgNPs against human fibroblast isolated from skin (MSU-1.1) as well as human endothelial cells isolated from skin (HSkMEC.2) was tested in three different concentrations of AgNPs, that is, 0.01, 1, and 5 $\mu g \cdot mL^{-1}$. No cytotoxic effect of AgNPs even for the highest concentration of 5 $\mu g \cdot mL^{-1}$ toward any normal cells of skin origin was observed.

The IC_{50} (inhibitory concentration, the concentration at which half of cells are necrotic) values were 7.8, 6.8, 4.3, and 6.6 $\mu g \cdot mL^{-1}$ for Gr4–Gr7, respectivly. This suggests that the melanoma cells were more sensitive to the solutions of Ag(I) ions before pm-rf-APGD treatment (Gr6) than to the solutions containing AgNPs. Overall, these data were consistent with the AgNPs synthesized by pm-rf-APGD inducing necrosis in human melanoma cancer cells, suggesting they may serve as an effective therapeutic agent for cancer treatment. The loss of cell viability following the AgNP treatment is believed to have been mediated through the release of Ag(I) ions within the tumor cells [57]. It is therefore not particularly surprising that treatment of the tumor cells with either AgNPs or free Ag(I) ions led to a strong reduction in cell viability, a result observed by both us and others [58]. The advantage of AgNP application lies in their selectivity toward tumor cells [59]. Whereas Ag(I) ions can display high toxicity to both cancerous and healthy cells, AgNPs can show greater specificity toward tumor cells, as the more acidic nature of their cytoplasm results in an elevated rate of Ag(I) ion release from the AgNPs relative to healthy cells [58,59]. It is important to consider that to fully determine the biological activity of nanoparticles, the correlation between material surface properties and cell functions must also be taken into account to eliminate undesired toxic effects of the nanoparticles [60–63].

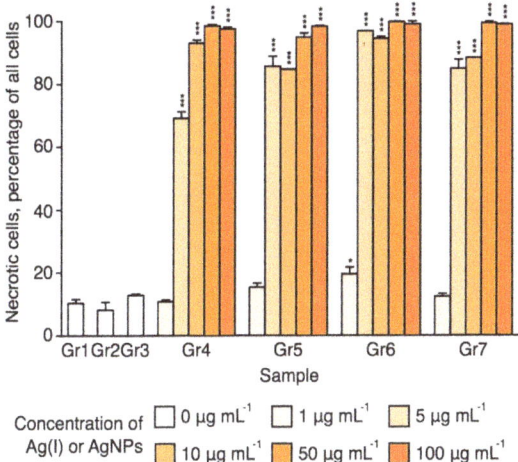

Figure 8. Percentage of necrotic human melanoma Hs 294T cells. Human melanoma (Hs 294T) cancer cells were treated with 1, 5, 10, 50, and 100 µg·mL^{-1} silver nanoparticles (AgNPs) or Ag(I) ions for 24 h or were treated with culture medium as a control (see Table 2 for a description of the groups). Percentages of necrotic cells were calculated as means ± the standard error of the mean of three independent experiments, each performed with triplicate wells for each treatment group. * $p < 0.05$; *** $p < 0.0001$.

4. Conclusions

In summary, we have developed a simple, rapid, and versatile pm-rf-APGD-based method for the size-defined synthesis of stable-in-time AgNPs. As a result of the continuous characteristic of the investigated plasma-reaction system, as well as the low-cost of its utilization, this method provides an appealing alternative to those that are presently applied for the production of high amounts of long-term stable Ag nanostructures. We believe further development of this plasma-reaction system could lead to a high-volume AgNPs-synthesis method. The possibility of controlling the properties of AgNPs should allow for further applications, not only in the necrosis of human melanoma cancer cell lines, but also, for example, in the inactivation of pathogenic bacteria.

Author Contributions: All authors planned the experiments. A.D. and J.M. performed the pm-rf-APGD-based synthesis of AgNPs. P.P. carried out the statistical analyses. A.D. performed the detailed characterization of the obtained Ag nanostructures by UV/Vis, DLS, TEM, SAED, and EDS. A.B.-P. carried out all the biological experiments. A.D., A.B.-P., G.C.d., P.J., and P.P. summarized all acquired results. G.C.d. provided the graphical support. P.P., A.D., A.B.-P., and G.C.d. wrote the presented manuscript. P.J. and A.K. supervised all work and took part in discussions.

Funding: A.D., P.J., and P.P. are thankful to the National Science Centre, Poland for providing the financial support for their research project (UMO-2014/13/B/ST4/05013). Furthermore, A.D. is supported by the Foundation for Polish Science (FNP), program START 022.2018. In addition, this work was financed by a statutory activity subsidy from the Polish Ministry of Science and Higher Education for the Faculty of Chemistry of Wroclaw University of Technology. G.C.d. is supported by a Natural Sciences and Engineering Research Council of Canada Post-Doctoral Fellowship.

Conflicts of Interest: The authors declare no conflict of interest. The founding sponsors had no role in the design of the study; in the collection, analyses, or interpretation of data; in the writing of the manuscript; or in the decision to publish the results.

References

1. Lansdown, A.B. Silver I: Its antibacterial properties and mechanism of action. *J. Wound Care* **2002**, *11*, 125–130. [CrossRef] [PubMed]
2. Braun, E.; Eichen, Y.; Sivan, U.; Ben-Yoseph, G. DNA-templated assembly and electrode attachment of a conducting silver wire. *Nature* **1998**, *391*, 775. [CrossRef] [PubMed]
3. Buzzi, S.; Galli, M.; Agio, M.; Loffler, J.F. Silver high-aspect-ratio micro-and nanoimprinting for optical applications. *Appl. Phys. Lett.* **2009**, *94*, 223115. [CrossRef]
4. Son, W.K.; Youk, J.H.; Lee, T.S.; Park, W.H. Preparation of antimicrobial ultrafine cellulose acetate fibers with silver nanoparticles. *Macromol. Rapid Commun.* **2004**, *25*, 1632–1637. [CrossRef]
5. Stamplecoskie, K.G.; Scaiano, J.C.; Tiwari, V.S.; Anis, H. Optimal size of silver nanoparticles for surface-enhanced Raman spectroscopy. *J. Phys. Chem. C* **2011**, *115*, 1403–1409. [CrossRef]
6. Xia, B.; He, F.; Li, L. Metal-enhanced fluorescence using aggregated silver nanoparticles. *Colloids Surf. A* **2014**, *444*, 9–14. [CrossRef]
7. Kulthong, K.; Srisung, S.; Boonpavanitchakul, K.; Kangwansupamonkon, W.; Maniratanachote, R. Determination of silver nanoparticle release from antibacterial fabrics into artificial sweat. *Part. Fibre Toxicol.* **2010**, *7*, 8. [CrossRef] [PubMed]
8. Wang, K.; Huang, Q.; Qiu, F.; Sui, M. Non-viral delivery systems for the application in p53 cancer gene therapy. *Curr. Med. Chem.* **2015**, *22*, 4118–4136. [CrossRef] [PubMed]
9. Zhang, B.; Wang, K.; Si, J.; Sui, M.; Shen, Y. *Charge-Reversal Polymers for Biodelivery*; Wiley-VCH Verlag GmbH & Co. KGaA: Weinheim, Germany, 2014; pp. 223–242.
10. Banti, C.N.; Hadjikakou, S.K. Anti-proliferative and anti-tumor activity of silver(I) compounds. *Metallomics* **2013**, *5*, 569–596. [CrossRef] [PubMed]
11. Zhang, X.F.; Liu, Z.G.; Shen, W.; Gurunathan, S. Silver nanoparticles: Synthesis, characterization, properties, applications, and therapeutic approaches. *Int. J. Mol. Sci.* **2016**, *17*, 1534. [CrossRef] [PubMed]
12. Yezhelyev, M.V.; Gao, X.; Xing, Y.; Al-Hajj, A.; Nie, S.; O'Regan, R.M. Emerging use of nanoparticles in diagnosis and treatment of breast cancer. *Lancet Oncol.* **2006**, *7*, 657–667. [CrossRef]
13. Gopinath, P.; Gogoi, S.K.; Chattopadhyay, A.; Ghosh, S.S. Implications of silver nanoparticle induced cell apoptosis for in vitro gene therapy. *Nanotechnology* **2008**, *19*, 075104. [CrossRef] [PubMed]
14. Ortega, F.G.; Fernandez-Baldo, M.A.; Fernandez, J.G.; Serrano, M.J.; Sanz, M.I.; Diaz-Mochon, J.J.; Lorente, J.A.; Raba, J. Study of antitumor activity in breast cell lines using silver nanoparticles produced by yeast. *Int. J. Nanomed.* **2015**, *10*, 2021–2031.
15. Zielinska, E.; Zauszkiewicz-Pawlak, A.; Wojcik, M.; Inkielewicz-Stepniak, I. Silver nanoparticles of different sizes induce a mixed type of programmed cell death in human pancreatic ductal adenocarcinoma. *Oncotarget* **2017** *9*, 4675–4697. [CrossRef]
16. De Lima, R.; Seabra, A.B.; Duran, N. Silver nanoparticles: A brief review of cytotoxicity and genotoxicity of chemically and biogenically synthesized nanoparticles. *J. Appl. Toxicol.* **2012**, *32*, 867–879. [CrossRef] [PubMed]
17. Akter, M.; Sikder, M.T.; Rahman, M.M.; Ullah, A.K.M.A.; Hossain, K.F.B.; Banik, S.; Hosokawa, T.; Saito, T.; Kurasaki, M. A systematic review on silver nanoparticles-induced cytotoxicity: Physicochemical properties and perspectives. *J. Adv. Res.* **2018**, *9*, 1–16. [CrossRef]
18. Franci, G.; Falanga, A.; Galdiero, S.; Palomba, L.; Rai, M.; Morelli, G.; Galdiero, M. Silver nanoparticles as potential antibacterial agents. *Molecules* **2015**, *18*, 8856–8874. [CrossRef] [PubMed]
19. Dzimitrowicz, A.; Motyka, A.; Jamroz, P.; Lojkowska, E.; Babinska, W.; Terefinko, D.; Pohl, P.; Sledz, W. Application of silver nanostructures synthesized by cold atmospheric pressure plasma for inactivation of bacterial phytopathogens from the genera *Dickeya* and *Pectobacterium*. *Materials* **2018**, *11*, 331. [CrossRef] [PubMed]
20. Akolkar, R.; Sankaran, R.M. Charge transfer processes at the interface between plasmas and liquids. *J. Vac. Sci. Technol. A* **2013**, *31*, 050811. [CrossRef]
21. Mariotti, D.; Sankaran, R.M. Microplasmas for nanomaterials synthesis. *J. Phys. D Appl. Phys.* **2010**, *43*, 323001. [CrossRef]

22. Dzimitrowicz, A.; Jamroz, P.; Pogoda, D.; Nyk, M.; Pohl, P. Direct current atmospheric pressure glow discharge generated between a pin-type solid cathode and a flowing liquid anode as a new tool for silver nanoparticles production. *Plasma Process. Polym.* **2017**, *14*, e1600251. [CrossRef]
23. De Vos, C.; Baneton, J.; Witzke, M.; Dille, J.; Godet, S.; Gordon, M.J.; Sankaran, R.M.; Reniers, F. A comparative study of the reduction of silver and gold salts in water by a cathodic microplasma electrode. *J. Phys. D Appl. Phys.* **2017**, *50*, 105206. [CrossRef]
24. Thong, Y.L.; Chin, O.H.; Ong, B.H.; Huang, N.M. Synthesis of silver nanoparticles prepared in aqueous solutions using helium DC microplasma jet. *Jpn. J. Appl. Phys.* **2016**, *55*, 01AE19. [CrossRef]
25. Ghosh, S.; Bishop, B.; Morrison, I.; Akolkar, R.; Scherson, D.; Sankaran, R.M. Generation of a direct-current, atmospheric-pressure microplasma at the surface of a liquid water microjet for continuous plasma-liquid processing. *J. Vac. Sci. Technol. A* **2015**, *33*, 021312. [CrossRef]
26. Tochikubo, F.; Shimokawa, Y.; Shirai, N.; Uchida, S. Chemical reactions in liquid induced by atmospheric-pressure dc glow discharge in contact with liquid. *Jpn. J. Appl. Phys.* **2014**, *53*, 126201. [CrossRef]
27. Tochikubo, F.; Shirai, N.; Uchida, S. Liquid-phase reactions induced by atmospheric pressure glow discharge with liquid electrode. *J. Phys. Conf. Ser.* **2014**, *565*, 012010. [CrossRef]
28. Yan, T.; Zhong, X.; Rider, A.E.; Lu, Y.; Furman, S.; Ostrikov, K. Microplasma-chemical synthesis and tunablereal-time plasmonic responses of alloyed Au Ag nanoparticles. *ChemComm* **2014**, *50*, 3144–3147.
29. Wang, R.; Zuo, S.; Zhu, W.; Zhang, J.; Zhu, W.; Becker, K.; Fang, J. Microplasma-assisted synthesis of colloidal gold nanoparticles and their use in the detection of cardiac troponin I (cTn-I). *Plasma Process. Polym.* **2014**, *12*, 380–891. [CrossRef]
30. Huang, X.Z.; Zhong, X.X.; Lu, Y.; Li, Y.S.; Rider, A.E.; Furman, S.A.; Ostrikov, K. Plasmonic Ag nanoparticles via environment-benign atmospheric microplasma electrochemistry. *Nanotechnology* **2013**, *24*, 095604. [CrossRef] [PubMed]
31. Chiang, W.H.; Richmonds, C.; Sankaran, R.M. Continuous-flow, atmospheric-pressure microplasmas: A versatile source for metal nanoparticle synthesis in the gas or liquid phase. *Plasma Sources Sci. Technol.* **2010**, *19*, 034011. [CrossRef]
32. Richmonds, C.; Sankaran, R.M. Plasma-liquid electrochemistry: Rapid synthesis of colloidal metal nanoparticles by microplasma reduction of aqueous cations. *Appl. Phys. Lett.* **2008**, *93*, 131501. [CrossRef]
33. Chang, F.C.; Richmonds, C.; Sankaran, R.M. Microplasma-assisted growth of colloidal Ag nanoparticles for point-of-use surface-enhanced Raman scattering applications. *J. Vac. Sci. Technol. A* **2010**, *28*, L5. [CrossRef]
34. Santosh, V.S.; Kondeti, K.; Gangal, U.; Yatom, S.; Bruggeman, P.J. Ag^+ reduction and silver nanoparticle synthesis at the plasma–liquid interface by an RF driven atmospheric pressure plasma jet: Mechanisms and the effect of surfactant. *J. Vac. Sci. Technol. A* **2017**, *35*, 061302.
35. Ameer, F.S.; Varahagiri, S.; Benza, D.W.; Willett, D.R.; Wen, Y.; Wang, F.; Chumanov, G.; Anker, J.N. Tuning localized surface plasmon resonance wavelengths of silver nanoparticles by mechanical deformation. *J. Phys. Chem. C* **2016**, *120*, 20886–20895. [CrossRef] [PubMed]
36. Calabrese, I.; Merli, M.; Turco-Liveri, M.L. Deconvolution procedure of the UV-vis spectra. A powerful tool for the estimation of the binding of a model drug to specific solubilisation loci of bio-compatible aqueous surfactant-forming micelle. *Spectrochim. Acta A Mol. Biomol. Spectrosc.* **2015**, *142*, 150–158. [CrossRef] [PubMed]
37. Dzimitrowicz, A.; Lesniewicz, T.; Greda, K.; Jamroz, P.; Nyk, M.; Pohl, P. Production of gold nanoparticles using atmospheric pressure glow microdischarge generated in contact with a flowing liquid cathode—A design of experiments study. *RSC Adv.* **2015**, *5*, 90534–90541. [CrossRef]
38. Dzimitrowicz, A.; Greda, K.; Lesniewicz, T.; Jamroz, P.; Nyk, M.; Pohl, P. Size-controlled synthesis of gold nanoparticles by a novel atmospheric pressure glow discharge system with a metallic pin electrode and a flowing liquid electrode. *RSC Adv.* **2016**, *6*, 80773–80783. [CrossRef]
39. Bursac, Z.; Gauss, C.H.; Williams, D.K.; Hosmer, D.W. Purposeful selection of variables in logistic regression. *Source Code Biol. Med.* **2008**, *3*, 17. [CrossRef] [PubMed]
40. Sleeper, A. *Minitab®DeMYSTiFieD*; Mc Graw Hill: New York, NY, USA, 2012.
41. Thanh, N.T.K.; Maclean, N.; Mahiddine, S. Mechanisms of nucleation and growth of nanoparticles in solution. *Chem. Rev.* **2014**, *114*, 7610–7630. [CrossRef] [PubMed]

42. Patel, J.; Nemcova, L.; Maguire, P.; Graham, W.G.; Mariotti, D. Synthesis of surfactant-free electrostatically stabilized gold nanoparticles by plasma-induced liquid chemistry. *Nanotechnolgoy* **2013**, *24*, 245604. [CrossRef] [PubMed]
43. Dzimitrowicz, A.; Jamroz, P.; Greda, K.; Nowak, P.; Nyk, M.; Pohl, P. The influence of stabilizers on the production of gold nanoparticles by direct current atmospheric pressure glow microdischarge generated in contact with liquid flowing cathode. *J. Nanopart. Res.* **2015**, *17*, 185. [CrossRef] [PubMed]
44. Mariotti, D.; Patel, J.; Svrcek, V.; Maguire, P. Plasma-liquid interactions at atmospheric pressure for nanomaterials synthesis and surface engineering. *Plasma Process. Polym.* **2012**, *9*, 1074–1085. [CrossRef]
45. Mie, G. Beitrage zur optik truber medien, speziell kolloidaler metallosungen. *Ann. Phys.* **1908**, *25*, 377–445. [CrossRef]
46. Greda, K.; Swiderski, K.; Jamroz, P.; Pohl, P. Flowing liquid anode atmospheric pressure glow discharge as an excitation source for optical emission spectrometry with the improved detectability of Ag, Cd, Hg, Pb, Tl, and Zn. *Anal. Chem.* **2016**, *88*, 8812–8820. [CrossRef] [PubMed]
47. Jamroz, P.; Greda, K.; Pohl, P.; Zyrnicki, W. Atmospheric pressure glow discharges generated in contact with flowing liquid cathode: Production of active species and application in wastewater purification processes. *Plasma Chem. Plasma Process.* **2014**, *34*, 25–37. [CrossRef]
48. Pereira-Lachataignerais, J.; Pons, R.; Panizza, P.; Courbin, L.; Rouch, J.; Lopez, O. Study and formation of vesicle systems with low polydispersity index by ultrasound method. *Chem. Phys. Lipids* **2006**, *140*, 88–97. [CrossRef] [PubMed]
49. Nobbmann, U. Polydispersity—What Does It Mean for DLS and Chromatography? Available online: http://www.materials-talks.com/blog/2014/10/23/polydispersity-what-does-it-mean-for-dls-and-chromatography/ (accessed on 1 June 2018).
50. Tomaszewska, E.; Soliwoda, K.; Kadziola, K.; Tkacz-Szczesna, B.; Celichowski, G.; Cichomski, M.; Szmaja, W.; Grobelny, J. Detection Limits of DLS and UV-Vis Spectroscopy in Characterization of Polydisperse Nanoparticles Colloids. *J. Nanomater.* **2013**, *2013*, 60. [CrossRef]
51. Kaasalainen, M.; Aseyev, V.; von Haartman, E.; Karaman, D.S.; Makila, E.; Tenhu, H.; Rosenholm, J.; Salonen, J. Size, stability, and porosity of mesoporous nanoparticles characterized with light scattering. *Nanoscale Res. Lett.* **2017**, *12*, 74. [CrossRef] [PubMed]
52. Kora, A.J.; Beedu, S.R.; Jayaraman, A. Size-controlled green synthesis of silver nanoparticles mediated by gum ghatti (*Anogeissus latifolia*) and its biological activity. *Org. Med. Chem. Lett.* **2012**, *2*, 17. [CrossRef] [PubMed]
53. The American Cancer Society, Key Statistics for Melanoma Skin Cancer. Available online: https://www.cancer.org/cancer/melanoma-skin-cancer/about/key-statistics.html (accessed on 1 June 2018).
54. Rosenberg, S.A.; Dudley, M.E. Adoptive cell therapy for the treatment of patients with metastatic melanoma. *Curr. Opin. Immunol.* **2009**, *21*, 233–240. [CrossRef] [PubMed]
55. Sierra-Rivera, C.A.; Franco-Molina, M.A.; Mendoza-Gamboa, E.; Zapata-Benavides, P.; Tamez-Guerra, R.S.; Rodriguez-Padilla, C. Potential of colloidal or silver nanoparticles to reduce the growth of B16F10 melanoma tumors. *Afr. J. Microbiol. Res.* **2013**, *7*, 2745–2750. [CrossRef]
56. Aftab, S.; Shah, A.; Nadhman, A.; Kurbanoglu, S.; Aysıl Ozkan, S.; Dionysiou, D.D.; Shukla, S.S.; Aminabhavi, T.M. Nanomedicine: An effective tool in cancer therapy. *Int. J. Pharm.* **2018**, *540*, 132–149. [CrossRef] [PubMed]
57. Yuan, Y.G.; Peng, Q.L.; Gurnathan, S. Silver nanoparticles enhance the apoptotic potential of gemcitabine in human ovarian cancer cells: Combination therapy for effective cancer treatment. *Int. J. Nanomed.* **2017**, *12*, 6487–6502. [CrossRef] [PubMed]
58. Greulich, C.; Braun, D.; Peetsch, A.; Diendorf, J.; Siebers, B.; Epple, M.; Koller, M. The toxic effect of silver ions and silver nanoparticles towards bacteria and human cells occurs in the same concentration range. *RSC Adv.* **2012**, *2*, 6981–6987. [CrossRef]
59. Urbanska, K.; Pajak, B.; Orzechowski, A.; Sokolowska, J.; Grodzik, M.; Sawosz, E.; Szmidt, M.; Sysz, P. The effect of silver nanoparticles (AgNPs) on proliferation and apoptosis of in ovo cultured glioblastoma multiforme (GBM) cells. *Nanoscale Res. Lett.* **2015**, *10*, 98. [CrossRef] [PubMed]
60. Zielinska, E.; Zauszkiewicz-Pawlak, A.; Wojcik, M.; Inkielewicz-Stepniak, I. Silver nanoparticles of different sizes induce a mixed type of programmed cell death in human pancreatic ductal adenocarcinoma. *Oncotarget* **2017**, *9*, 4675–4697. [CrossRef] [PubMed]

61. Wang, K.; He, X.; Linthicum, W.; Mezan, R.; Wang, L.; Rojanasakul, Y.; Wen, Q.; Yang, Y. Carbon nanotubes induced fibrogenesis on nanostructured substrates. *Environ. Sci. Nano* **2017**, *4*, 689–699. [CrossRef] [PubMed]
62. Zhang, L.; Webster, T. Nanotopography of biomaterials for controlling cancer cell function. In *Biomaterials for Cancer Therapeutics, Diagnosis, Prevention and Therapy*; Park, K., Ed.; Woodhead Publishing: Oxford, UK, 2013; pp. 461–487.
63. Wang, K.; Bruce, A.; Mezan, R.; Kadiyala, A.; Wang, L.; Dawson, J.; Rojanasakul, Y.; Yang, Y. Nanotopographical modulation of cell function through nuclear deformation. *Appl. Mater. Interfaces* **2016**, *8*, 5082–5092. [CrossRef] [PubMed]

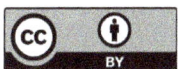

© 2018 by the authors. Licensee MDPI, Basel, Switzerland. This article is an open access article distributed under the terms and conditions of the Creative Commons Attribution (CC BY) license (http://creativecommons.org/licenses/by/4.0/).

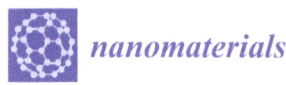

Article

Treatment of Nanocellulose by Submerged Liquid Plasma for Surface Functionalization

Denis Mihaela Panaitescu [1,*], Sorin Vizireanu [2,*], Cristian Andi Nicolae [1], Adriana Nicoleta Frone [1], Angela Casarica [3], Lavinia Gabriela Carpen [2] and Gheorghe Dinescu [2]

1. Department of Polymer, National Institute for Research and Development in Chemistry and Petrochemistry, 202 Spl. Independentei, 060021 Bucharest, Romania; cristian.nicolae@icechim-pd.ro (C.A.N.); ciucu_adriana@yahoo.com (A.N.F.)
2. National Institute for Laser, Plasma and Radiation Physics, Atomistilor 409, Magurele-Bucharest, 077125 Ilfov, Romania; lavinia.carpen@infim.ro (L.G.C.); dinescug@infim.ro (G.D.)
3. National Institute for Chemical—Pharmaceutical Research and Development, 112 Calea Vitan, 031299 Bucharest, Romania; angelacasarica@yahoo.com
* Correspondence: panaitescu@icechim.ro (D.M.P.); s_vizi@infim.ro (S.V.); Tel.: +40-021-316-3068 (D.M.P.)

Received: 24 May 2018; Accepted: 22 June 2018; Published: 26 June 2018

Abstract: Tailoring the surface properties of nanocellulose to improve the compatibility of components in polymer nanocomposites is of great interest. In this work, dispersions of nanocellulose in water and acetonitrile were functionalized by submerged plasmas, with the aim of increasing the quality of this reinforcing agent in biopolymer composite materials. Both the morphology and surface chemistry of nanocellulose were influenced by the application of a plasma torch and filamentary jet plasma in a liquid suspension of nanocellulose. Depending on the type of plasma source and gas mixture the surface chemistry was modified by the incorporation of oxygen and nitrogen containing functional groups. The treatment conditions which lead to nanocellulose based polymer nanocomposites with superior mechanical properties were identified. This work provides a new eco-friendly method for the surface functionalization of nanocellulose directly in water suspension, thus overcoming the disadvantages of chemical treatments.

Keywords: nanocellulose; plasma treatment; dielectric barrier discharge; submerged liquid plasma; polymer nanocomposite

1. Introduction

Nanocellulose (NC) is a very attractive material due to its unique properties, i.e., lightweight, strength, flexibility, biodegradability and biocompatibility, wide availability and cost efficiency of the sources [1–3]. The increasingly severe environmental policies and the exceptional properties of NC promote it as a valuable material for a wide range of applications. NC can be extracted from a multitude of primary sources, such as wood, plants, algae, and sea animals (tunicates) as well as from secondary sources or wastes resulting from the industrial processing of wood, bast fiber crops, vegetables or fruits, etc. [3–8]. In order to obtain NC, mechanical, chemical, enzymatic processes or a combination of the above are, generally, used. A promising approach to prepare NC is from bacterial cellulose (BC), which is biosynthesized by some bacteria as an extracellular material [8–13]. By applying mechanical disintegration [8,10,11] or chemical treatments (acid hydrolysis, 2,2,6,6-tetramethylpiperidine-N-oxyl (TEMPO) catalyzed oxidation) [9,12,13], BC membranes may release nanofibers.

For most applications, the surface properties of cellulose must be improved by physical or chemical treatments. Although BC has OH groups on the surface, which may react with other groups, it is not easy to be functionalized. This is caused by its high purity compared to plant cellulose which undergoes multiple treatments to remove other components (lignin, hemicellulose, pectin) and its high crystallinity (generally over 80% [10]). For example, the morphology and arrangement of BC nanofibers in the 3D structure of BC membranes were not changed by TEMPO oxidation [14] and a lower rate was noticed in the TEMPO-mediated oxidation of BC compared to cellulose from other sources [13].

Several attempts to surface functionalize BC by chemical routes have been reported [15–18]. Wet BC membranes were grafted with (3-aminopropyl)triethoxysilane (APTES) in ethanol and showed increased hydrophobicity and antibacterial properties [15]. However, a slight decrease of cell viability was reported for BC-g-APTES membranes with the increase of grafting yield [15]. Dried BC membranes were grafted with two organosilanes, octadecyltrichlorosilane and APTES in hexane showing increased hydrophobicity in the first case and improved cell attachment and spreading in the case of APTES treatment [16]. Carboxymethylated cellulose was obtained starting from water suspension of BC, previously homogenized with a blender, which was solvent-exchanged to isopropanol and carboxymethylated [18]. The degree of substitution was tailored by controlling the reaction conditions.

It is worth noting that the use of chemical solvents and reagents to adjust the properties of BC may remove some of its above-mentioned benefits and may also raise environmental issues. Therefore, plasma treatments are more suited when food industry and biomedical applications are foreseen. Cold plasma is now seen as an environmentally safe and more efficient technique compared to "chemical" processing for many fields, especially for textile, food packaging, and biomedicine.

Plasma treatment of cellulose has been intensively studied for the textile and paper industry and other fields, for different purposes like cleaning, sterilization, activation, increased hydrophilicity or hydrophobicity [19–25]. Plasma pretreatment is very efficient for the activation of textile surfaces [19,20]. For example, the surface of cellulose-based textiles was modified using nitrogen plasma which ensured new active and binding sites for the attachment of silver nanoparticles [19]. Plasma and silver treated textiles showed good antibacterial activity even after 15 laundering cycles [19]. Plasma treatment with a helium/oxygen mixture was applied to grey cotton knitted fabric to remove surface impurities [20]. The plasma treatment was efficient in cleaning the textile and enhancing the wettability but the yellowness was not reduced probably because of the thermal oxidation. Recent study has shown that the microwave Ar plasma conditions influenced the properties of cotton fabric in different directions, i.e., applying maximum gas pressure and minimum power led to increased hydrophobicity and crystallinity and a smooth surface [21]. High hydrophobicity and water repellency of 100% cotton fabric were obtained by Ar plasma treatment followed by immersion in an ethanol solution of oleic acid [22] or by surface treatment with helium/1,3-butadiene plasma at atmospheric pressure [23].

Cellulose films or sheets have also been plasma treated for different purposes. For example, films of regenerated cellulose treated by low pressure oxygen plasma showed different surface chemistry and topography [24]. Similarly, dielectric barrier discharge (DBD) plasma treatment of a cellulose film at atmospheric pressure using N_2/NH_3 (90/10) gas mixture led to surface functionalization with amine and amide groups, which promoted cell differentiation [25]. Natural terpenes (limonene and myrcene) grafted on cellulose sheets using vacuum plasma modified the cellulose substrate from highly hydrophilic to hydrophobic [26] and fatty acids (butyric acid and oleic acid) grafted on unbleached and bleached kraft pulp using vacuum plasma increased the hydrophobicity of cellulose fibers [27]. Conversely, O_2 plasma treatment of bacterial cellulose membranes led to a decrease of the effective pore area and water flux and to increased hydrophilicity, which are important for filtration [28]. On the other hand, lyophilized bacterial cellulose sheets treated with nitrogen plasma under vacuum showed increased porosity and enhanced adhesion of endothelial and neuroblast cells due to the functional nitrogen groups grafted on the surface of cellulose [29].

The application of DBD plasma for the surface modification of cellulose fibers or textiles has been extensively studied [19,30,31] but in the case of cellulose nanofibers/nanocrystals treated by DBD, the literature is extremely scarce. Only in a recent study [32], cellulose nanofibers from water suspension were deposited on glass and the resulted coatings were treated by DBD plasma in helium gas. The treatment increased the content of carbonyl and carboxyl groups on the nanocellulose coatings and their roughness. However, the plasma treated nanocellulose obtained by this method cannot be re-dispersed in water or other solvents due to hornification [33] and it cannot be used in dried form as a reinforcing agent, for enhancing the properties of polymers [10].

Submerged liquid plasma (SLP) is a recent hot topic and a valuable method to obtain or modify nanostructured materials [34,35]. So far, SLP has mainly been used as a low energy synthesis method to produce nanostructured carbon materials. Thus, nitrogen-functionalized graphene was produced by applying a high electric potential between graphite and Pt electrodes in acetonitrile solvent [35]. This product showed a good dispersibility in both hydrophilic and hydrophobic solvents. SLP treatments produce several active agents, highly reactive species, radicals, charged particles, ozone, ultraviolet radiation, and shockwaves in the aqueous suspension [36] which may lead to the surface functionalization of nanocellulose. It is expected that the application of cold plasma directly to the water suspension of cellulose nanofibers is much more suited to obtain cellulose nano-reinforcements with a modified surface for polymer composites. Besides the advantages of using plasma sources at atmospheric pressure (without vacuum components, no chamber limitation and easy operation at low cost), plasma treatments in liquid have the great advantage of enabling the treatment of nanoparticles or nanofibers as suspensions in liquids.

In this work, the nanocellulose liquid suspensions were treated by using two types of non-thermal plasma sources developed for surface treatment, which are conceptually different: (i) a filamentary plasma jet based on dielectric barrier discharge (DBD) [37,38] and (ii) a plasma torch [39]. To the best of our knowledge, this is the first example of the use of SLP for the surface treatment of nanocellulose and the first time a filamentary jet discharge with dielectric barrier is used submerged in liquid. DBD filamentary jets were previously used for polymer deposition [40] but not immersed in the liquid where the material to be treated is dispersed. Both sources can be operated at low radiofrequency power (around 100 W) in continuous Ar flow. These atmospheric pressure plasma sources were previously used for the surface treatment of polymers [41], decomposition of dye solutions [42] or functionalization of graphene suspensions [43]. These plasma sources work properly both in open atmosphere and completely immersed in various liquid media, such as nanocellulose water suspensions or graphene suspensions. The aim of this work was to investigate the effect of these plasma sources in different operating conditions on the surface properties of nanocellulose (NC) obtained by mechanical disintegration of BC membranes and designed as reinforcing agent in biopolymers. NC surface changes were examined by Fourier transform infrared spectroscopy (FTIR), X-ray photoelectron spectroscopy (XPS), and thermogravimetric analysis (TGA). Plasma treated NC samples were tested as reinforcing agents in a biopolymer matrix, poly (3-hydroxybutyrate) (PHB).

2. Materials and Methods

2.1. Materials

Bacterial strain Gluconacetobacter Xylinus DSM 2004, purchased from Leibniz Institute DSMZ (German Collection of Microorganisms and Cell Cultures, Braunschweig, Germany), was used for the biosynthesis of bacterial cellulose (BC) membranes. Acetonitrile 99% (ACN) was purchased from Fluka (Buchs, Switzerland) and used as received. PHB type P304 with a tensile strength of 28 MPa (ISO 527, 50 mm/min) and a Charpy impact strength of 60 kJ/m^2 (ISO 179, 23 °C) was purchased from Biomer (Krailling, Germany). All the other chemicals were of analytical grade and were purchased from Sigma-Aldrich (St. Louis, MI, USA).

2.2. Production of BC Membranes; Defibrillation of BC Membranes to Obtain Nanocellulose

The culture medium used for the fermentation of Gluconacetobacter Xylinus contained 7.5% glucose equivalents from poor quality apples extract, 2% glycerol, 0.2% ammonium sulfate, and 0.5%

citric acid. This culture media (50 mL) was autoclaved at 121 °C, for 15 min and, after cooling, it was inoculated with 10% (*v*/*v*) stock culture (Gluconacetobacter Xylinus on Schramm–Hestrin medium). BC membranes were produced under static conditions at 30 °C for 14 days. After the treatment with sodium hydroxide and sodium azide for cell lysis and reduction of microbial contamination, the BC membranes were neutralized with 1% acetic acid and washed several times with distilled water. NC was obtained from fresh BC membranes by mechanical defibrillation (Figure 1) using a blender and a colloid mill, as described in [10].

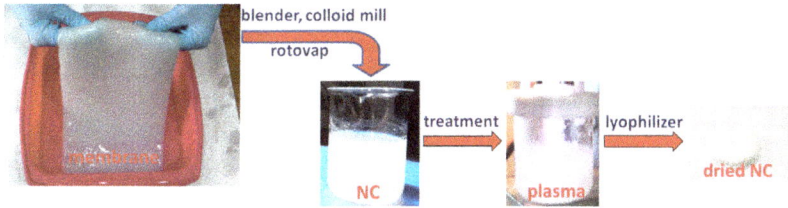

Figure 1. Schematic representation of defibrillation and plasma treatment of nanocellulose.

The diluted suspension of NC in water was concentrated using a rotary evaporator (Heidolph, Schwabach, Germany) and then plasma treated. Following this step, different treated NC suspensions were lyophilized using a FreeZone 2.5 L (Labconco, Kansas City, MO, USA) resulting in dried surface-treated NC.

2.3. Plasma Treatment of NC

The two types of plasma sources that were used for the surface functionalization of NC are shown in Figure 2. The DBD plasma source with floating electrode is shown in Figure 2a whilst the plasma torch (E) with the expanding plasma jet in contact with electrodes is presented in Figure 2b. Both sources are capacitively coupled with a radiofrequency (RF, 13.56 MHz) power supply and may produce an external jet of over 40 mm, depending on the operation parameters (gas flow, RF power). Both discharges are initiated in open atmosphere and, then, the jets are completely immersed in the water suspension for the surface functionalization of NC. The conditions used for the plasma treatments are shown in Table 1. Both plasma sources were designed for atmospheric pressure [39,40] and the plasma torch was previously tested completely immersed in liquid for the functionalization of graphene [43].

A typical experiment for the surface treatment of NC consists of the ignition of a plasma operating at atmospheric pressure in a 3000 sccm argon (Ar) flow and a power of 100 W, injecting the reactive gases (oxygen, nitrogen or ammonia) and immersing the plasma jet in the liquid suspension (50 mL) for 15–30 min. The concentration of NC in the liquid suspension was 1 wt %. Acetonitrile was also introduced into the water suspension of NC, the rest of the process parameters being identical. Droplets from the plasma treated NC suspensions were dried on silicon substrates for further investigations (XPS, FTIR). Plasma treated NC suspensions were lyophilized to obtain dried NC with a modified surface. Due to the characteristics of the second plasma source type, more nitrogen was used for the surface treatment of NC and a higher RF power (Table 1, E15 and E30). Dried surface-treated NC samples were used in small concentration (0.2 wt %) as reinforcement in PHB. The nanocomposites were obtained in the mixing chamber of a Brabender LabStation (Duisburg, Germany) at 165 °C for 10 min, rotor speed of 50 min^{-1}. For mechanical characterization, films with the thickness of about 200 μm were obtained by compression molding in an electrically heated press (Dr. Collin, Ebersberg, Germany) at 175 °C, with 120 s of preheating (5 bar) and 75 s under pressure (100 bar). The films were quickly cooled down in a cooling cassette.

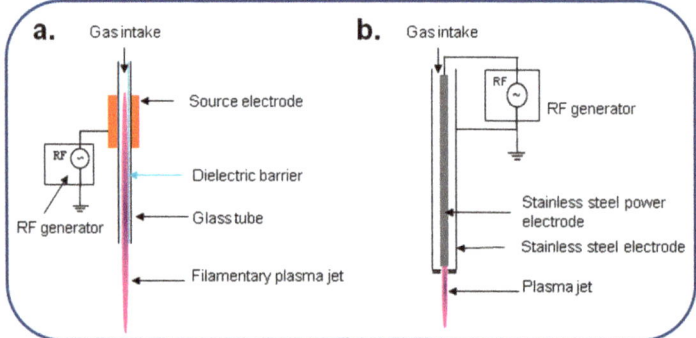

Figure 2. Configuration of plasma jet sources: dielectric barrier discharge (DBD) (**a**) and plasma torch (E) (**b**).

Table 1. Conditions for dielectric barrier discharge (DBD) and plasma torch (E) plasma treatments of nanocellulose (NC).

Samples	Ar flow (sccm)	Reactive Gas/Liquid	RF Power (W)	Treatment Time (min)
NC Ar	3000	-	100	30
NC Ar/O$_2$	3000	O$_2$ (5 sccm)	100	30
NC Ar/N$_2$	3000	N$_2$ (10 sccm)	100	30
NC Ar/N$_2$ (E15)	2000	N$_2$ (1500 sccm)	250	15
NC Ar/N$_2$ (E30)	2000	N$_2$ (1500 sccm)	250	30
NC Ar/NH$_3$	3000	NH$_3$ (5 sccm)	100	30
NC Ar-ACN	3000	ACN 30% in water	100	30

2.4. Characterization

Scanning electron microscopy (SEM) images of NC were obtained using a Quanta Inspect F scanning electron microscope (FEI-Philips, Hillsboro, OR, USA)) with a field emission gun at an accelerating voltage of 30 kV with a resolution of 1.2 nm. NC samples were directly mounted on the adhesive tape and sputter-coated with gold for 30 s before examination. Plasma treated NC films deposited on silicon substrates were examined by atomic force microscopy (AFM) using a Bruker MultiMode 8 (Santa Barbara, CA, USA) in Peak Force QNM (Quantitative Nanomechanical Mapping) mode. The images were captured using a silicon tip with the spring constant of 40 N/m and a resonant frequency of 300 kHz at a scanning rate of 0.9 Hz. Tensor 37 spectrometer with attenuated total reflectance (ATR) setup from Bruker Optics (Ettlingen, Germany) was used to examine the surface chemistry changes and to record the Fourier transform infrared spectroscopy (FTIR) spectra of the NC films deposited on silicon substrates. The spectra were collected in duplicate, at room temperature, from 4000 to 400 cm^{-1}. All the spectra were the average of 16 scans at a spectral resolution of 4 cm^{-1}. The NC treated under different experimental conditions, deposited on silicon substrates was also analyzed by X-ray photoelectron spectroscopy (XPS) using a ESCALAB™ XI+ spectrometer (Thermo Scientific, Waltham, MA, USA) with a monochromatic Al Kα source at 1486.6 eV. The XPS spectra were recorded as survey spectra with the pass energy of 100 eV (for 10 scans) and the high-resolution scans in the C1s, O1s and N1s regions, with the pass energy of 20 eV and resolution 0.1 eV (for 20 scans). Thermogravimetric analysis (TGA) of both plasma treated NC and nanocomposites was performed on a TA-Q5000 V3.13 (TA Instruments Inc., New Castle, DE, USA) using nitrogen as the purge gas at a flow rate of 40 mL/min. A heating cycle from 25 °C to 700 °C at a heating rate of 10 °C/min was applied. The experimental error was less than ±0.5 °C for all the characteristic temperatures. Tensile properties of PHB/NC nanocomposites were measured according to ISO 527, at room temperature, on five specimens for each nanocomposite, using an Instron

3382 universal testing machine (Instron Corporation, Norwood, MA, USA) and a crosshead speed of 2 mm/min.

3. Results and Discussion

3.1. NC Morphology before and after Plasma Treatments

The nanometric dimensions of cellulose fibers obtained by the disintegration of BC pellicles provide a high surface area for plasma treatment. Indeed, in the SEM image of dried NC (Figure 3) it is shown that BC pellicles were disintegrated resulting in a sparse network of cellulose nanofibers with thickness between 40 and 100 nm.

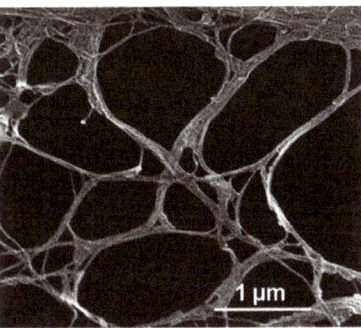

Figure 3. Scanning electron microscopy (SEM) image of nanocellulose (NC) from defibrillated membranes showing a sparse network of nanofibers.

NC films deposited on silicon substrates were examined by AFM before and after the plasma treatments (Figure 4).

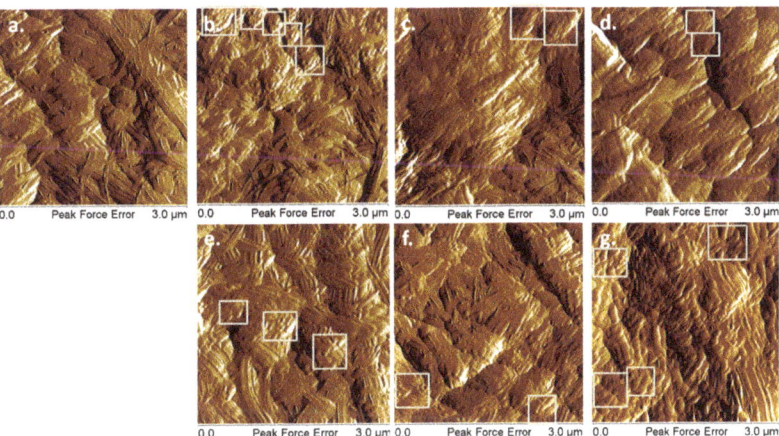

Figure 4. Atomic force microscopy (AFM) images (peakforce error) of untreated (**a**) and plasma treated NC: Ar (**b**); Ar/O$_2$ (**c**); Ar/N$_2$ (**d**); Ar/N$_2$ (E30) (**e**); Ar/NH$_3$ (**f**); Ar-ACN (**g**); Regions of interest showing small-length nanofibers agglomerations are framed in squares.

Both individual nanofibers and fibers bundles were noticed in the AFM images on the surface of all the films, regardless of the treatment, but with different surface morphologies and arrangement of the nanofibers. For example, more small-length nanofibers were observed after plasma treatments which allow a more dense arrangement. These nanofibers were noticed as heaps containing agglomerations of small fibers on the surface of the films and they were framed with squares in Figure 4. More such regions of interest were noted on the surface of Ar treated NC and NC Ar-ACN samples, suggesting a more efficient treatment. This may be due to the plasma treatments, which led to the detachment of nanofibers from the network and their breaking. Similarly, mechanical treatments, acid hydrolysis or ultrasonic treatments led to the decrease in cellulose fiber size [44,45].

More information can be extracted from the higher magnification AFM images shown in Figure 5. Before plasma treatment, the NC mostly appears as individual tapes longer than 1 µm, and with a smooth surface. After Ar treatment, both individual twisted tapes and small size fragmented fibers were noticed. Such fragments, similar to nanoparticles, were observed in the bottom right corner of Figure 5b. Ar/O_2, Ar/N_2, Ar/N_2 (E30), and Ar/NH_3 treatments led to more agglomerated and fragmented NC tapes compared to Ar treatment. The smallest fibers in this series were observed after DBD plasma treatment with Ar/NH_3 and torch plasma in Ar/N_2 (Figure 5e,f). However, Ar-ACN treatment was the most efficient in lowering the size of NC and mostly NC particles and fragmented tapes were observed on the surface of this film (Figure 5g).

For a quantitative analysis, the root mean square roughness (R_{RMS}) of the NC films surface was measured with the NanoScope software. Three different locations of square shape (3 × 3 µm) were analyzed for each sample and the R_{RMS} was an average of these values. The R_{RMS} of the NC Ar/N2 (E30) and NC Ar surfaces was 58 ± 3 nm and 48 ± 4 nm, respectively, lower than that of the other films which varied from 70 ± 3 (for the reference) to 78 ± 4 for NC Ar/N_2 and NC Ar/O_2. This suggests a more compact arrangement of the fibers on the surface of the first samples.

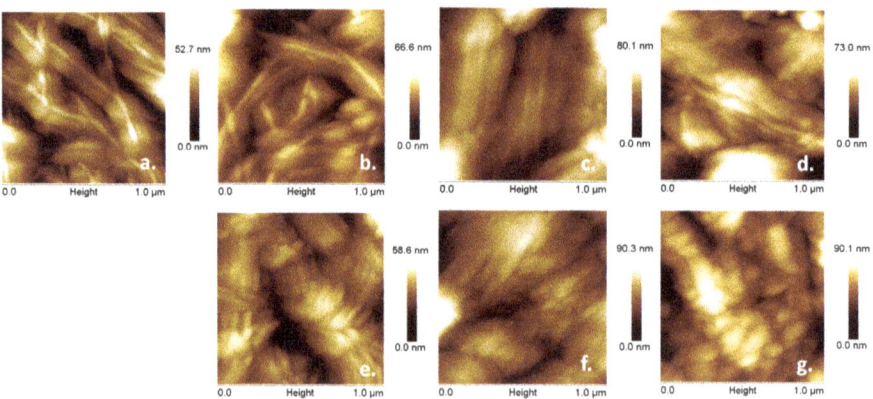

Figure 5. AFM topographic images of untreated (a) and plasma treated NC: Ar (b); Ar/O_2 (c); Ar/N_2 (d); Ar/N_2 (E30) (e); Ar/NH_3 (f); Ar-ACN (g).

Morphological investigation on the surface of plasma treated NC deposited as films on silicon substrates emphasize the different effects of plasma treatments depending on the type of the source (DBD plasma jet or torch), the reactivity of the gas (Ar, N_2, O_2, NH_3) or the liquid (water or ACN).

3.2. Thermal Analysis of NC before and after the Treatments

Thermal analysis may give valuable information on the structural changes of NC after plasma treatments due to the fact that these changes are reflected in a different thermal behavior. The different conditions of plasma treatment influenced the thermal behavior of NC as shown in Figure 6a,b. The temperature at the maximum degradation rate (T_{max}), the onset degradation temperature (T_{on}), and the temperature at 10% weight loss ($T_{10\%}$) as well as the residue at 700 °C (R) and the residue after the first decomposition step (R_I) are summarized in Table 2.

Table 2. Thermogravimetric analysis (TGA) results for plasma treated NC.

Samples	$T_{10\%}$ (°C)	T_{on} (°C)	T_{max} (°C)	R_I (%)	T'_{max} (°C)	R (%)
NC	244.0	284.1	332.1	-	-	10.6
NC Ar	278.6	310.2	350.3	-	-	5.5
NC Ar/O_2	228.5	261.0	309.0	22.5	436.9	7.6
NC Ar/N_2	261.4	294.3	350.1	-	-	8.1
NC Ar/N_2 (E15)	250.4	290.2	343.6	23.8	474.5	4.1
NC Ar/N_2 (E30)	241.9	282.6	340.2	31.8	486.4	6.5
NC Ar/NH_3	237.3	268.4	323.6	20.4	436.6	6.9
NC Ar-ACN	241.2	289.0	333.8	-	-	8.3

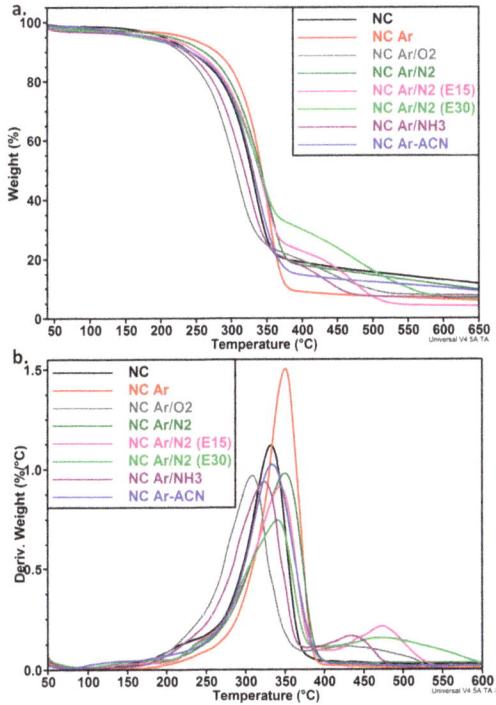

Figure 6. Thermogravimetric analysis (TGA) spectra (**a**) and derivative thermogravimetric (DTG) overlapped curves (**b**) of plasma treated NC.

Pristine NC and DBD plasma treated NC with Ar (in water or water–ACN) and with Ar/N_2 gases showed only a one-step degradation process and a T_{max} at 330–350 °C. This peak (Figure 6b) is commonly attributed to the dehydration and depolymerization of the cyclic structures of cellulose [46]. DBD plasma treatment using more reactive gases (O_2 or NH_3 in Ar) and the treatment in Ar/N_2 mixture using plasma torch and harsher conditions, characteristic of this plasma source, led to a two-step degradation pattern. The different degradation processes highlighted by TGA correspond to different structures. A good correlation between TGA results and cross-linking was previously reported [47]. Cellulose cross-linked with epichlorohydrin at variable levels showed the main decomposition events at different temperatures depended on the cross-linking degree, the higher temperature events being attributed to covalent bond cleavage of the polymer network. Thus, it may be presumed that the second degradation process around 437 °C in the case of NC Ar/O_2 and NC Ar/NH_3 or around 475 °C and 486 °C, for NC Ar/N_2 (E15) and NC Ar/N_2 (E30), respectively, may be assigned to the cross-linked cellulose. Hydroxyl radicals, electrons, and ions were formed during these treatments which may break the cyclic structures and favor the cross-linking reactions.

The concentration of the cross-linked polymer may be roughly estimated from the residue after the first decomposition step, 20%–23% for 30 min of DBD plasma exposure and 24% or 32% when plasma torch was used for 15 or 30 min. This means that the changes induced by the treatments depend both on the type of the source and time of exposure. A small shoulder occurred only for unmodified NC, at about 225 °C; it is usually associated with the release of water or other low molecular weight fractions from defibrillated BC [48]. No shoulder was detected in this temperature range for NC after plasma treatment. This may lead to the conclusion that the treatment with filamentary plasma jet and plasma torch in Ar or gas mixtures was able to remove the bond water and low molecular weight impurities from NC. In addition to removing water, the plasma torch treatment may cause some chemical changes which led to the release of a small concentration (6%–7%) of low molecular weight fractions around 240 °C.

The DBD plasma treatment in Ar and Ar/N_2 mixture significantly increased the T_{on} value of NC, with 35 °C and 17 °C, respectively. An increase of the characteristic temperatures was also observed in the case of plasma torch for NC Ar/N_2 (E15) (Table 2). The higher thermal stability may be caused by the removal of less thermally stable components, including low molecular weight fractions and impurities. The release of water and slight cross-linking may also be caused by the milder conditions of the filamentary plasma treatment and the plasma torch for small duration. A slight increase of T_{on} with 3 °C was reported for Quiscal fibers after atmospheric DBD plasma treatment [31]. An increase of the decomposition temperature with about 20 °C was also observed for jute fibers treated with Ar plasma under vacuum [49]. However, natural fibers like Quiscal or jute fibers contain hemicelluloses and lignin in a high proportion which greatly influence the thermal stability during the plasma treatment. Generally, the literature regarding the influence of plasma treatment on the thermal stability of cellulose is rather scarce and no information regarding nanocellulose is available.

No significant change in T_{on} and T_{max} values was noticed for NC Ar-ACN and NC Ar/N_2 (E30) plasma treatments compared to untreated nanocellulose, however a decrease of the characteristic temperatures was obvious for the plasma treatment with more reactive gases, O_2 or NH_3 in Ar (Table 2). Although used in small amount in the Ar flow, NH_3 and, especially, O_2 decrease the T_{on} with 16 °C and 24 °C, respectively. A slight decrease of the thermal stability was observed for vacuum plasma treated Arundo fibers exposed to a plasma power of 150 W for 120 s [50]. In contrast, a decrease of the final degradation temperature with 107 °C was observed for air plasma treated gray linen compared to the untreated sample [51]. Again, the non-cellulosic components of natural fibers have definitely influenced the thermal stability. It is worth mentioning that all the treatments led to a lower residue, which highlights the efficiency of these treatments in cleaning the nanocellulose from low molecular weight impurities.

3.3. Surface Analysis by ATR-FTIR

The FTIR spectra of NC before and after plasma treatments are shown in Figure 7a. For comparison, all FTIR spectra were normalized using the C–H stretching vibration from 2897 cm^{-1} [52]. Regarding the crystalline structure, NC is a mixture of Iα and Iβ allomorphs with Iα the predominant crystal form [10] since it was obtained from BC by mechanical disintegration. The presence of the two allomorphs was detected in all the samples, untreated and plasma treated, at 750 cm^{-1} (assigned to the contribution of cellulose Iα) and at 710 cm^{-1} (corresponding to cellulose Iβ) [10,53]. No significant change in the intensity ratio and position of the bands corresponding to the two allomorphs was observed after the plasma treatments, regardless of the source or conditions (Figure 5b); this shows that the crystalline phase in NC is resistant to the plasma attack.

The O–H groups in cellulose are hydrogen bonded and the overlap of several O–H stretching modes leads to a broad peak as that observed in Figure 7, between 3000 and 3600 cm^{-1}. The most important vibrations were noticed at about 3242 cm^{-1} for cellulose Iα and were assigned to intra-chain hydrogen-bonded 2OH [54] and between 3300 and 3350 cm^{-1} for coupled vibrations corresponding to inter and intra-chain hydrogen bonded 2OH, 3OH, and 6OH groups [54]. The OH peak position is shifted to a lower wavenumber because of hydrogen bonding [54,55]. The assignment of OH absorption bands is complicated by the contribution from N–H stretching vibrations in amide groups, knowing that BC may contain a small amount of proteins. The main peak shifted from about 3340 cm^{-1} for NC and NC Ar, to 3343 cm^{-1} for NC Ar/O_2 and NC Ar-ACN, to 3342 cm^{-1} for NC Ar/N_2 and NC Ar/NH_3 and to 3341 cm^{-1} for NC Ar/N_2 (E30). This slight shift to higher wavenumber is an indication of the decrease of hydrogen bonding due to cross-linking or participation of OH in other bonds [54,56] and, possibly, due to the presence of N–H vibration from newly created bonds [57].

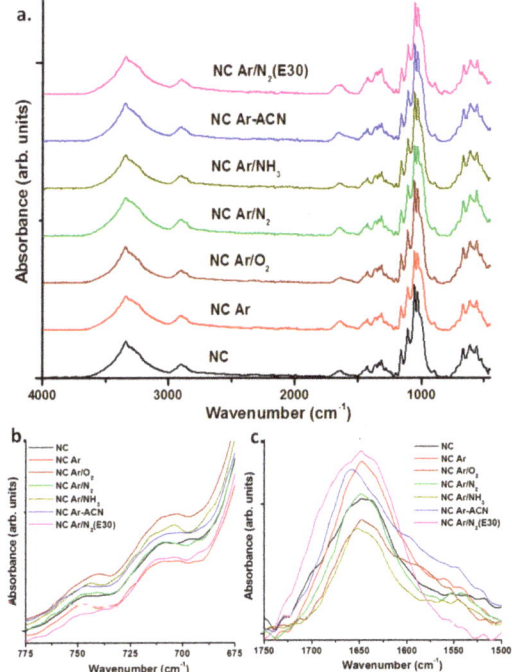

Figure 7. Fourier transform infrared spectroscopy (FTIR) spectra of untreated and plasma treated NC (**a**); zoomed-in regions (775–675 cm^{-1}) (**b**) and (1750–1500 cm^{-1}) (**c**) of the same spectra.

The FTIR spectra in the range from 1500 to 1750 cm^{-1} show important differences (Figure 7c). This is a region where several vibrations overlap. For example, H–O–H bending absorption [58] and C=O stretching vibration in amide I [59] are assigned at 1635–1650 cm^{-1}, N–H and C–N vibrations in amide II at about 1550 cm^{-1} [59,60], aliphatic and aromatic C=C stretching and C=N stretching vibrations in the range 1600–1660 cm^{-1} [61–63]. It is worth mentioning that the peak at 1647–1648 cm^{-1} in pristine NC and plasma treated NC with Ar, Ar/N_2 and Ar/O_2 is shifted to a higher wavenumber in the case of Ar/NH_3 (1651 cm^{-1}) and Ar-ACN (1658 cm^{-1}) treatments. This may be due to the formation of new C=O or C=C bonds in the case of the last two treatments. In addition to the peak at 1648 cm^{-1}, the NC treated with plasma torch (E30) shows a wide shoulder stretching from 1660 to

1700 cm^{-1}, with a local peak at about 1665 cm^{-1}. This shoulder may be assigned to C=O stretching vibration and C=N stretching in imines and oximes [63].

The shoulder at 1550 cm^{-1} which is generally associated with N–H and C–N vibrations in amide II [59,60] is hardly visible for pristine NC, because of the low content in amide from the protein residues of the bacterial cells, but in the case of Ar/N$_2$ and Ar/NH$_3$ treatments this is obvious. Likewise, a wide shoulder is observed in the range from 1500 to 1600 cm^{-1} in the case of Ar, Ar/O$_2$ and, especially, Ar-ACN plasma treated samples (Figure 7c). Considering the shift of the main peak and the new shoulders which appear after plasma treatments it may be concluded that both DBD and torch plasma sources led to nitrogen containing groups on the surface of NC. However, the assignment of vibration modes is difficult because of the overlapping of vibrations and XPS analysis was undertaken to obtain more information on the type of nitrogen containing bonds on the surface of cellulose.

3.4. Surface Analysis by XPS

The surface chemistry of pristine NC and submerged plasma treated samples were investigated by XPS. Carbon, oxygen, and small amount of nitrogen were identified in the general XPS spectra. The relative atomic concentration of elements and oxygen/carbon and nitrogen/carbon ratio are presented in Table 3.

From the survey spectra, one can see the tendency of NC oxidation after plasma treatment. Regarding oxidation efficiency, DBD filamentary jet in pure Ar is more efficient (O/C = 0.57) compared with similar treatments performed in Ar/O$_2$, Ar/N$_2$, and Ar/NH$_3$ mixtures (O/C lower than 0.55), but DBE treatments produce by far the highest oxidation; the O/C ratio increased from an initial 0.55 value to 0.61 after 15 min and 0.63 after 30 min of DBE treatment. Concerning N incorporation, the highest N/C ratio was observed for the Ar-ACN treatment with the DBD source.

Table 3. Relative atomic concentrations of carbon, oxygen, and nitrogen.

Samples	C1s (%)	O1s (%)	N1s (%)	O/C	N/C
NC	63.8	35.0	1.2	0.55	0.02
NC Ar	62.9	36.2	0.9	0.57	0.01
NC Ar/O2	63.5	35.1	1.4	0.55	0.02
NC Ar/N2	64.6	33.9	1.5	0.52	0.02
NC Ar/N2 (E15)	61.4	37.5	1.1	0.61	0.02
NC Ar/N2 (E30)	61.0	38.2	0.8	0.63	0.01
NC Ar/NH3	65.4	33.2	1.4	0.51	0.02
NC Ar-ACN	63.2	34.4	2.4	0.54	0.04

The presence of nitrogen in untreated NC comes from the biosynthesis and is caused by the proteins from cell debris. Slight change of N 1s% between samples was observed, with a clear increase of nitrogen content in the case of filamentary plasma in Ar submerged in ACN.

In order to evaluate the elemental bonding states at the samples surface, high resolution spectra were measured for C1s, O1s, and N1s regions. Each C1s spectrum (Figure 8) was deconvoluted in four components which were assigned according to the binding energy to: (i) C–C and C–H bonds for C1s at about 284.6 ± 0.1 eV (C1), (ii) single bonded C in C–O (ether, hydroxyl) or C–N at 286.3 ± 0.1 eV (C2), (iii) double bonded C in C=O (carbonyl) or O–C–O (acetal) at about 287.9 ± 0.1 eV (C3), O–C=O (carboxyl or ester) at 289.5 ± 0.1 eV (C4). Similarly, the O1s regions contain three sub-peaks centered on the binding energy of 531.0 ± 0.1 eV (O1: O=C in carbonyl and ketone), 532.9 ± 0.1 eV (O2: single bonded O, in hydroxyl or epoxy), and 534.9 ± 0.1 eV (O3: attributed to carboxyl or ester groups). The percentage of each component, with respect to the C1s and O1s peak areas, are presented in Table 4.

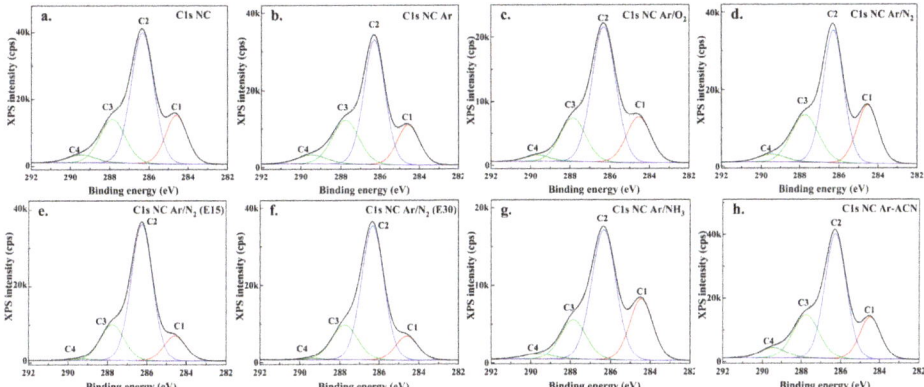

Figure 8. High resolution spectra of C1s region with deconvolution (different colored C1–C4 components) for pristine NC (**a**) and plasma treated NC: NC-Ar (**b**); NC Ar/O$_2$ (**c**); NC Ar/N$_2$ (**d**); NC Ar/N$_2$ (E15) (**e**); NC Ar/N$_2$ (E30) (**f**); NC Ar/NH$_3$ (**g**), and NC Ar-ACN (**h**).

Table 4. Percentage of components from the total amount of carbon C1s and O1s.

Samples	C1s Components				O1s Components		
	C1 (%)	C2 (%)	C3 (%)	C4 (%)	O1 (%)	O2 (%)	O3 (%)
NC	19.7	55.3	20.7	4.2	2.9	87.5	9.6
NC Ar	17.9	53.2	23.5	5.4	3.1	85.2	11.7
NC Ar/O2	20.2	56.8	20.1	2.9	3.1	88.9	8.1
NC Ar/N2	23.1	49.4	23.6	4.0	4.0	85.0	11.0
NC Ar/N2 (E15)	12.5	66.9	19.7	0.8	2.2	96.1	1.7
NC Ar/N2 (E30)	12.1	66.9	20.3	0.7	1.9	96.4	1.8
NC Ar/NH3	24.9	54.5	17.6	2.9	3.6	88.0	8.4
NC Ar-ACN	18.3	53.6	22.6	5.6	3.4	82.7	13.9

In the C1s region, the predominant peaks correspond to C–O (C2 sub-peak). The percentage of C2 components varies between 49.4% and 66.9%, depending on the treatment. From the high-resolution spectra in the carbon region one can observe that all the treatments induced changes and reorganization of chemical groups on the NC surface. The filamentary DBD treatments mostly led to diminished C2 component, while plasma torch to increased C2 component with respect to pristine NC.

Regarding the C1 component, i.e., assigned to low molecular weight fractions and impurities, one can observe a reduction of C–C/C–H bonds (cleaning of NC) by the Ar plasma and, especially, torch treatments. In addition to NC cleaning process, torch treatments (E15 and 30 samples) also led to the decrease of C3 and C4 components and, therefore, the increase of C–O bonds at the expense of C–C/C–H (C1) and O–C=O (C4) bonds was noticed. It is likely that the contaminant carbon, rich in alkyl and carboxyl groups, was removed by plasma torch treatments. Still, an increase of the C4 component was observed in the case of Ar and Ar-ACN DBD treatments, possibly due to a higher affinity to water molecules and oxidation. This fact was also confirmed in the O1s region.

Regarding the concentration of O1, O2, and O3 components (see Table 4) one can observe that the majority of oxygen (O2 peak) is distributed in relation to C2 component and only few percentages in combination to C1 and C3. The results confirm the purification of NC after torch treatments where O2 component reaches a maximum of 96.1%–96.4%.

From the N1s region (Figure 9), it is seen that the untreated NC presents two types of nitrogen bonds, with binding energies at 401.8 eV (N1) and 399.9 eV (N2).

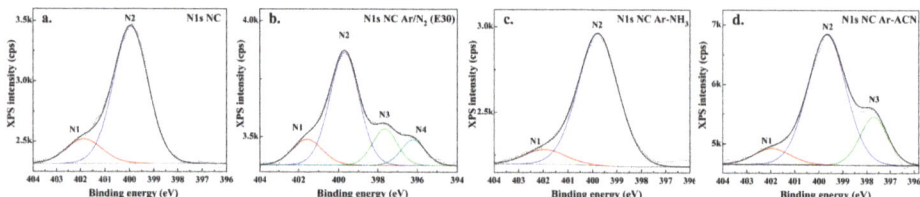

Figure 9. High resolution N1s spectra with deconvolution (different colored N1–N4 components) of pristine NC (**a**); NC Ar/N$_2$ (E30) (**b**); NC Ar/NH$_3$ (**c**), and NC Ar-ACN sample (**d**).

The N1 (15.8%) and N2 (84.2%) peaks on NC are associated to: protonated amines or lactam [64] and to amides, alkylamides or amines, respectively [65,66]. We observed that all treated samples keep the native nitrogen, with a slight variation of the total percentage. In addition, the introduction of new nitrogen bond types was noticed. Compared to pristine NC, the torch treatment in N$_2$ for 30 min and the DBD in NH$_3$ and ACN produced the largest changes. New peaks occurred after these treatments leading to changes of the percentage of bonds; the treatment in acetonitrile modified the percentage of N1 (8.4%) and N2 (71.6%) components, by introducing new nitrogen containing bonds at about 398 eV, with a relative concentration of 20%, assigned to the iminic group [67] (component N3). Another additional peak was observed after nitrogen treatment by torch (E30), at around 396.5 eV, assigned to the pyridinic C=N [68] (component N4). The concentration of N1, N2, N3, and N4 components for samples (E30) were 11%, 16.1%, 59.2%, and 13.7%, respectively. Ammonia plasma even increase the content of amine groups N2 (89.8%) at the expense of N1 component (10.2%) with respect to untreated NC. Therefore, the source type and the gas mixture as well as the liquid medium influenced the functionalization of the nanocellulose surface.

3.5. Effect of Plasma Treated NC on PHB Properties

The analysis of submerged liquid plasma treated NC samples by FTIR, XPS, and TGA showed that nanocellulose was surface functionalized by oxidation and bonding of nitrogen containing groups. The effect of these functionalized NC samples on the thermal stability and mechanical properties of a biopolymer with high expectations for biomedicine (i.e., PHB) was also studied. To differentiate the effect of each NC surface modification, a low concentration (0.2 wt %) of submerged liquid plasma functionalized NC was used in the melt compounded PHB nanocomposites. The thermal degradation of PHB nanocomposite containing pristine NC is a two-step process (Figure 10a,b), with a small shoulder at 215–220 °C, characteristic to the decomposition of NC and a main degradation step at about 282 °C, characteristic of PHB.

PHB containing plasma functionalized NC showed similar thermal behavior compared to that of PHB-NC. Similar T_{on} and T_{max} values for the nanocomposites with NC, NC Ar/N$_2$ (E30) and NC Ar-ACN are shown in Table 5. Slightly lower values were obtained for the rest of the samples. However, the shift of the characteristic temperatures was less than 9 °C. The efficiency of a reinforcing fiber is decisively influenced by the fiber–polymer interface, a good interface adhesion leading to a better stress transfer from the polymer to the fiber and to a higher strength [69]. The mechanical properties of PHB nanocomposites were measured in tensile mode (Table 5). Although used in a small amount in PHB, plasma functionalized NC induced an increase of the tensile strength, with 10%–15%, compared to the nanocomposite with the same amount of pristine NC. This shows the enhancement of the adhesion between PHB and surface treated NC probably because of the new functionalities on the fiber surface induced by plasma treatments and emphasized by FTIR and XPS.

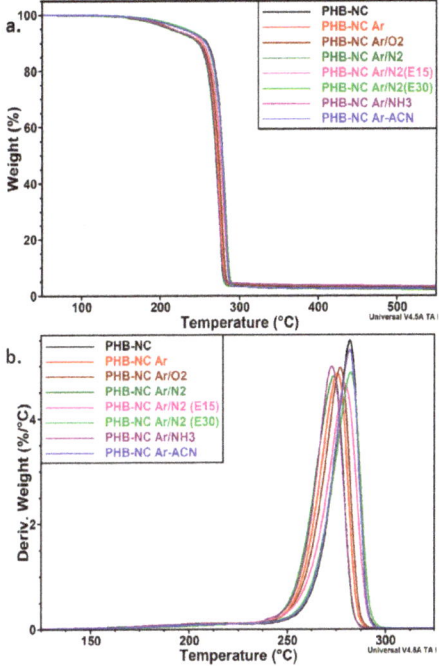

Figure 10. TGA (**a**) and DTG (**b**) curves for poly (3-hydroxybutyrate) (PHB) nanocomposites containing plasma functionalized NC.

Table 5. Thermal (T_{on} and T_{max}) and mechanical characteristics (tensile strength and Young's modulus) of PHB-NC nanocomposites.

Nanocomposites	Tensile Strength (MPa)	Young's Modulus (MPa)	T_{on} (°C)	T_{max} (°C)
PHB-NC	26.0 ± 1.4	1324 ± 62	269.0	281.9
PHB-NC Ar	29.5 ± 0.7	1358 ± 49	262.2	276.0
PHB-NC Ar/O2	29.0 ± 1.1	1387 ± 59	263.6	277.2
PHB-NC Ar/N2	28.5 ± 0.6	1395 ± 30	260.2	273.8
PHB-NC Ar/N2 (E15)	29.1 ± 0.5	1307 ± 41	265.5	279.5
PHB-NC Ar/N2 (E30)	29.8 ± 0.5	1309 ± 55	268.9	282.5
PHB-NC Ar/NH3	29.2 ± 0.9	1402 ± 55	260.8	273.0
PHB-NC Ar-ACN	30.6 ± 0.3	1408 ± 22	269.1	281.9

The Young's modulus is measured using the stress and strain values in the elastic region, where the deformation is small and, therefore, it is less influenced by the adhesion at the fiber–polymer interface [70]. The values of Young's modulus in Table 5 also show smaller influence of the different treatments compared to the tensile strength. The cumulative analysis of thermal and mechanical behaviors shows that Ar treatment of NC in ACN-water suspension has the best influence on the properties of PHB, an increase of the tensile strength with 18%, a slight increase (6%) of Young's modulus and good thermal stability, similar to that of PHB and PHB-NC. It is worth mentioning that there is a good correlation between these results and the structural analyses (FTIR and XPS) and morphological investigation of the Ar-ACN treated NC.

4. Conclusions

This study demonstrated that the application of a plasma torch and filamentary jet plasma modified the morphology and surface chemistry of nanocellulose fibers dispersed in a liquid phase. The plasmas were operated in Ar or mixtures of Ar with O_2, N_2, NH_3, while the liquid was water or ACN in water. The treatment with filamentary plasma jet and plasma torch in Ar or gas mixtures was able to remove the bond water and low molecular weight impurities from NC. All the treatments led to a lower residue, which highlights the efficiency of these treatments in cleaning the nanocellulose. Individual small length nanofibers in higher proportion were formed after the plasma treatments which may favor a more homogeneous dispersion in nanocomposites. However, the intensity of this effect was different depending on the type of the source and gas mixture. FTIR and XPS measurements showed that both oxygen and nitrogen functional groups were formed on the surface of NC depending upon conditions. The functionalization with oxygen moieties was more effective in the case of the plasma torch system in water and the functionalization with nitrogen moieties was most effective using the filamentary jet in ACN media. Both functionalization types can promote the adhesion of components in nanocomposites. Indeed, small proportion of plasma functionalized NC using the filamentary jet led to 10%–15% increase of the tensile strength, compared to the nanocomposite with the same amount of untreated NC. This work provides a new eco-friendly method for the surface functionalization of nanocellulose directly in its water suspension which overcomes the disadvantages of polluting, time consuming, and complex chemical treatments.

Author Contributions: D.M.P., G.D., and S.V. conceived and designed the experiments; A.C. prepared the BC membranes. L.G.C. performed the plasma experiments; A.N.F. contributed to the preparation of composites, tensile tests, and FTIR; C.A.N. performed the thermal characterization; interpretation of XPS results was performed by S.V., G.D., and D.M.P.; D.M.P contributed to the interpretation of the thermal and mechanical results; D.M.P., S.V., and G.D. wrote the paper. The manuscript was read and approved by all the authors.

Funding: This work was supported by a grant of the Romanian National Authority for Scientific Research and Innovation, CNCS/CCCDI—UEFISCDI, project number PN-III-P2-2.1-PED-2016-0287 (122/2017 CELLAB-SLP), within PNCDI III.

Acknowledgments: The authors gratefully acknowledge Veronica Satulu for XPS measurements, Roxana Trusca for SEM investigation of bacterial cellulose nanofibers, Maximilian Teodorescu and Eusebiu Rosini Ionita for their contribution to the achievement of the plasma sources.

Conflicts of Interest: The authors declare no conflict of interest.

References

1. Grishkewich, N.; Mohammed, N.; Tang, J.; Tam, K.C. Recent advances in the application of cellulose nanocrystals. *Curr. Opin. Colloid Interface Sci.* **2017**, *29*, 32–45. [CrossRef]
2. Sindhu, K.A.; Prasanth, R.; Thakur, V.K. Medical applications of cellulose and its derivatives: Present and future. In *Nanocellulose Polymer Nanocomposites. Fundamentals and Applications*; Thakur, V.K., Ed.; Wiley-Scrivener: Hoboken, NJ, USA, 2015; pp. 461–462.
3. Nechyporchuk, O.; Belgacem, M.N.; Bras, J. Production of cellulose nanofibrils: A review of recent advances. *Ind. Crops Prod.* **2016**, *93*, 2–25. [CrossRef]
4. García, A.; Gandini, A.; Labidi, J.; Belgacem, N.; Bras, J. Industrial and crop wastes: A new source for nanocellulose biorefinery. *Ind. Crops Prod.* **2016**, *93*, 26–38. [CrossRef]
5. Karimi, S.; Tahir, P.M.; Karimi, A.; Dufresne, A.; Abdulkhani, A. Kenaf bast cellulosic fibers hierarchy: A comprehensive approach from micro to nano. *Carbohydr. Polym.* **2014**, *101*, 878–885. [CrossRef] [PubMed]
6. Leao, R.M.; Mileo, P.C.; Maia, J.M.L.L.; Luz, S.M. Environmental and technical feasibility of cellulose nanocrystal manufacturing from sugarcane bagasse. *Carbohydr. Polym.* **2017**, *175*, 518–529. [CrossRef] [PubMed]
7. Frone, A.N.; Chiulan, I.; Panaitescu, D.M.; Nicolae, C.A.; Ghiurea, M.; Galan, A.M. Isolation of cellulose nanocrystals from plum seed shells, structural and morphological characterization. *Mater. Lett.* **2017**, *194*, 160–163. [CrossRef]

8. Dima, S.-O.; Panaitescu, D.-M.; Orban, C.; Ghiurea, M.; Doncea, S.-M.; Fierascu, R.C.; Nistor, C.L.; Alexandrescu, E.; Nicolae, C.-A.; Trică, B.; et al. Bacterial nanocellulose from side-streams of Kombucha beverages production: Preparation and physical-chemical properties. *Polymers* **2017**, *9*, 374. [CrossRef]
9. Martinez-Sanz, M.; Lopez-Rubio, A.; Lagaron, J.M. Optimization of the nanofabrication by acid hydrolysis of bacterial cellulose nanowhiskers. *Carbohydr. Polym.* **2011**, *85*, 228–236. [CrossRef]
10. Panaitescu, D.M.; Frone, A.N.; Chiulan, I.; Casarica, A.; Nicolae, C.A.; Ghiurea, M.; Trusca, R.; Damian, C.M. Structural and morphological characterization of bacterial cellulose nano-reinforcements prepared by mechanical route. *Mater. Des.* **2016**, *110*, 790–801. [CrossRef]
11. Ruka, D.R.; Simon, G.P.; Dean, K. Harvesting fibrils from bacterial cellulose pellicles and subsequent formation of biodegradable poly-3-hydroxybutyrate nanocomposites. *Cellulose* **2014**, *21*, 4299–4308. [CrossRef]
12. Vasconcelos, N.F.; Feitosa, J.P.A.; Gama, F.M.P.; Morais, J.P.S.; Andrade, F.K.; Filho, M.M.S.; Rosa, M.F. Bacterial cellulose nanocrystals produced under different hydrolysis conditions: Properties and morphological features. *Carbohydr. Polym.* **2017**, *155*, 425–431. [CrossRef] [PubMed]
13. Lai, C.; Zhang, S.; Sheng, L.; Liao, S.; Xi, T.; Zhang, Z. TEMPO-mediated oxidation of bacterial cellulose in a bromide-free system. *Colloid Polym. Sci.* **2013**, *291*, 2985–2992. [CrossRef]
14. Luo, H.; Xiong, G.; Hu, D.; Ren, K.; Yao, F.; Zhu, Y.; Gao, C.; Wan, Y. Characterization of TEMPO-oxidized bacterial cellulose scaffolds for tissue engineering applications. *Mater. Chem. Phys.* **2013**, *143*, 373–379. [CrossRef]
15. Shao, W.; Wu, J.; Liu, H.; Ye, S.; Jiang, L.; Liu, X. Novel bioactive surface functionalization of bacterial cellulose membrane. *Carbohydr. Polym.* **2017**, *178*, 270–276. [CrossRef] [PubMed]
16. Taokaew, S.; Phisalaphong, M.; Newby, B.Z. Modification of bacterial cellulose with organosilanes to improve attachment and spreading of human fibroblasts. *Cellulose* **2015**, *22*, 2311–2324. [CrossRef] [PubMed]
17. Stumpf, T.R.; Yang, X.; Zhang, J.; Cao, X. In situ and ex situ modifications of bacterial cellulose for applications in tissue engineering. *Mater. Sci. Eng. C* **2018**, *82*, 372–383. [CrossRef] [PubMed]
18. Casaburi, A.; Rojo, U.M.; Cerrutti, P.; Vazquez, A.; Foresti, M.L. Carboxymethyl cellulose with tailored degree of substitution obtained from bacterial cellulose. *Food Hydrocoll.* **2018**, *75*, 147–156. [CrossRef]
19. Ibrahim, N.A.; Eid, B.M.; Abdel-Aziz, M.S. Effect of plasma superficial treatments on antibacterial functionalization and coloration of cellulosic fabrics. *Appl. Surf. Sci.* **2017**, *392*, 1126–1133. [CrossRef]
20. Kan, C.; Lam, C. Atmospheric pressure plasma treatment for grey cotton knitted fabric. *Polymers* **2018**, *10*, 53. [CrossRef]
21. Prabhu, S.; Vaideki, K.; Anitha, S. Effect of microwave argon plasma on the glycosidic and hydrogen bonding system of cotton cellulose. *Carbohydr. Polym.* **2017**, *156*, 34–44. [CrossRef] [PubMed]
22. Cabrales, L.; Abidi, N. Microwave plasma induced grafting of oleic acid on cotton fabric surfaces. *Appl. Surf. Sci.* **2012**, *258*, 4636–4641. [CrossRef]
23. Samanta, K.K.; Joshi, A.G.; Jassal, M.; Agrawal, A.K. Study of hydrophobic finishing of cellulosic substrate using He/1,3-butadiene plasma at atmospheric pressure. *Surf. Coat. Technol.* **2012**, *213*, 65–76. [CrossRef]
24. Calvimontes, A.; Mauersberger, P.; Nitschke, M.; Dutschk, V.; Simon, F. Effects of oxygen plasma on cellulose surface. *Cellulose* **2011**, *18*, 803–809. [CrossRef]
25. Flynn, C.N.; Byrne, C.P.; Meenan, B.J. Surface modification of cellulose via atmospheric pressure plasma processing in air and ammonia–nitrogen gas. *Surf. Coat. Technol.* **2013**, *233*, 108–118. [CrossRef]
26. Gaiolas, C.; Belgacem, M.N.; Silva, L.; Thielemans, W.; Costa, A.P.; Nunes, M.; Silva, M.J.S. Green chemicals and process to graft cellulose fibers. *J. Colloid Interface Sci.* **2009**, *330*, 298–302. [CrossRef] [PubMed]
27. Popescu, M.C.; Totolin, M.; Tibirna, C.M.; Sdrobis, A.; Stevanovic, T.; Vasile, C. Grafting of softwood kraft pulps fibers with fatty acids under cold plasma conditions. *Int. J. Biol. Macromol.* **2011**, *48*, 326–335. [CrossRef] [PubMed]
28. Bhanthumnavin, W.; Wanichapichart, P.; Taweepreeda, W.; Sirijarukula, S.; Paosawatyanyong, B. Surface modification of bacterial cellulose membrane by oxygen plasma treatment. *Surf. Coat. Technol.* **2016**, *306*, 272–278. [CrossRef]
29. Pertile, R.A.N.; Andrade, F.K.; Alves, C., Jr.; Gama, M. Surface modification of bacterial cellulose by nitrogen-containing plasma for improved interaction with cells. *Carbohydr. Polym.* **2010**, *82*, 692–698. [CrossRef]

30. Vander Wielen, L.C.; Ostenson, M.; Gatenholm, P.; Ragauskas, A.J. Surface modification of cellulosic fibers using dielectric-barrier discharge. *Carbohydr. Polym.* **2006**, *65*, 179–184. [CrossRef]
31. Relvas, C.; Castro, G.; Rana, S.; Fangueiro, R. Characterization of physical, mechanical and chemical properties of Quiscal fibres: The influence of atmospheric DBD plasma treatment. *Plasma Chem. Plasma Process.* **2015**, *35*, 863–878. [CrossRef]
32. Kusano, Y.; Madsen, B.; Berglund, L.; Aitomäki, Y.; Oksman, K. Dielectric barrier discharge plasma treatment of cellulose nanofibre surfaces. *Surface Eng.* **2017**. [CrossRef]
33. Weise, U.; Maloney, T.; Paulapuro, H. Quantification of water in different states of interaction with wood pulp fibres. *Cellulose* **1996**, *3*, 189–202. [CrossRef]
34. Senthilnathan, J.; Weng, C.-C.; Liao, J.-D.; Yoshimura, M. Submerged liquid plasma for the synthesis of unconventional nitrogen polymers. *Sci. Rep.* **2013**, *3*, 2414. [CrossRef] [PubMed]
35. Senthilnathan, J.; Sanjeeva Rao, K.; Yoshimura, M. Submerged liquid plasma—Low energy synthesis of nitrogen-doped graphene for electrochemical applications. *J. Mater. Chem. A* **2014**, *2*, 3332–3337. [CrossRef]
36. Anpilov, A.M.; Barkhudarov, E.M.; Bark, Y.B.; Zadiraka, Y.V.; Christofi, M.; Kozlov, Y.N.; Kossyi, I.A.; Kop'ev, V.A.; Silakov, V.P.; Taktakishvili, M.I.; Temchin, S.M. Electric discharge in water as a source of UV radiation, ozone and hydrogen peroxid. *J. Phys. D Appl. Phys.* **2011**, *34*, 993–999. [CrossRef]
37. Kogelschatz, U. Dielectric-barrier discharges: Their History, Discharge Physics, and Industrial Applications. *Plasma Chem. Plasma Process.* **2003**, *23*, 1–46. [CrossRef]
38. Teodorescu, M.; Bazavan, M.; Ionita, E.R.; Dinescu, G. Characteristics of a long and stable filamentary argon plasma jet generated in ambient atmosphere. *Plasma Sources Sci. Technol.* **2015**, *24*, 025033. [CrossRef]
39. Dinescu, G.; Ionita, E.R.; Luciu, I.; Grisolia, C. Flexible small size radiofrequency plasma torch for Tokamak wall cleaning. *Fusion Eng. Des.* **2007**, *82*, 2311–2317. [CrossRef]
40. Tsai, T.C.; Staack, D. Low-temperature polymer deposition in ambient air using a floating-electrode dielectric barrier discharge jet. *Plasma Process. Polym.* **2011**, *8*, 523–534. [CrossRef]
41. Ionita, E.R.; Ionita, M.D.; Stancu, E.C.; Teodorescu, M.; Dinescu, G. Small size plasma tools for material processing at atmospheric pressure. *Appl. Surf. Sci.* **2009**, *225*, 5448–5452. [CrossRef]
42. Stancu, E.C.; Piroi, D.; Magureanu, M.; Dinescu, G. Decomposition of methylene blue by a cold atmospheric pressure plasma jet source. In Proceedings of the 20th International Symposium on Plasma Chemistry, Philadelphia, PA, USA, 24–29 July 2011; p. 375.
43. Ionita, M.D.; Vizireanu, S.; Stoica, S.D.; Ionita, M.; Pandele, A.M.; Cucu, A.; Stamatin, I.; Nistor, L.C.; Dinescu, G. Functionalization of carbon nanowalls by plasma jet in liquid treatment. *Eur. Phys. J. D* **2016**, *70*, 31. [CrossRef]
44. Shaheen, T.I.; Emam, H.E. Sono-chemical synthesis of cellulose nanocrystals from wood sawdust using acid hydrolysis. *Int. J. Biol. Macromol.* **2018**, *107*, 1599–1606. [CrossRef] [PubMed]
45. Fatah, I.Y.A.; Khalil, H.P.S.A.; Hossain, M.S.; Aziz, A.A.; Davoudpour, Y.; Dungani, R.; Bhat, A. Exploration of a Chemo-Mechanical Technique for the Isolation of Nanofibrillated Cellulosic Fiber from Oil Palm Empty Fruit Bunch as a Reinforcing Agent in Composites Materials. *Polymers* **2014**, *6*, 2611–2624. [CrossRef]
46. Amin, M.C.I.M.; Abadi, A.G.; Katas, H. Purification, characterization and comparative studies of spray-dried bacterial cellulose microparticles. *Carbohydr. Polym.* **2014**, *99*, 180–189. [CrossRef] [PubMed]
47. Udoetok, I.A.; Dimmick, R.M.; Wilson, L.D.; Headley, J.V. Adsorption properties of cross-linked cellulose-epichlorohydrin polymers in aqueous solution. *Carbohydr. Polym.* **2016**, *136*, 329–340. [CrossRef] [PubMed]
48. Kiziltas, E.E.; Kiziltas, A.; Gardner, D.J. Synthesis of bacterial cellulose using hot water extracted wood sugars. *Carbohydr. Polym.* **2015**, *124*, 131–138. [CrossRef] [PubMed]
49. Morshed, M.M.; Alam, M.M.; Daniels, S.M. Moisture removal from natural jute fibre by plasma drying process. *Plasma Chem. Plasma Process.* **2012**, *32*, 249–258. [CrossRef]
50. Scalici, T.; Fiore, V.; Valenza, A. Effect of plasma treatment on the properties of Arundo Donax, L. leaf fibres and its bio-based epoxy composites: A preliminary study. *Compos. Part B* **2016**, *94*, 167–175. [CrossRef]
51. Sadova, S.F.; Pankratova, E.V. Low-temperature plasma surface modification of textiles made from natural fibers and advanced technologies. *High Energy Chem.* **2009**, *43*, 234–240. [CrossRef]
52. Lindh, J.; Ruan, C.; Strømme, M.; Mihranyan, A. Preparation of porous cellulose beads via introduction of diamine spacers. *Langmuir* **2016**, *32*, 5600–5607. [CrossRef] [PubMed]

53. Yamamoto, H.; Horii, F.; Hirai, A. In situ crystallization of bacterial cellulose II. Influences of different polymeric additives on the formation of celluloses Iα and Iβ at the early stage of incubation. *Cellulose* **1996**, *3*, 229–242. [CrossRef]
54. Lee, C.M.; Kubicki, J.D.; Fan, B.; Zhong, L.; Jarvis, M.C.; Kim, S.H. Hydrogen-bonding network and OH stretch vibration of cellulose: Comparison of computational modeling with polarized IR and SFG spectra. *J. Phys. Chem. B* **2015**, *119*, 15138–15149. [CrossRef] [PubMed]
55. Turki, A.; El Oudiani, A.; Msahli, S.; Sakli, F. Investigation of OH bond energy for chemically treated alfa fibers. *Carbohydr. Polym.* **2018**, *186*, 226–235. [CrossRef] [PubMed]
56. Sun, Y.; Lin, L.; Deng, H.; Li, J.; He, B.; Sun, R.; Ouyang, P. Structural changes of bamboo cellulose in formic acid. *BioResources* **2008**, *3*, 297–315.
57. Gu, J.; Hu, C.; Zhong, R.; Tu, D.; Yun, H.; Zhang, W.; Leu, S.-Y. Isolation of cellulose nanocrystals from medium density fiberboards. *Carbohydr. Polym.* **2017**, *167*, 70–78. [CrossRef] [PubMed]
58. Chatjigakis, A.K.; Pappas, C.; Proxenia, N.; Kalantzi, O.; Rodis, P.; Polissiou, M. FT-IR Spectroscopic Determination of the Degree of Esterification of Cell Wall Pectins from Stored Peaches and Correlation to Textural Changes. *Carbohydr. Polym.* **1998**, *37*, 395–408. [CrossRef]
59. Chen, N.; Lin, Q.; Rao, J.; Zeng, Q.; Luo, X. Environmentally friendly soy-based bio-adhesive: Preparation, characterization, and its application to plywood. *BioResources* **2012**, *7*, 4273–4283.
60. Nashy, E.H.A.; Osman, O.; Mahmoud, A.A.; Ibrahim, M. Molecular spectroscopic study for suggested mechanism of chrome tanned leather. *Spectrochim. Acta Pt. A Mol. Biomol. Spectrosc.* **2012**, *88*, 171–176. [CrossRef] [PubMed]
61. Keplinger, T.; Cabane, E.; Chanana, M.; Hass, P.; Merk, V.; Gierlinger, N.; Burgert, I. A versatile strategy for grafting polymers to wood cell walls. *Acta Biomater.* **2015**, *11*, 256–263. [CrossRef] [PubMed]
62. Caschera, D.; Mezzi, A.; Cerri, L.; de Caro, T.; Riccucci, C.; Ingo, G.M.; Padeletti, G.; Biasiucci, M.; Gigli, G.; Cortese, B. Effects of plasma treatments for improving extreme wettability behavior of cotton fabrics. *Cellulose* **2014**, *21*, 741–756. [CrossRef]
63. Kumar, S.S.; Manoj, P.; Giridhar, P. Fourier transform infrared spectroscopy (FTIR) analysis, chlorophyll content and antioxidant properties of native and defatted foliage of green leafy vegetables. *J. Food Sci. Technol.* **2015**, *52*, 8131–8139. [CrossRef] [PubMed]
64. Liao, B.; Long, P.; He, B.; Yi, S.; Ou, B.; Shen, S.; Chen, J. Reversible fluorescence modulation of spiropyran functionalized carbon nanoparticles. *J. Mater. Chem. C* **2013**, *1*, 3716–3721. [CrossRef]
65. Jansen, R.J.J.; van Bekkum, H. XPS of nitrogen-containing functional groups on activated carbon. *Carbon* **1995**, *33*, 1021–1027. [CrossRef]
66. Qaiser, A.A.; Hyland, M.M. X-ray photoelectron spectroscopy characterization of polyaniline-cellulose ester composite membranes. *Mater. Sci. Forum* **2010**, *657*, 35–45. [CrossRef]
67. Desimoni, E.; Brunetti, B. X-Ray Photoelectron Spectroscopic Characterization of Chemically Modified Electrodes Used as Chemical Sensors and Biosensors: A Review. *Chemosensors* **2015**, *3*, 70–117. [CrossRef]
68. Zhu, P.; Song, J.; Lv, D.; Wang, D.; Jaye, C.; Fischer, D.A.; Wu, T.; Chen, Y. Mechanism of enhanced carbon cathode performance by nitrogen doping in lithium–sulfur battery: An X-ray absorption spectroscopic study. *J. Phys. Chem. C* **2014**, *118*, 7765–7771. [CrossRef]
69. Wang, F.; Zhou, S.; Yang, M.; Chen, Z.; Ran, S. Thermo-Mechanical Performance of Polylactide Composites Reinforced with Alkali-Treated Bamboo Fibers. *Polymers* **2018**, *10*, 401. [CrossRef]
70. Lu, Y.; Jiang, N.; Li, X.; Xu, S. Effect of inorganic–organic surface modification of calcium sulfate whiskers on mechanical and thermal properties of calcium sulfate whisker/poly(vinyl chloride) composites. *RSC Adv.* **2017**, *7*, 46486–46498. [CrossRef]

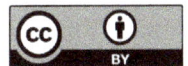

© 2018 by the authors. Licensee MDPI, Basel, Switzerland. This article is an open access article distributed under the terms and conditions of the Creative Commons Attribution (CC BY) license (http://creativecommons.org/licenses/by/4.0/).

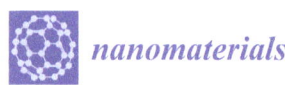

Article

Atmospheric Pressure Plasma-Mediated Synthesis of Platinum Nanoparticles Stabilized by Poly(vinylpyrrolidone) with Application in Heat Management Systems for Internal Combustion Chambers

Anna Dzimitrowicz [1,*], Piotr Cyganowski [2], Pawel Pohl [1], Dorota Jermakowicz-Bartkowiak [2], Dominik Terefinko [1] and Piotr Jamroz [1]

[1] Department of Analytical Chemistry and Chemical Metallurgy, Faculty of Chemistry, Wroclaw University of Science and Technology, Wybrzeze St. Wyspianskiego 27, 50-370 Wroclaw, Poland; pawel.pohl@pwr.edu.pl (P.P.); terefinko.dominik@gmail.com (D.T.); piotr.jamroz@pwr.edu.pl (P.J.)
[2] Department of Polymer and Carbonaceous Materials, Faculty of Chemistry, Wroclaw University of Science and Technology, Wybrzeze St. Wyspianskiego 27, 50-370 Wroclaw, Poland; piotr.cyganowski@pwr.edu.pl (P.C.); dorota.jermakowicz-bartkowiak@pwr.edu.pl (D.J.-B.)
* Correspondence: anna.dzimitrowicz@pwr.edu.pl; Tel.: +48-71-320-24-94

Received: 25 July 2018; Accepted: 13 August 2018; Published: 15 August 2018

Abstract: Poly(vinylpyrrolidone)-stabilized Pt nanoparticles (PVP-PtNPs) were produced in a continuous-flow reaction-discharge system by application of direct current atmospheric pressure glow discharge (dc-APGD) operated between the surface of a flowing liquid anode (FLA) and a pin-type tungsten cathode. Synthesized PVP-PtNPs exhibited absorption across the entire UV/Vis region. The morphology and elemental composition of PVP-PtNPs were determined with transmission electron microscopy (TEM) and energy dispersive X-ray scattering (EDX), respectively. As assessed by TEM, PVP-PtNPs were approximately spherical in shape, with an average size of 2.9 ± 0.6 nm. EDX proved the presence of Pt, C, and O. Dynamic light scattering (DLS) and attenuated total reflectance Fourier transform-infrared spectroscopy (ATR FT-IR) confirmed PtNPs functionalization with PVP. As determined by DLS, the average size of PtNPs stabilized by PVP was 111.4 ± 22.6 nm. A fluid containing resultant PVP-PtNPs was used as a heat conductive layer for a spiral radiator managing heat generated by a simulated internal combustion chamber. As compared to water, the use of PVP-PtNPs enhanced efficiency of the system, increasing the rate of heat transfer by 80% and 30% during heating and cooling, respectively.

Keywords: direct current atmospheric pressure glow discharge; heat transfer; nanostructures; plasma–liquid interactions; stabilizer

1. Introduction

Plasma is one of the four states of matter [1]. Due to the unique properties of atmospheric pressure plasmas (APPs), for example, their highly non-equilibrium state, this type of plasma has been used in many fields of science. These applications include, for example, treatment of skin diseases or tissue engineering in biomedicine [2–4], detection of elements in analytical chemistry [5], activation of seeds to stimulate plant growth in agriculture [6], decomposition of diluted organic compounds in air in environmental protection [7], and fabrication of nanomaterials in nanotechnology and material engineering [1,8,9]. One area of application in material engineering is synthesis of inorganic nanoparticles (NPs), such as platinum nanoparticles (PtNPs), which display special physicochemical, thermal, and catalytic properties [10]. PtNPs are widely utilized as catalysts in numerous chemical reactions, such as conversion of hydrocarbons [11] and oxygen reduction reactions [12].

Application of APP-mediated methods for production of PtNPs has numerous advantages. These methods rely on generation of reactive oxygen and nitrogen species (RONS), solvated electrons, as well as UV radiation and heat. All these factors facilitate formation of NPs through reduction of metallic precursor compounds, eliminating the need for additional reducing agents, such as hydrazine [13] or sodium borohydrate [14]. To the best of our knowledge, only a few research groups have attempted to synthesize PtNPs by APP [15–20]. Koo et al. [15] and Shim et al. [16] produced Pt nanostructures using atmospheric pressure alternating current (ac) H_2/He discharge generated in contact with a solution of H_2PtCl_6. Synthesized PtNPs exhibited an average size of 2 nm and 3–5 nm, respectively [15,16]. Hu et al. [17] synthesized carbon-supported PtNPs by plasma sputtering in water. Similar to PtNPs obtained by Koo et al. [15], PtNPs produced by Hu et al. [17] were 2 nm in size. Comparable results were obtained by Sato et al. [18], who produced PtNPs of 3–10 nm in size by applying microwave-induced plasma generated in liquid. Ichin et al. [19] reported deposition of PtNPs on carbon nanoballs in an aqueous solution of H_2PtCl_6 using poly(vinylpyrrolidone) (PVP) or sodium dodecyl sulfate (SDS) as protection agents. The size of PtNPs produced with the aid of PVP and SDS were, on average, 17.5 and 23.0 nm, respectively. Finally, Dao et al. [20] applied radio frequency (rf) atmospheric pressure discharge operated in Ar for production of nanomaterials for flexible dye-sensitized solar cells. Designed nanomaterials consisted of 2–3 nm PtNPs synthesized by a two-step protocol. In the first step, the PtNPs precursor was partially reduced by alcoholic reduction to Pt atoms, following which the reduction process was completed with the aid of APP [20].

The main limitation of all abovementioned reaction-discharge systems used for production of PtNPs is that they worked in a non-continuous-flow mode. To increase the rate of production of metallic nanostructures, our group has developed continuous-flow reaction-discharge systems. These systems relied on either direct current atmospheric pressure glow discharge (dc-APGD) or pulse-modulated radio frequency atmospheric pressure glow discharge (pm-rf-APGD) as APP sources. Both types of APP were operated between the surface of solutions of flowing liquid electrodes and pin-type tungsten electrodes [8,9,21–23].

A necessary consideration in synthesis of NPs is to ensure that they are highly stable in the dispersing medium. Aggregation, agglomeration, and coalescence are inconvenient processes that commonly result from short interparticle distances between NPs, leading them to attract each other through van der Waals interactions [24]. To prevent these phenomena, repulsive forces in the colloidal phase are necessary to counter van der Waals interactions and increase the stability of isolated NPs [24]. This can be accomplished through selection of a proper capping agent.

Successfully stabilized PtNPs can be used as nanofluids (NFs) for improved transfer of energy in heat management systems (HMSs) [25,26]. HMSs are applied in internal combustion engines, where combustion chambers must operate at extremely high temperatures, reaching 2500 K [27], which result in the oxidation and degradation of the materials used in engines [28]. HMSs can help protect engines by dissipating all waste heat, or by recovering it by transformation into yet another form of energy.

The most popular HMS, used for cooling internal combustion chambers, involves application of a cooling liquid that circulates between header tanks and a radiator [29]. Performance of this type of HMS is achieved by passing the cooling liquid through the combustion chamber block and a set of narrow channels, where it is air-cooled. To increase efficiency of this system, the surface of heat exchange has to be increased; however, this approach is limited because the radiator has to be compact. An alternative route is to apply water-based cooling liquids of improved heat transfer, including NFs [30,31]. For instance, Al_2O_3 or CuNPs might facilitate cooling of the internal combustion block by increasing waste heat transfer from 45% to 80%, as compared to water [29,32]. This increased heat transfer efficiency results in increased combustion efficiency and decreased fuel consumption. However, the volume of NF-based cooling liquid required to manage heat of internal combustion engines often exceeds 5 L, while the volume needed to manage heat of internal combustion chambers in power plants can be counted in tens of thousands of liters. This may raise serious problems related to the large scale of such systems and their proper sealing that can prevent potential emission of NPs to the environment. For this reason, a suitable HMS should be characterized by great efficiency and a limited concentration of NPs present in cooling liquid. The answer to these problems may be application of NFs containing NPs of noble metals, because they are extremely effective heat conductors even at ultra-low concentrations, i.e., 0.001% [26,33]. In our previous work, it was demonstrated that polymer-supported AuNPs facilitated heat transfer at a 300% higher rate than water [8]. It could be believed that application of PtNPs could also provide enhanced heat transfer, while their stabilization with PVP would make suitable NFs for cooling combustion chambers. Since the price of Pt is relatively high, PtNPs-based NFs seems to not be suitable for application as cooling liquids on a large scale. Therefore, a HMS is proposed in the present study, where the NF is used not as a mobile phase but as a heat conductive layer, immobilized and sealed within a radiator.

The main objective of this work was to develop a fast and effective plasma-mediated method for synthesis of stable-in-time and monodisperse PVP-coated PtNPs on the basis of dc-APGD, generated between the surface of a flowing liquid anode (FLA) solution and a pin-type tungsten cathode, and operated in a continuous-flow reaction-discharge system. Synthesized PtNPs were characterized by UV/Vis absorption spectrophotometry (UV/Vis) and transmission electron microscopy (TEM) supported by energy-dispersive X-ray scattering (EDX). To confirm surface functionalization of resultant PtNPs by PVP, dynamic light scattering (DLS) and attenuated total reflectance Fourier transform-infrared spectroscopy (ATR FT-IR) were used. PVP-PtNPs were then applied in the form of a NF in a HMS of simulated internal combustion chambers. The NF was used as a conductive layer for dissipating heat from a circulating liquid used for two scenarios: (i) managing heat of the simulated combustion chamber, and (ii) emergency cooling thereof. To the best of our knowledge, this is the first work in which PVP-PtNPs were produced by dc-APGD generated in a continuous-flow reaction discharge-system and then applied in the HMS for internal combustion chambers.

2. Materials and Methods

2.1. Reagents and Solutions

Chloroplatinic acid hydrate ($H_2PtCl_6 \cdot H_2O$, Sigma-Aldrich, Steinheim, Germany) was used to prepare a stock solution of 1000 mg L^{-1} of Pt(IV) ions. A working solution of 50 mg L^{-1} of Pt(IV) ions was prepared by appropriately diluting the stock solution. Next, 0.25 g of solid poly(vinylpyrrolidone) (PVP, MW = 40,000, Sigma-Aldrich, Steinheim, Germany) was mixed with 1000 mL of the working solution of Pt(IV) ions, giving a final PVP concentration of 0.25% (m/v). All reagents were of analytical grade or better. Re-distilled water was used throughout.

2.2. One-Step Synthesis of PVP-PtNPs

The mixed working solution of the PtNPs precursor (as Pt(IV) ions at 50 mg L^{-1}) and PVP (at 0.25%) was treated by dc-APGD operated in the continuous-flow reaction-discharge system previously reported by Dzimitrowicz et al. [21]. To find the optimal concentration of PVP, the effect of three concentrations of this polymer were examined, i.e., 0.10, 0.25, and 0.50% (m/v). It was observed that in the presence of PVP at 0.10% (m/v), visible sedimentation of PtNPs occurred. On the other hand, at 0.50% (m/v) of PVP, even aggregates occurred. At 0.25% (m/v) of PVP, no sedimentation, aggregation, nor coalescence of produced PtNPs was observed. Stable dc-APGD was sustained between the surface of the FLA solution and the sharpened pin-type tungsten cathode (Figure 1) in a 90 mm (height) by 40 mm (radial) quartz chamber. The gap between both electrodes was ~5.0 mm. A dc-HV supply (Dora Electronics Equipment, Wroclaw, Poland) was used to provide a HV-positive potential (1100–1300 V) to liquid electrode. The discharge current was maintained at a constant value of 55 mA by applying a ballast resistor with resistance of 10 kΩ (Tyco Electronics, Berwyn, IL, USA). The mixed working solution was introduced to the reaction-discharge system through a quartz-graphite tube at a flow rate of 3.0 mL min^{-1} by using a four-channel peristaltic pump (Masterflex L/S, Cole-Parmer, Vernon Hills, IL, USA), and dc-APGD-treated solutions overflowing the quartz-graphite tube were collected for subsequent analyses.

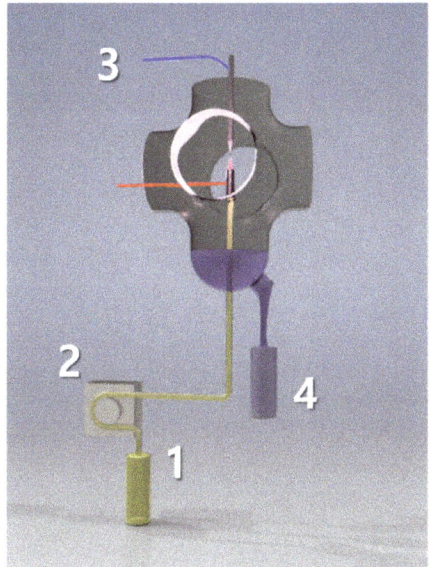 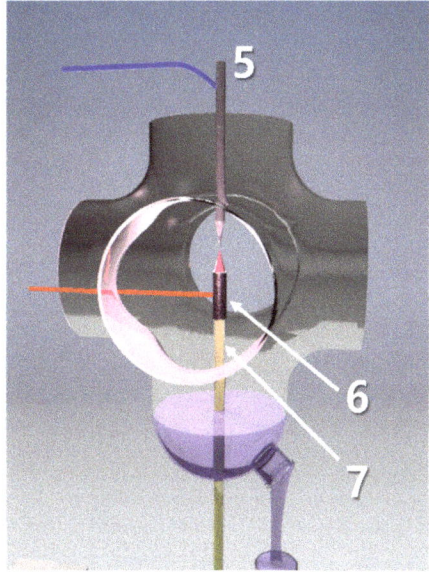

Figure 1. A continuous-flow reaction-discharge system for synthesis of poly(vinylpyrrolidone)-stabilized Pt nanoparticles (PVP-PtNPs); (**1**) the mixed working solution containing the PtNPs precursor and the PVP capping agent (FLA), (**2**) a four-channel peristaltic pump, (**3**) high-voltage wires, (**4**) a collector for the direct current atmospheric pressure glow discharge (dc-APGD)-treated solution, (**5**) a tungsten cathode, (**6**) graphite, and (**7**) quartz tubes.

Detailed characteristics of the plasma reaction-discharge system with APP generated in contact with a FLA are given elsewhere [34]. The rotational temperature of N_2 molecules, determined in the liquid-discharge interfacial zone, was considered an approximation of kinetic gas temperature and was about 1400 K, while the vibrational temperature of N_2 molecules (~5300 K) and the excitation temperature of H atoms (~5200 K) were considerably higher. Differences between temperatures indicated that the developed APGD-based reaction-discharge system was in a high non-equilibrium state. In the spectral range of 200–800 nm, NO, N_2, N_2^+, and OH species were easily excited. Additionally, H and O atomic lines were identified.

2.3. Characterization of PVP-PtNPs

Optical properties of PVP-PtNPs present in dc-APGD treated solutions were determined using a Specord 210 (Analytic Jena AG, Jena, Germany) spectrophotometer. The UV/Vis spectra were acquired in the spectral range from 350 to 700 nm at a scanning speed of 20 nm s^{-1} and a step of 0.2 nm. These spectra were recorded 24 h after dc-APGD treatment of mixed working solutions.

Granulometric properties (size, shape, and elemental composition) of synthesized PVP-PtNPs were assessed using a Tecnai G^{2}20 X-TWIN TEM instrument (FEI, Hillsboro, OR, USA), equipped with an EDX microanalyzer (FEI, Hillsboro, OR, USA). TEM and EDX measurements were carried out as follows: one drop of dc-APGD-treated solution was placed onto a Cu grid (CF400-Cu-UL, Electron Microscopy Sciences, Hatfield, PA, USA) and left to dry on air. The average size of PVP-PtNPs was calculated on the basis of the diameters of 100 single nanostructures using FEI Software (version 3.2 SP6 build 421, FEI, Hillsboro, OR, USA).

2.4. Surface Functionalization of PtNPs by PVP

To confirm surface functionalization of PtNPs by PVP, plasma-synthesized Pt nanostructures included in collected solutions were characterized using DLS and ATR FT-IR. DLS measurements were performed applying a Zetasizer Nano-ZS instrument (Malvern Instrument, Malvern, UK) with an optical arrangement of the detector at 173° (backscatter angle) and a HeNe laser (633 nm). DLS analyses were carried out in optically homogenous polystyrene cuvettes at temperature of 25 °C. Results (size by number) were evaluated using the ZetaSizer Software (Malvern Dispersion Technology Software, version 7.11) and averaged for three independent runs. ATR FT-IR spectra were acquired in the range from 4000 to 400 cm^{-1}, with resolution of 4 cm^{-1} and 64 scans by using a Vertex 70v FTIR spectrophotometer (Bruker, Bremen, Germany). The instrument was equipped with a diamond ATR accessory.

2.5. Application of PVP-PtNPs in the HMS

The NF containing PVP-PtNPs at a concentration of 0.0008% (m/m) was used as a conductive layer within a radiator to cool a liquid circulating between the radiator and a simulated internal combustion block. Figure 2 schematically shows the designed HMS.

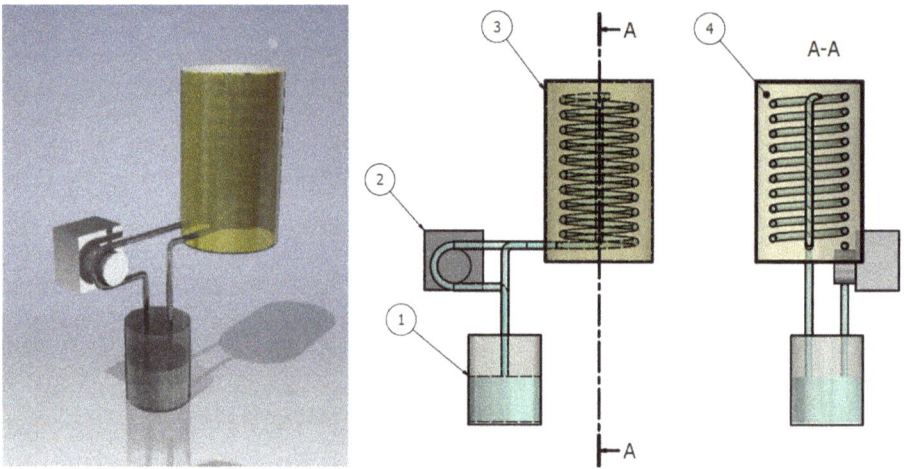

Figure 2. A 3D model of the heat management system (HMS) composed of (**1**) a cooling liquid reservoir, (**2**) a peristaltic pump, (**3**) a spiral radiator filled with (**4**) a conductive layer (the NF containing PVP-PtNPs or water).

The system, as displayed in Figure 2, was composed of a container with cooling liquid (100 mL), a peristaltic pump, and a radiator (150 mm long, diameter 22.5 mm) containing 60 mL of a heat conductive layer (water or the NF). To simulate cooling of the internal combustion block, the container with the liquid was placed on an IKA MAG HS 7 heating plate (Warsaw, Poland), which played the role of the internal combustion chamber, and transferred heat to the liquid. The heating plate was set at a constant power of 200 W, as preliminary tests indicated that this value was sufficient to heat the system to 80 °C. The heated liquid was circulated within the system by a peristaltic pump at a flow rate of 50 mL min^{-1}. To monitor the simulated HMS, the procedure was divided into two parts: (i) assessment of the system to control temperature of the cooling liquid at a constant power of the combustion chamber, and (ii) emergency cooling thereof. In the case of heat management, a container filled with water was placed on a heating plate and heated to 80 °C, which was defined as a theoretical border after which a further increase in temperature could cause overheating of the system. Therefore, when the system reached 80 °C, the peristaltic pump was turned on to simulate the HMS. This caused water to be circulated through the system, and resulted in cooling down of the heated water. When it was heated back up to 80 °C, the second part of the procedure was initiated, i.e., emergency cooling. In this case, after the system returned to 80 °C, the heating plate was immediately turned off, and a fan attached to the radiator was turned on to simulate emergency cooling of the internal combustion block. Water was circulated until it was cooled down to 30 °C. The procedure was carried out at ambient temperature (25 °C). Temperatures of water and the heat conductive layer (either the NF or water) were constantly monitored. Recorded temperatures and duration of heating/cooling were used as variables in a simplified version of Newton's relation between temperatures of the heated/cooled liquid and the surrounding environment [35], defined as $dT(t)/dt = k(h/c) \cdot \Delta T(t)$—where $T(t)$ is temperature at a given time; $k(h/c)$ is the rate of temperature changes, i.e., heating or cooling (s^{-1}); and $\Delta T(t)$ is a difference in temperature over time t.

3. Results and Discussion

3.1. Application of dc-APGD for Synthesis of PVP-PtNPs

The first evidence that dc-APGD operated between the surface of the FLA solution and the pin-type tungsten cathode effectively led to continuous-flow synthesis of PVP-PtNPs was the change in color of the mixed working solution treated by the discharge in the studied reaction-discharge system. In these conditions, the solution was observed to change from colorless to black (Figure 3A). According to Wang et al., it was likely associated with formation of PtNPs nuclei in this solution [36]. Moreover, neither aggregation, agglomeration, nor sedimentation of resultant Pt nanostructures was observed (Figure 3A). This first visual observation confirmed successful production of PtNPs stabilized by PVP in the continuous-flow reaction-discharge system used.

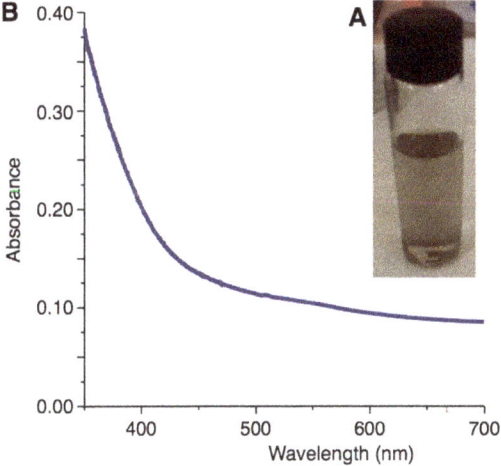

Figure 3. dc-APGD-mediated synthesis of PVP-PtNPs. (**A**) Color exhibited by the mixed working solution after dc-APGD treatment and related to production of PVP-PtNPs; (**B**) the UV/Vis spectrum of PVP-PtNPs.

3.2. Characterization of PVP-PtNPs

Figure 3B displays the UV/Vis absorption spectrum of the mixed working solution treated by dc-APGD. As can be seen, it presents typical features for Pt nanostructures, i.e., the absorption band occurred across the entire UV/Vis region. Furthermore, absorption increased as the wavelength decreased. As was suggested by Yang et al., this was consistent with the optical properties of PtNPs, and hence, supported the presence of Pt nanostructures synthesized due to plasma-liquid interactions (PLIs) [37].

The morphology and element composition of PVP-PtNPs was determined using TEM and EDX, respectively. On the basis of TEM measurements, the average size of PtNPs was 2.92 nm with a relatively narrow size distribution, i.e., 0.6 nm as standard deviation. TEM images also indicated that the PVP-PtNPs formed were monodisperse, and approximately spherical in shape (Figure 4A–C). Based on the EDX spectrum, the presence of Pt, C, O, and Cu was identified (Figure 4D). Occurrence of metallic Pt resulted from reduction of $PtCl_6^{2-}$ ions to Pt(0) of nanometric size by dc-APGD-mediated processes in the applied continuous-flow reaction-discharge system. Detection of C and O was likely associated with the chemical structure of PVP. Occurrence of Cu was due to deposition of samples on Cu grids prior to TEM analysis. All these data confirmed that it was possible to produce small (average size of approximately 2 nm) PtNPs through PLIs in the studied reaction-discharge system. This was coincident with results reported by others, who produced PtNPs of ~2 nm in size using different types of APPs [15,17,20]. Nevertheless, the unquestionable advantage of the plasma-based method developed here over other APP-based methods reported in the literature was its continuous-flow character, resulting in high production efficiency of PVP-PtNPs. Accordingly, it was possible to produce 180 mL of PVP-PtNPs per hour in the proposed continuous-flow reaction-discharge system.

Surface functionalization of PtNPs with PVP was examined using DLS and ATR FT-IR. Size measurements of resultant Pt nanostructures, as determined by DLS, were much larger than those calculated on the basis of TEM micrographs; the average size by number was 111.4 ± 22.6 nm (Figure 5). This discrepancy in the size of PVP-PtNPs determined using both mentioned techniques was consistent with successful functionalization of Pt nanostructures with PVP [38]. This was because DLS enabled measurement of the hydrodynamic diameter of entire structures, i.e., PtNPs plus attached compounds, whereas TEM measurements were solely based on metallic cores of Pt nanostructures. ATR FT-IR further supported surface functionalization of PtNPs (Figure 6). A sharp, intensive absorption band at 1677 cm^{-1} was observed in the spectrum, and was attributed to C=O stretching vibrations ν from the carbonyl group. Absorption bands at 2950, 1423, and 1286 cm^{-1} were assigned to CH_2 asymmetric stretching vibrations of the aliphatic methylene group and C–N stretching vibrations ν of the PVP ring, respectively [39–41]. Furthermore, occurrence of the absorption band at 845 cm^{-1} was previously recognized as indicative of the PVP ring oriented towards PtNPs [36]. Moreover, all absorption bands observed in the ATR FT-IR spectrum were shifted by about 20 cm^{-1} in relation to standard charts used for evaluation of characteristic groups and moieties [41]. This effect was already observed [39] and explained by coordination of metallic species by PVP [42]. All these observations confirmed the presence of PVP in Pt NPs, and the role of this capping agent in steric stabilization and functionalization of plasma-synthesized PtNPs.

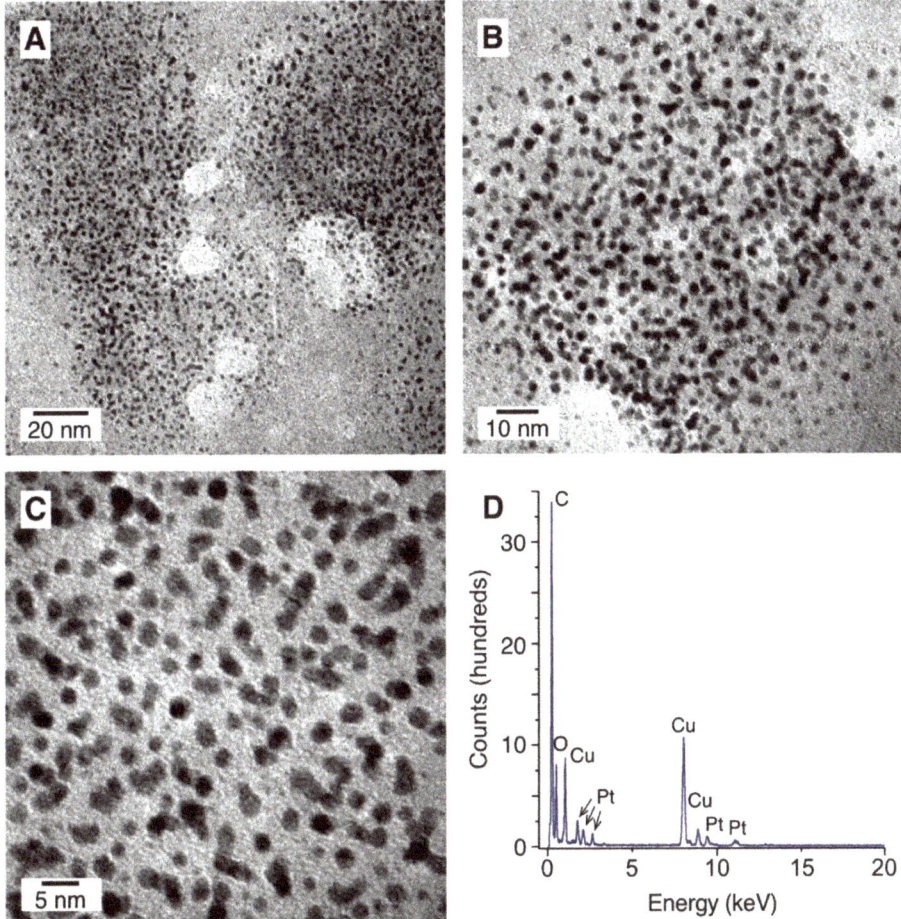

Figure 4. Granulometric properties of PVP-PtNPs synthesized with the aid of dc-APGD. (**A**–**C**) Representative TEM photomicrographs; (**D**) the EDX spectrum.

TEM micrographs further suggested that the PVP matrix could encapsulate PtNPs. In this case, PtNPs seemed to be purposely dispersed, that is, grouped in approximately spherical regions of over 60 nm in diameter. Formation of PVP capsules containing PtNPs, as opposed to formation of individual PtNPs coated with PVP, could also partly explain differences in the size as measured by TEM and DLS. DLS could measure the size of entire capsules, whereas TEM would reveal the size of individual PtNPs within these capsules. Formation of capsules might be related to physicochemical properties of PVP. This polymer contains N and O atoms bearing free electron pairs that could have ability to chelate surface-active compounds such PtNPs [39,43].

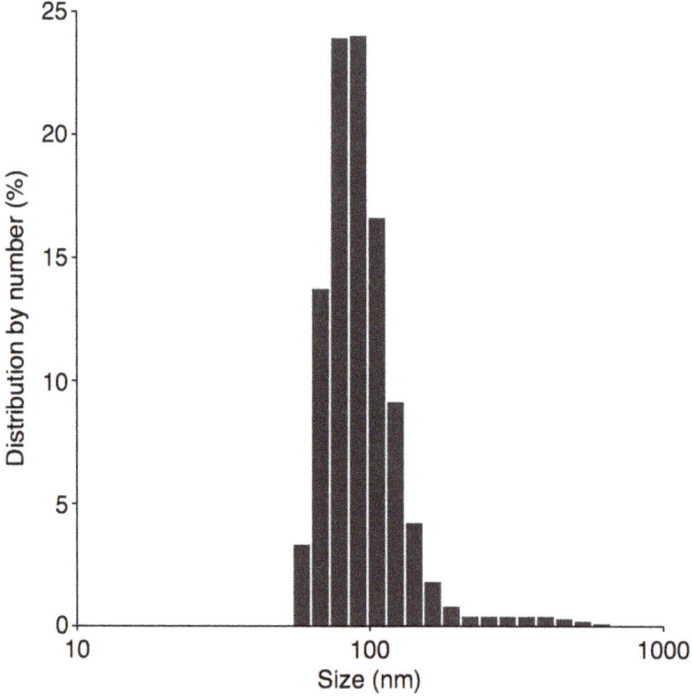

Figure 5. A histogram displaying size by number distribution of PVP-PtNPs as determined by DLS.

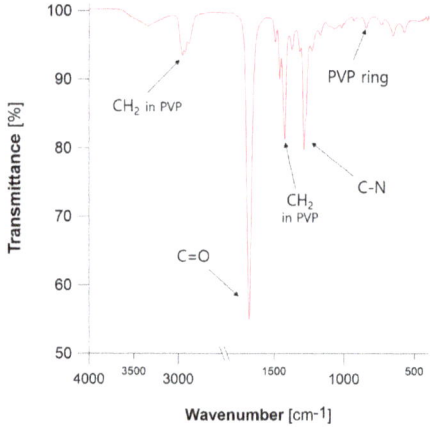

Figure 6. The ATR FT-IR spectrum of PVP-PtNPs.

3.3. Mechanism of PtNPs Formation

The use of dc-APGD generated in contact with liquid for synthesis of PtNPs is extremely rarely reported in literature. Only Koo et al. and Shim et al. reported to use ac-APGDs operated with the aid of H_2/He jets in contact with bulky solution reservoirs containing $PtCl_6^{2-}$ ions for plasma-mediated synthesis of PtNPs [15,16]. These authors hypothesized that $PtCl_6^{2-}$ ions were possibly reduced by H atoms formed in the solution. This could only be partly correct because much more reactive species, capable of reducing the PtNPs precursor, would be formed as a result of PLIs [44]. In the present work, dc-APGD, fully sustained in surrounding air atmosphere (with no additional gas) and operated in contact with the FLA solution, was used for continuous-flow reduction of $PtCl_6^{2-}$ ions and synthesis of PtNPs through PLIs. Detailed characteristics of this reaction-discharge system have been previous published, and the produced reactive species characterized [34], allowing us to provide a putative mechanism for the formation of PtNPs. In case of the reaction-discharge system proposed in the present work, there was no voltage fall at the liquid surface and hence, a large flux of electrons from the discharge column bombarded the surface of the FLA solution, leading to production of a very high concentration of interfacial solvated electrons (e_{aq}^-) [45]. These electrons are both highly reactive, and have an anomalously high diffusion constant [45]. Therefore, they could take part in direct reduction of $PtCl_6^{2-}$ ions in the FLA solution (e.g., $PtCl_6^{2-} + 4e_{aq}^- = Pt^0 + 6Cl^-$), resulting in formation of a large number of Pt^0 nuclei in a very short period of time. Such large number of Pt seeds reached in the FLA solution certainly helped in obtaining smaller in size NPs, as indicated by their morphology as assessed by TEM. Other reactive species could also be formed due to the decomposition of water molecules (in the interfacial zone as well as in the liquid phase, i.e., the FLA solution), including H atoms, OH radicals, or H_2O_2 molecules. However, yields of reactions leading to formation of these species should be much lower than observed for the liquid cathode, as reported for dc-APGDs operated using gaseous jets in contact with ionic liquids (ILs) [46].

The role of PVP in the stabilization of the small-sized PtNPs synthesized could be related to their adhesion to nanoparticles through charge-transfer interactions between pyrrolidone rings and the surface of Pt atoms, and formation of >C=O–Pt coordination bonds [47,48]. In this way, PVP-capped PtNPs could be stabilized in two different ways, that is, a polymeric shell could be formed, leading to a structure that prevents further growth and/or agglomeration [47]; in addition, charge transfer could occur [48], making PtNPs negatively charged, and hence, repulsing them in the solution.

3.4. Enhanced HMS

To the best of our knowledge, no research on the evaluation of the suitability of NFs containing noble metal NPs for cooling internal combustion chambers have been reported so far. For that reason, a HMS composed of a cooling liquid (water) circulating between a reservoir and a spiral radiator within a layer of the NF containing PVP-PtNPs synthesized by dc-APGD (see Figure 2 for more details) was proposed, and studied in detail. Design of the HMS used in the present work corresponded to common designs of popular liquid-cooling systems applied for managing temperature of combustion blocks [29]. The HMS examined here particularly simulated two scenarios, i.e., (i) suppression of an increase in temperature of the cooling liquid, and (ii) emergency cooling of the internal combustion chamber (see Section 2.4 for more details). The temperature of heating/cooling (T) was measured as a function of time (t), and plotted as shown in Figure 7, for both the cooling liquid (water) and the heat conductive layer (water or the NF with PVP-PtNPs).

When the cooling liquid reached a temperature of 80 °C, the medium of the conductive layer began to circulate within the system, resulting in a decrease in temperature of the cooling liquid. Circulation was continued until the cooling liquid was heated back up to 80 °C. As a result, temperature of the medium of the conductive layer in the radiator also increased; this is shown in Figure 7A,C. As can be seen in Figure 7C, initial temperature (80 °C) within the water reservoir rapidly decreased at the beginning of circulation, because the medium of the conductive layer initially had room temperature. The same phenomenon usually takes place in internal combustion engines, however, valves placed between internal and external circuits of the circulation system allow for proper control of the extent of cooling. Afterwards, the temperature of the cooling liquid was increased, as it is done by internal combustion chambers. As can be seen in Figure 7C, if the medium of the conductive layer in the radiator was water, the cooling liquid in the reservoir was heated back to 80 °C within 25 min. By contrast, when the medium of the conductive layer was the NF containing synthesized PVP-PtNPs, the system was unable to reach 80 °C (provided by a heating plate at 200 W), and instead of this, it reached equilibrium at 78 °C within 43 min. Similar differences were also observed for temperature of the medium of the conductive layer. When the temperature of the circulating cooling liquid increased, the temperature of water in the radiator leveled at 75 °C while temperature of the NF of PVP-PtNPs reached just 67 °C.

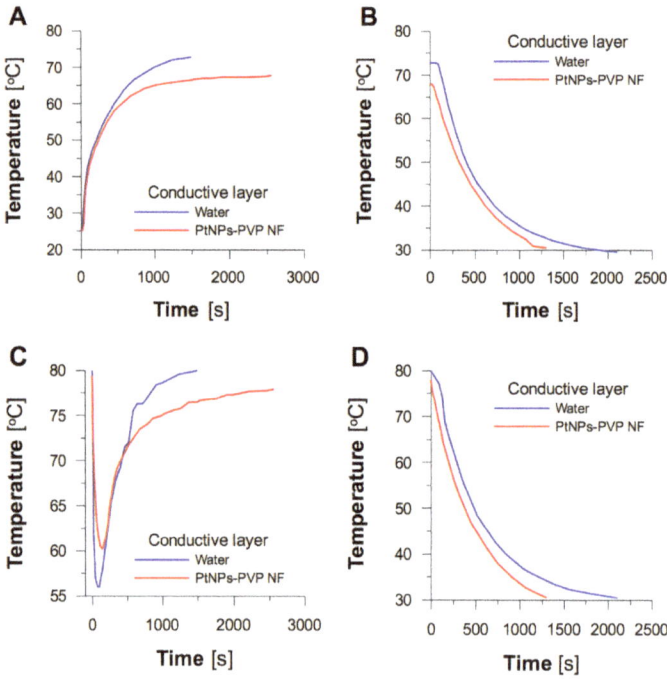

Figure 7. Time-dependent changes of temperature obtained for (**A**) heating, and (**B**) cooling of the conductive layer; (**C**) heating, and (**D**) cooling of the circulating liquid.

When the artificial overheating border was reached, the procedure of emergency cooling was engaged (see Section 2.5 for more details). Although the system with the NF containing PVP-PtNPs did not reach this temperature, the procedure of cooling was initiated at its equilibrium temperature of 78 °C. As can be seen in Figure 7D, the cooling liquid circulating in the system was cooled down to 30 °C within 21 min when the NF containing PVP-PtNPs was applied. This was 14 min faster than when water was used as the medium of the conductive layer. The same tendency was observed when monitoring temperature of water and the NF placed within the radiator (see Figure 7B). All these observations indicated that application of the NF as the conductive layer in the spiral radiator prevented overheating of the system in a fast and effective way. Certainly, the NF-containing PVP-PtNPs displayed an increased heat conductivity within the radiator, as compared to water. To evaluate the efficiency of the system, rate constants of heating (k_h) and cooling (k_c) of the liquid circulating within the system were assessed (see Table 1).

Table 1. Rate constants of heating (k_h) and cooling (k_c) of the circulating liquid.

Medium of the Conductive Layer	Rate Constants [$\times 10^{-3}$ s^{-1}]	
	k_h	k_c
Water	4.88	2.55
PVP-PtNPs	2.70	3.41

When the NF containing PVP-PtNPs was used as the conductive layer, the rate constant responsible for the increase of temperature (k_h) was almost half the value of this assessed for water, i.e., 2.70×10^3 s^{-1} versus 4.88×10^3 s^{-1}. This meant that the presence of the NF significantly extended operation of the system against overheating, as compared to water placed in the radiator. On the other hand, the rate constant of cooling (k_c) was greater when the NF of PVP-PtNPs was used instead of water, which was responsible for the reduced time needed to cool down the whole system. These differences were certainly reflected by ability of the system to operate within safe temperature. The circulating liquid cooled by water placed in the radiator achieved overheating temperature within 25 min, while the NF containing PVP-PtNPs conveniently prevented overheating of the system.

Based on all observations, it appeared that application of PVP-PtNPs would efficiently facilitate both temperature control of the cooling liquid circulating in the internal combustion block, and emergency cooling thereof. It was previously reported that application of a NF containing 1.5% of Cu and Al_2O_3 NPs led to increased heat exchange up to 80%, as compared to water [29,32]. As found in the present work, utilization of the NF containing 0.0008% of PVP-PtNPs resulted in increasing efficiency of the system by 80% during heating, and 30% during cooling, as compared to water. However, it must be remembered that the medium containing PVP-PtNPs was used only as the heat-conductive layer located in the radiator, not as the cooling liquid itself. This significantly reduced the required amount of the NF; hence, the expense for such a system might meet economic requirements. The applied approach overcame two barriers of such systems. Firstly, (1) application of PtNPs led to a significant reduction in the concentration of NPs in the NF needed to successfully manage heat, as compared to already reported systems. Secondly, (2) stabilization of PtNPs by PVP allowed for sealing and immobilization of NF in the radiator; this led to a reduction of the volume of the NF, addressing a potential issue with emission of NPs into the environment.

4. Conclusions

It was established that the action of dc-APGD, completely operated in surrounding air only, onto the continuously flowing solution of $PtCl_6^{2-}$ ions with admixed PVP, led to on-line formation of monodisperse and nearly spherical PVP-capped PtNPs in the liquid phase, with the average diameter of 2.9 ± 0.6 nm. Since the solution of the PtNPs precursor was positively charged and acted as the FLA, it was supposed that solvated electrons were the most important species responsible for reduction of $PtCl_6^{2-}$. Functionalization of the surface of reduced Pt by PVP resulted in high stability of continuously synthesized and uniformly sized PtNPs. It was also found that the NF containing just 0.0008% of PVP-capped PtNPs could serve as a very promising heat conductive medium for a spiral radiator that efficiently manages heat generated by a simulated combustion chamber. As compared to water, the NF containing PVP-PtNPs resulted in increasing efficiency of such system by 80% and 30% during heating and cooling, respectively.

Author Contributions: A.D. and P.C. planned all experiments; A.D. and D.T. carried out dc-APGD-based synthesis of PVP-PtNPs; A.D. described characterization of obtained nanostructures and summarized all acquired data; A.D. and P.C. analyzed all data associated with PtNPs surface functionalization by PVP; P.P. described plasma-liquid interactions involved in PtNPs synthesis; P.C. performed experiments related to application of PtNPs in HMSs for internal combustion chambers; P.P., D.J.-B., and P.J. supervised all work and took part in discussion; A.D. and P.C. prepared the draft of the manuscript.

Funding: A.D., P.C., P.J., and P.P. are thankful to the National Science Centre, Poland (agreements nos. UMO-2014/13/B/ST4/05013 and 2017/01/X/ST5/01666) for co-founding the present project. In addition, this work was financed by a statutory activity subsidy from the Polish Ministry of Science and Higher Education for the Faculty of Chemistry of Wroclaw University of Science and Technology. A.D. is supported by the Foundation for Polish Science (FNP), program START 022.2018 and by Wroclaw Centre of Biotechnology, the program Leading National Research Centre (KNOW) for years 2014–2018.

Conflicts of Interest: The authors declare no conflict of interest. Furthermore, founding sponsors had no role in design of the study; in collection, analyses, or interpretation of data; in writing of the manuscript, and in decision to publish these results.

References

1. d'Agostino, R.; Favia, P.; Oehr, C.; Wertheimer, M.R. Low-temperature plasma processing of materials: past, present, and future. *Plasma Process. Polym.* **2005**, *2*, 7–15. [CrossRef]
2. Weltmann, K.D.; von Woedtke, T. Plasma medicine—Current state of research and medical application. *Plasma Phys. Control. Fusion* **2017**, *59*, 014031. [CrossRef]
3. Weltmann, K.D.; Kindel, E.; von Woedtke, T.; Hahnel, M.; Stieber, M.; Brandenburg, R. Atmospheric-pressure plasma sources: Prospective tools for plasma medicine. *Pure Appl. Chem.* **2010**, *82*, 1223–1237. [CrossRef]
4. Lu, X.; Xiong, Z.; Zhao, F.; Xian, Y.; Xiong, Q.; Gong, W.; Zou, C.; Jiang, Z.; Pan, Y. A simple atmospheric pressure room-temperature air plasma needle device for biomedical applications. *Appl. Phys. Lett.* **2009**, *95*, 181501. [CrossRef]
5. Jamroz, P.; Greda, K.; Pohl, P. Development of direct-current, atmospheric-pressure, glow discharges generated in contact with flowing electrolyte solutions for elemental analysis by optical emission spectrometry. *TrAC Trends Anal. Chem.* **2012**, *41*, 105–121. [CrossRef]
6. Zhou, Z.; Huang, Y.; Yang, S.; Chen, W. Introduction of a new atmospheric pressure plasma device and application on tomato seeds. *J. Agric. Sci.* **2011**, *2*, 23–27. [CrossRef]
7. Oda, T. Non-thermal plasma processing for environmental protection: Decomposition of dilute vocs in air. *J. Electrostat.* **2003**, *57*, 293–311. [CrossRef]
8. Cyganowski, P.; Dzimitrowicz, A.; Jamroz, P.; Jermakowicz-Bartkowiak, D.; Pohl, P. Polymerization-driven immobilization of dc-APGD synthesized gold nanoparticles into a quaternary ammonium-based hydrogel resulting in a polymeric nanocomposite with heat-transfer applications. *Polymers* **2018**, *10*, 377. [CrossRef]
9. Dzimitrowicz, A.; Bielawska-Pohl, A.; diCenzo, G.; Jamroz, P.; Macioszczyk, J.; Klimczak, A.; Pohl, P. Pulse-modulated radio-frequency alternating-current-driven atmospheric-pressure glow discharge for continuous-flow synthesis of silver nanoparticles and evaluation of their cytotoxicity toward human melanoma cells. *Nanomaterials* **2018**, *8*, 398. [CrossRef] [PubMed]
10. Rioux, R.; Song, H.; Grass, M.; Habas, S.; Niesz, K.; Hoefelmeyer, J.; Yang, P.; Somorjai, G. Monodisperse platinum nanoparticles of well-defined shape: Synthesis, characterization, catalytic properties and future prospects. *Top. Catal.* **2006**, *39*, 167–174. [CrossRef]
11. Choi, K.M.; Na, K.; Somorjai, G.A.; Yaghi, O.M. Chemical environment control and enhanced catalytic performance of platinum nanoparticles embedded in nanocrystalline metal–organic frameworks. *J. Am. Chem. Soc.* **2015**, *137*, 7810–7816. [CrossRef] [PubMed]
12. Cheng, N.; Banis, M.N.; Liu, J.; Riese, A.; Li, X.; Li, R.; Ye, S.; Knights, S.; Sun, X. Extremely stable platinum nanoparticles encapsulated in a zirconia nanocage by area-selective atomic layer deposition for the oxygen reduction reaction. *Adv. Mater.* **2015**, *27*, 277–281. [CrossRef] [PubMed]
13. Yadav, O.; Palmqvist, A.; Cruise, N.; Holmberg, K. Synthesis of platinum nanoparticles in microemulsions and their catalytic activity for the oxidation of carbon monoxide. *Colloids Surf. A Physicochem. Eng. Asp.* **2003**, *221*, 131–134. [CrossRef]
14. Nagao, H.; Ichiji, M.; Hirasawa, I. Synthesis of platinum nanoparticles by reductive crystallization using polyethyleneimine. *Chem. Eng. Technol.* **2017**, *40*, 1242–1246. [CrossRef]
15. Koo, I.G.; Lee, M.S.; Shim, J.H.; Ahn, J.H.; Lee, W.M. Platinum nanoparticles prepared by a plasma-chemical reduction method. *J. Mater. Chem.* **2005**, *15*, 4125–4128. [CrossRef]
16. Shim, J.; Joung, K.J.; Ahn, J.H.; Lee, W.M. Carbon-supported platinum nanoparticles synthesized by plasma-chemical reduction method for fuel cell applications. *J. Electrochem. Soc.* **2007**, *154*, B165–B169. [CrossRef]

17. Hu, X.; Takai, O.; Saito, N. Simple synthesis of platinum nanoparticles by plasma sputtering in water. *Jpn. J. Appl. Phys.* **2013**, *52*, 01AN05. [CrossRef]
18. Sato, S.; Mori, K.; Ariyada, O.; Atsushi, H.; Yonezawa, T. Synthesis of nanoparticles of silver and platinum by microwave-induced plasma in liquid. *Surf. Coat. Technol.* **2011**, *206*, 955–958. [CrossRef]
19. Ichin, Y.; Mitamura, K.; Saito, N.; Takai, O. Characterization of platinum catalyst supported on carbon nanoballs prepared by solution plasma processing. *J. Vac. Sci. Technol. A* **2009**, *27*, 826–830. [CrossRef]
20. Dao, V.-D.; Tran, C.Q.; Ko, S.-H.; Choi, H.-S. Dry plasma reduction to synthesize supported platinum nanoparticles for flexible dye-sensitized solar cells. *J. Mater. Chem. A* **2013**, *1*, 4436–4443. [CrossRef]
21. Dzimitrowicz, A.; Greda, K.; Lesniewicz, T.; Jamroz, P.; Nyk, M.; Pohl, P. Size-controlled synthesis of gold nanoparticles by a novel atmospheric pressure glow discharge system with a metallic pin electrode and a flowing liquid electrode. *RSC Adv.* **2016**, *6*, 80773–80783. [CrossRef]
22. Dzimitrowicz, A.; Jamroz, P.; Pogoda, D.; Nyk, M.; Pohl, P. Direct current atmospheric pressure glow discharge generated between a pin-type solid cathode and a flowing liquid anode as a new tool for silver nanoparticles production. *Plasma Process. Polym.* **2017**, *14*, 1600251. [CrossRef]
23. Dzimitrowicz, A.; Motyka, A.; Jamroz, P.; Lojkowska, E.; Babinska, W.; Terefinko, D.; Pohl, P.; Sledz, W. Application of silver nanostructures synthesized by cold atmospheric pressure plasma for inactivation of bacterial phytopathogens from the genera Dickeya and Pectobacterium. *Materials* **2018**, *11*, 331. [CrossRef] [PubMed]
24. Polte, J. Fundamental growth principles of colloidal metal nanoparticles–a new perspective. *CrystEngComm* **2015**, *17*, 6809–6830. [CrossRef]
25. Das, S.K.; Choi, S.U.S.; Patel, H.E. Heat transfer in nanofluids—A review. *Heat Transfer Eng.* **2006**, *27*, 3–19. [CrossRef]
26. Patel, H.E.; Das, S.K.; Sundararajan, T.; Sreekumaran Nair, A.; George, B.; Pradeep, T. Thermal conductivities of naked and monolayer protected metal nanoparticle based nanofluids: Manifestation of anomalous enhancement and chemical effects. *Appl. Phys. Lett.* **2003**, *83*, 2931–2933. [CrossRef]
27. Wang, P.; Lv, J.; Bai, M.; Li, G.; Zeng, K. The reciprocating motion characteristics of nanofluid inside the piston cooling gallery. *Powder Technol.* **2015**, *274*, 402–417. [CrossRef]
28. Kajiwara, H.; Fujioka, Y.; Negishi, H. Prediction of temperatures on pistons with cooling gallery in diesel engines using CFD tool. *SAE Tech. Pap.* **2003**, *1*, 0986.
29. Hatami, M.; Ganji, D.; Gorji-Bandpy, M. A review of different heat exchangers designs for increasing the diesel exhaust waste heat recovery. *Renew. Sustain. Energy Rev.* **2014**, *37*, 168–181. [CrossRef]
30. Xuan, Y.; Li, Q. Heat transfer enhancement of nanofluids. *Int. J. Heat Fluid Flow* **2000**, *21*, 58–64. [CrossRef]
31. Kakac, S.; Pramuanjaroenkij, A. Review of convective heat transfer enhancement with nanofluids. *Int. J. Heat Mass Transf.* **2009**, *52*, 3187–3196. [CrossRef]
32. Moghaieb, H.S.; Abdel-Hamid, H.M.; Shedid, M.H.; Helali, A.B. Engine cooling using Al_2O_3/water nanofluids. *Appl. Therm. Eng.* **2017**, *115*, 152–159. [CrossRef]
33. Tsai, C.Y.; Chien, H.T.; Ding, P.P.; Chan, B.; Luh, T.Y.; Chen, P.H. Effect of structural character of gold nanoparticles in nanofluid on heat pipe thermal performance. *Mater. Lett.* **2004**, *58*, 1461–1465. [CrossRef]
34. Greda, K.; Swiderski, K.; Jamroz, P.; Pohl, P. Flowing liquid anode atmospheric pressure glow discharge as an excitation source for optical emission spectrometry with the improved detectability of Ag, Cd, Hg, Pb, Tl, and Zn. *Anal. Chem.* **2016**, *88*, 8812–8820. [CrossRef] [PubMed]
35. Burmeister, L.C. Solutions manual. In *Convective Heat Transfer*; John Wiley & Sons, Incorporated: New York, NY, USA, 1993.
36. Wang, C.; Daimon, H.; Onodera, T.; Koda, T.; Sun, S. A general approach to the size-and shape-controlled synthesis of platinum nanoparticles and their catalytic reduction of oxygen. *Angew. Chem. Int. Ed.* **2008**, *47*, 3588–3591. [CrossRef] [PubMed]
37. Yang, W.; Ma, Y.; Tang, J.; Yang, X. "Green synthesis" of monodisperse Pt nanoparticles and their catalytic properties. *Colloids Surf. A Physicochem. Eng. Asp.* **2007**, *302*, 628–633. [CrossRef]
38. Chytil, S.; Glomm, W.R.; Vollebekk, E.; Bergem, H.; Walmsley, J.; Sjoblom, J.; Blekkan, E.A. Platinum nanoparticles encapsulated in mesoporous silica: Preparation, characterisation and catalytic activity in toluene hydrogenation. *Microporous Mesoporous Mater.* **2005**, *86*, 198–206. [CrossRef]
39. Abdelghany, A.; Mekhail, M.S.; Abdelrazek, E.; Aboud, M. Combined DFT/FTIR structural studies of monodispersed PVP/Gold and silver nano particles. *J. Alloys Compd.* **2015**, *646*, 326–332. [CrossRef]

40. Song, Y.-J.; Wang, M.; Zhang, X.-Y.; Wu, J.-Y.; Zhang, T. Investigation on the role of the molecular weight of polyvinyl pyrrolidone in the shape control of high-yield silver nanospheres and nanowires. *Nanoscale Res. Lett.* **2014**, *9*, 17. [CrossRef] [PubMed]
41. Long, D.A. Infrared and Raman characteristic group frequencies. Tables and charts George Socrates John Wiley and sons, ltd, chichester, third edition, 2001. *J. Raman Spectrosc.* **2004**, *35*, 905. [CrossRef]
42. Kim, J.H.; Min, B.R.; Kim, C.K.; Won, J.; Kang, Y.S. Spectroscopic interpretation of silver ion complexation with propylene in silver polymer electrolytes. *J. Phys. Chem. B* **2002**, *106*, 2786–2790. [CrossRef]
43. Cyganowski, P.; Lesniewicz, A.; Polowczyk, I.; Checmanowski, J.; Kozlecki, T.; Pohl, P.; Jermakowicz-Bartkowiak, D. Surface-activated anion exchange resins for synthesis and immobilization of gold and palladium nano- and microstructures. *React. Funct. Polym.* **2018**, *124*, 90–103. [CrossRef]
44. Chen, C.; Li, J.S.; Li, Y.F. A review of plasma-liquid interactions for nanomaterials synthesis. *J. Phys. D Appl. Phys.* **2015**, *48*, 424005. [CrossRef]
45. Bruggeman, P.J.; Kushner, M.J.; Locke, B.R.; Gardeniers, J.G.E.; Graham, W.G.; Graves, D.B.; Hofman-Caris, R.C.H.M; Maric, D.; Reid, J.P.; et al. Plasma-liquid interactions: A review and roadmap. *Plasma Sources Sci. Technol.* **2016**, *25*, 053002. [CrossRef]
46. Hofft, O.; Endres, F. Plasma electrochemistry in ionic liquids: An alternative route to generate nanoparticles. *Phys. Chem. Chem. Phys.* **2011**, *13*, 13472–13478. [CrossRef] [PubMed]
47. Borodko, Y.; Habas, S.E.; Koebel, M.; Yang, P.; Frei, H.; Somorjai, G.A. Probing the interaction of poly(vinylpyrrolidone) with platinum nanocrystals by UV-Raman and FTIR. *J. Phys. Chem. B* **2006**, *110*, 23052–23059. [CrossRef] [PubMed]
48. Qiu, L.; Liu, F.; Zhao, L.Z.; Yang, W.S.; Yao, J.N. Evidence of a unique electron donor-acceptor property for platinum nanoparticles as studied by XPS. *Langmuir* **2006**, *22*, 4480–4482. [CrossRef] [PubMed]

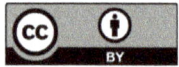

© 2018 by the authors. Licensee MDPI, Basel, Switzerland. This article is an open access article distributed under the terms and conditions of the Creative Commons Attribution (CC BY) license (http://creativecommons.org/licenses/by/4.0/).

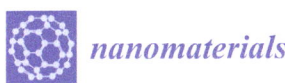

Article

Antibacterial Activity of Fructose-Stabilized Silver Nanoparticles Produced by Direct Current Atmospheric Pressure Glow Discharge towards Quarantine Pests

Anna Dzimitrowicz [1,†], Agata Motyka-Pomagruk [2,†], Piotr Cyganowski [3], Weronika Babinska [2], Dominik Terefinko [1], Piotr Jamroz [1], Ewa Lojkowska [2], Pawel Pohl [1,‡] and Wojciech Sledz [2,*,‡]

1. Department of Analytical Chemistry and Chemical Metallurgy, Faculty of Chemistry, Wroclaw University of Science and Technology, Wybrzeze St. Wyspianskiego 27, 50-370 Wroclaw, Poland; anna.dzimitrowicz@pwr.edu.pl (A.D.); dominik.terefinko@pwr.edu.pl (D.T.); piotr.jamroz@pwr.edu.pl (P.J.); pawel.pohl@pwr.edu.pl (P.P.)
2. Department of Biotechnology, Intercollegiate Faculty of Biotechnology University of Gdansk and Medical University of Gdansk, Abrahama 58, 80-307 Gdansk, Poland; agata.motyka@biotech.ug.edu.pl (A.M.-P.); weronikababinska29@gmail.com (W.B.); ewa.lojkowska@biotech.ug.edu.pl (E.L.)
3. Department of Polymer and Carbonaceous Materials, Faculty of Chemistry, Wroclaw University of Science and Technology, Wybrzeze St. Wyspianskiego 27, 50-370 Wroclaw, Poland; piotr.cyganowski@pwr.edu.pl
* Correspondence: wojciech.sledz@biotech.ug.edu.pl; Tel.: +48-58-523-63-29
† These authors contributed equally to this work.
‡ These authors contributed equally to this work.

Received: 24 August 2018; Accepted: 18 September 2018; Published: 21 September 2018

Abstract: Development of efficient plant protection methods against bacterial phytopathogens subjected to compulsory control procedures under international legislation is of the highest concern having in mind expensiveness of enforced quarantine measures and threat of the infection spread in disease-free regions. In this study, fructose-stabilized silver nanoparticles (FRU-AgNPs) were produced using direct current atmospheric pressure glow discharge (dc-APGD) generated between the surface of a flowing liquid anode (FLA) solution and a pin-type tungsten cathode in a continuous flow reaction-discharge system. Resultant spherical and stable in time FRU-AgNPs exhibited average sizes of 14.9 ± 7.9 nm and 15.7 ± 2.0 nm, as assessed by transmission electron microscopy (TEM) and dynamic light scattering (DLS), respectively. Energy dispersive X-ray spectroscopy (EDX) analysis revealed that the obtained nanomaterial was composed of Ag while selected area electron diffraction (SAED) indicated that FRU-AgNPs had the face-centered cubic crystalline structure. The fabricated FRU-AgNPs show antibacterial properties against *Erwinia amylovora*, *Clavibacter michiganensis*, *Ralstonia solanacearum*, *Xanthomonas campestris* pv. *campestris* and *Dickeya solani* strains with minimal inhibitory concentrations (MICs) of 1.64 to 13.1 mg L^{-1} and minimal bactericidal concentrations (MBCs) from 3.29 to 26.3 mg L^{-1}. Application of FRU-AgNPs might increase the repertoire of available control procedures against most devastating phytopathogens and as a result successfully limit their agricultural impact.

Keywords: atmospheric pressure plasma; nanostructures; phytopathogens; plant protection; quarantine; *Erwinia amylovora*; *Clavibacter michiganensis*; *Ralstonia solanacearum*; *Xanthomonas campestris* pv. *campestris*; *Dickeya solani*

1. Introduction

In recent decades, a rapid increase in the fabrication of noble metal nanoparticles (NPs) has been observed. Dynamic development in production of these inorganic nanostructures has been associated with their unique optical [1], chemical [2], and photothermal [3] properties, which are different from those of bulky samples made of the same material. Among noble metal nanostructures, the most studied and utilized are silver nanoparticles (AgNPs). Various methods have been developed for synthesis of AgNPs so far [4,5]. The most common are based on chemical [6], physicochemical [7], and biological [8] reduction of Ag(I) ions. Importantly, these methods are usually multi-step and, hence, time-consuming. Additionally, the chemical reduction approach often requires toxic reagents such as hydrazine [9]. For these reasons, several research groups applied atmospheric pressure plasmas (APPs) generated in contact with liquids and tried to use plasma-liquid interactions (PLIs) for the synthesis of stable in time AgNPs in a much faster and less complicated way [10–17]. In our group, several continuous-flow reaction-discharge systems based either on the operation of dc-APGD [18,19] or a pulse modified radio frequency version of this discharge (pm-rf-APGD) [20] were developed and used for the fabrication of AgNPs. In these systems, APP was operated between a flowing liquid electrode, which were the solutions of the AgNPs precursor and certain stabilizers and a pin-type solid tungsten electrode. The operation of APP resulted in the production of various reactive oxygen and nitrogen species (RONS) in addition to solvated electrons and hydrogen radicals (H·). Subsequently, all these species mediated reduction of Ag(I) ions and formation of AgNPs [18–20].

AgNPs have found many interesting applications for instance in degradation of organic dyes in catalysis [21], ultrasensitive DNA detection in biosensors [22], inactivation of bacteria in textile production [23], and treatment of human melanoma cancer in medicine [20]. Additionally, their possible implementation into agriculture has been suggested previously [18,24,25]. Having in mind synthesis of biocompatible, natural, and low-cost nanomaterials [26,27] for such a practice, several AgNPs synthesis methods based on reductive properties of plant extracts [28], natural biopolymers [29], agricultural wastes [30], or commercially available biocontrol agents [31] have been developed up to the present day. Importantly, AgNPs might be efficiently applied for direct eradication of fungal [32–35] and bacterial [18,24,25] phytopathogens. Considering that various formulations of fungicides are still successful in plant disease control [36] while costs of quarantine enforcement are quite high, the objective of the present study was to investigate the activity of plasma synthesized AgNPs against bacterial phytopathogens subjected to compulsory control measures, according to European Union legislation by a Council Directive 2000/29/EC and posterior directives (most recently Commission Implementing Directive 2017/1279) amending its annexes. For this research, we focused on *Erwinia amylovora* (Eam), *Clavibacter michiganensis* (Cm), *Ralstonia solanacearum* (Rsol), *Xanthomonas campestris* pv. *campestris* (Xcc), and *Dickeya solani* (Dsol) whose economic significance was further emphasized by either a place or honorable mentions on the top 10 list of plant pathogenic bacteria by Mansfield et al. [37].

Eam is a Gram(−) bacterial phytopathogen that causes fire blight on the *Rosaceae* family including mostly subfamilies *Maloideae* or *Pomoideae* [37]. Typical symptoms of the above-mentioned disease include flower necrosis, fruit rot, shepherd's crook in shoots, bacterial ooze, and cankers in woody tissue [38]. The highest economic losses are recorded on apples and pears and might result in disrupting orchard production for several years. To exemplify, the financial impact of Eam recorded in the north-west part of USA exceeded 68 million dollars in 1998 alone [39]. On the other hand, Cm of Gram(+) coryneform morphology is responsible for bacterial canker on tomato. Most recognizable diagnostic symptoms of this disorder involve wilting and bird's eye-spot lesions among less species-specific, but highly devastating being vascular discolorations, brown streaks opening as cankers, leaf necrosis, plant stunting and desiccation in addition to premature fruits fall. Substantial financial damage in tomato production might even reach $300,000 per grower in a single year [40]. On the contrary, Rsol is a Gram(−) soil-borne causative agent of bacterial wilt on several hundred plant species belonging to more than 44 families [41]. Notably, plant-specific names of this disease are frequently used, i.e., brown rot on potato and Moko disease on banana. The pathogen penetrating from soil into plant roots reaches the xylem where it multiplies and subsequently triggers systemic infection. Plants wilt, their stems soften and split while releasing bacterial exudates. Focusing on potatoes, browning of the tuber vascular ring characterizes an advanced stage of Rsol infection. High economic impact of this disease mainly results from wide geographic distribution and costly quarantine procedures. For instance, about 50% potato tuber losses caused by these bacteria are noted in India [42]. Concerning an etiological agent of black rot being a Gram(−) rod Xcc, its most important hosts include the members of the crucifer family *Brassicaceae* with cabbage, cauliflower, broccoli, radish, Brussels sprouts, and kale [43]. In the case of this disorder, contaminated plant tissues become necrotic and leaves fall prematurely while severe rotting leading to plant death follows systemic infection. V-shaped, chlorotic yellow lesions are typical symptoms. Black rot was detected on all continents and it is regarded as the most important disease of brassica worldwide [44]. Dsol, which is a Gram(−) rod-shaped bacterium not yet regarded as a quarantine microorganism outside Israel and North Africa countries, was subjected to a zero tolerance policy in Scotland [45]. This relatively new threat to European potato production has been efficiently spreading across the continent since 2005 [46]. Dsol causes blackening and softening of the stem base referred to as blackleg in addition to soft rot meaning maceration and collapse of the inner tuber tissue. Interestingly, the resultant disease symptoms besides their severity are indistinguishable from these caused by other species from the genera *Dickeya* or *Pectobacterium*. To illustrate, Tsror et al. [47] reported potato yield reduction of 20% to 25% when the disease incidence exceeded 15%.

Here, the dc-APGD-based continuous-flow reaction-discharge system was applied to produce uniform and monodisperse spherical AgNPs stabilized by fructose (FRU). Optical properties of the synthesized FRU-AgNPs were analyzed by using UV/Vis absorption spectrophotometry. Their granulometric properties were examined with the aid of transmission electron microscopy (TEM) supported by energy dispersive X-ray spectroscopy (EDX) and selected area electron diffraction (SAED). Dynamic light scattering (DLS) was further used to evaluate the size of the produced Ag nanostructures. To confirm surface functionalization of AgNPs by FRU, attenuated total Reflection-Fourier transformation infrared spectroscopy (ATR FT-IR) was applied. Lastly, antibacterial properties of the resultant FRU-AgNPs were studied against phytopathogenic microorganisms classified to Eam, Cm, Rsol, Xcc, and Dsol species.

2. Materials and Methods

2.1. Reagents and Solutions

A working solution of the AgNPs precursor (100 mg L^{-1} of Ag(I) ions with 0.25% (m/v) D-fructose) was prepared as follows: 0.0157 g of solid silver nitrate (AgNO$_3$, Avantor Performance Materials, Gliwice, Poland) and 0.25 g of D-fructose (Avantor Performance Materials, Gliwice, Poland) were dissolved in water. The concentration of the capping agent (0.25% (m/v) of FRU) in this solution was chosen in order to allow for stable operation of dc-APGD in the continuous-flow reaction-discharge system. All reagents were of analytical grade or higher purity. Re-distilled water was used throughout.

2.2. Production of FRU-AgNPs in the dc-APGD-based Reaction-Discharge System

FRU-AgNPs were synthesized in the dc-APGD-based continuous-flow reaction-discharge system previously described by Dzimitrowicz et al. [19]. The working solution of the AgNPs precursor was introduced to the system through a quartz capillary (OD = 4.0 mm, ID = 2.0 mm) onto which a graphite tube (OD = 6.0 mm, ID = 4.0 mm) was mounted (Figure 1). The flow rate of this solution was 2.0 mL min^{-1} and was maintained by applying a four-channel peristaltic pump (Masterflex L/S, Cole-Parmer, Vernon Hills, IL, USA). In these conditions, the working solution acted as the flowing liquid anode (FLA) while a solid tungsten (W) electrode was the cathode of this discharge system. dc-APGD was sustained and stably operated between the surface of this FLA solution and the sharpened tip of the W cathode (ID = 4.0 mm). Both electrodes were placed inside a 90 mm (height) by 40 mm (radial) quartz chamber. The distance between them was 5.0 mm to allow for stable operation of dc-APGD. To ignite dc-APGD, a high voltage (HV) of 1100–1300 V provided by a dc-HV supplier (Dora Electronics

Equipment, Wroclaw, Poland) was supplied to both electrodes. Stabilization of the discharge current (30 mA) was maintained by applying a ballast resistor of 10 kΩ (Tyco Electronics, Berwyn, IL, USA) situated in the anode circuit. The dc-APGD-treated working solution, which contained the synthesized FRU-AgNPs, was collected into 10 mL glass vials and kept for further analyses including determination of their optical, granulometric, and antibacterial properties.

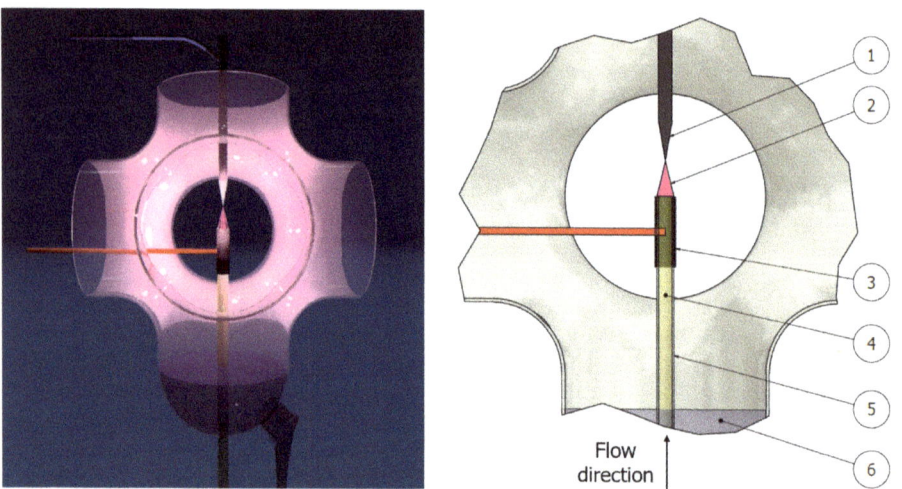

Figure 1. A schematic representation of the dc-APGD-based reaction-discharge system working in a continuous-flow mode. (1) A pin-type W cathode, (2) dc-APGD, (3) a graphite tube, (4) a working solution (with the AgNPs precursor and D-fructose) acting as a flowing liquid anode (FLA), (5) a quartz capillary, and (6) a compartment for the collection of the dc-APGD treated working solution containing the synthesized FRU-AgNPs.

2.3. Characterization of Optical and Granulometric Properties of FRU-AgNPs

To examine suitability of dc-APGD for the production of stable in time, spherical, monodisperse, and uniform in size FRU-AgNPs, their optical and granulometric properties were evaluated.

Optical properties of the produced Ag nanostructures were assessed by UV/Vis absorption spectrophotometry. UV/Vis absorption spectra were acquired by using a Specord 210 spectrophotometer (Analytik Jena AG, Jena, Germany) in the spectral range from 300 nm to 900 nm. The scanning speed was 20 nm s^{-1} and the step was 1 nm.

Granulometric properties (size, shape, elemental composition, and crystalline structure) of the fabricated FRU-AgNPs were determined by TEM (Tecnai G^{2}20 X-TWIN, FEI, Hillsboro, OR, USA). The measurements were performed in a bright field and in electron diffraction modes for direct imagining and SAED, respectively. For EDX analyses, the mode of energy dispersion of X-rays supported by an EDX detector was applied. To carry out all analyses according to the granulometric properties of the resultant FRU-AgNPs, one-drop of the dc-APGD-treated working solution was placed onto an ultra-thin carbon-copper grid (CF400-Cu-UL, Electron Microscopy Sciences, Hatfield, PA, USA). Then, the so-prepared sample was sequentially rinsed with re-distilled water and dried to remove sugar from it before the analysis. To analyze the collected data, the FEI software (version 3.2 SP6 build 421, FEI, Hillsboro, OR, USA) was applied. The size distribution of the FRU-AgNPs was determined from high-resolution TEM photomicrographs. Since removal of FRU resulted in the creation of a considerable number of agglomerates, the graphics were segmented by applying image thresholds that allow the detection of a single nanoparticle within an agglomerate. Then, the counted particles were analyzed by using Microsoft Excel (Richmond, VA, USA) Analysis Tool Pack add-in, which created an appropriate histogram. Size distribution by the number of FRU-AgNPs was also estimated by DLS and by applying a Photocor Complex instrument (Photocor Instruments, Tallin, Estonia) equipped with a 638 nm/25 mW^3 laser. Measurements were performed in round glass vials (ID = 14.8 mm) submerged in decalin at the scattering angle of 90°. Temperature during all tests was 21.96 °C and water viscosity was 0.9864 mPa·s^{-1}. DynaLS software (Alango Ltd., Tirat Carmel, Israel) was utilized for data evaluation.

2.4. Surface Functionalization of AgNPs by FRU

To confirm the stabilizing role of FRU during AgNPs production, ATR FT-IR spectroscopy was applied. Respective ATR FT-IR spectra were acquired for two samples: (i) the raw working solution prior to treatment with dc-APGD and (ii) the dc-APGD-treated working solution containing the produced FRU-AgNPs. All ATR FT-IR spectra were collected in the range from 4000 to 400 cm^{-1} using a Nicolet 6700 instrument (Thermo Fisher Scientific, Waltham, MA, USA) that was equipped with a Smart Orbit ATR accessory. Measurements were taken at a resolution of 4 cm^{-1} and the scans number was 64. All analyses were carried out under vacuum conditions.

2.5. Purification of FRU-AgNPs

In order to purify the fabricated FRU-AgNPs from unreacted Ag(I) ions, dialysis, as previously reported by Dzimitrowicz et al. [18], was used. A portion of the dc-APGD-treated working solution with the synthesized FRU-AgNPs was poured into a dialysis tube with a molecular weight cut-off of 14,000 Da (Sigma-Aldrich, Poznan, Poland) and immersed in 500 mL of re-distilled water in a glass beaker. Then, the glass beaker was placed onto a magnetic laboratory stirring plate (WIGO, Pruszkow, Poland) and its contents was subjected to stirring at 1000 rpm for 24 h.

2.6. Determination of the Concentration of the Purified FRU-AgNPs

To determine the concentration of the purified FRU-AgNPs (as Ag) after dialysis, flame atomic absorption spectrometry (FAAS) was used. The appropriate volume of the solution obtained after dialysis from the dialysis tube was poured into a 200-mL beaker and treated with a 65% (m/m) HNO$_3$ solution (Avantor Performance Materials, Gliwice, Poland). Afterwards, the resulting mixture was heated to boil for 30 min on a hot plate for digestion of FRU-AgNPs. Next, a PerkinElmer (Bodenseewerk Perkin-Elmer GmbH, Uberlingen, Germany) single-beam FAAS instrument, model 1100B with a deuterium lamp, was applied for quantification of the Ag concentration in the final sample solution.

2.7. Bacterial Strains and Their Culture Methods

Plant pathogenic bacteria investigated in this study are listed in Table 1. All microorganisms originated from the collection of bacterial phytopathogens of the Intercollegiate Faculty of Biotechnology University of Gdansk and Medical University of Gdansk (IFB UG & MUG) (Gdansk, Poland) and had been previously stored at −80 °C in 40% (*v*/*v*) glycerol. The tested microorganisms were recovered from frozen stocks by plating on optimal solid media (Table 1). 24 h of incubation at 28 °C followed. To obtain the overnight liquid cultures, a single bacterial colony per species was utilized for the inoculation of the proper liquid medium (Table 1) prior to 24 h of incubation at 28 °C.

Table 1. Studied strains of bacterial phytopathogens and the utilized growth media.

Species, Abbreviation	Strain Nos [a]	Disease Caused	Country, Year of Isolation	Host Plant	Growth Medium [b]	Reference
Erwinia amylovora, Eam	IFB9037, CL0640	Fireblight	Poland, 2011	*Pyrus* spp.	Levan [48]	CL collection
Clavibacter michiganensis, Cm	IFB9038, CL0335	Bacterial canker	Poland, 2005	*Lycopersicon esculentum*	NCP-88 [49]	CL collection
Dickeya solani, Dsol	IFB0099, LMG28824	Blackleg, Soft rot	Poland, 2005	*Solanum tuberosum*	TSA (BTL, Poland)	[50,51]
Ralstonia solanacearum, Rsol	IFB8019, NCPPB4156	Brown rot	The Netherlands, 2001	*Solanum tuberosum*	TZC [52]	NCPPB collection
Xanthomonas campestris pv. *campestris*, Xcc	IFB9022, LMG582	Black rot	Belgium, 1980	*Brassica* spp.	GF [53]	[51,54,55]

[a] IFB—Intercollegiate Faculty of Biotechnology University of Gdansk and Medical University of Gdansk (Gdansk, Poland), CL—Central Laboratory of Main Inspectorate of Plant Health and Seed Inspection (Torun, Poland), LMG—Belgian Coordinated Collections of Microorganisms (Gent, Belgium), NCPPB—National Collection of Plant Pathogenic Bacteria (London, UK). [b] To obtain the corresponding solid media, 15 g L^{-1} of agar was added.

2.8. Antibacterial Properties of FRU-AgNPs Against Bacterial Phytopathogens

Overnight liquid bacterial cultures were centrifuged for 10 min at 6000 rpm. The harvested cells were washed twice and subsequently suspended in a sterile 0.85% NaCl solution to reach the turbidity of 0.5 in the McFarland scale (McF) as measured by a DEN-1B densitometer (BioSan, Riga, Latvia). The purified FRU-AgNPs were dissolved in sterile re-distilled water to obtain 2×, 3×, 4×, 6×, 8×, 16×, and 32× dilutions. 10 µL of the 0.5 McF bacterial suspensions, 90 µL of the corresponding growth media (Table 1), and 100 µL of FRU-AgNPs dilutions or the concentrated stock solution were added to each well in sterile 96-well microplates. Appropriate negative controls (containing solely the respective growth media or these media supplemented with 0.85% NaCl or re-distilled water) and positive controls (the respective growth media inoculated with a given phytopathogen) were included. Optical densities at 600 nm (OD_{600}) of bacterial cultures within the microplates were measured by using an EnVision Multilabel Plate Reader (PerkinElmer, Waltham, MA, USA). Incubation at 28 °C for 24 h followed. Then, OD_{600} of the bacterial cultures were investigated again to state minimal inhibitory concentrations (MICs) of FRU-AgNPs to define the concentration of AgNPs potent enough to inhibit the growth of bacterial phytopathogens in liquid media [18,55]. The contents of 96-well microplates showing no visible bacterial growth were also plated on the appropriate solid growth media (Table 1) to establish minimal bactericidal concentrations (MBCs) as described previously [18,55]. The plates were incubated at 28 °C for 24 h. The resultant bacterial colonies were counted. The whole experiment was repeated in triplicate for each bacterial strain.

3. Results and Discussion

3.1. Optical Properties of FRU-AgNPs

It was possible to confirm the formation of Ag nanostructures as well as to estimate their optical properties based on UV/Vis absorption spectra of the dc-APGD-treated working solution (Figure 2). Spherical metallic nanostructures of different sizes are able to absorb and reflect light of unique wavelengths, which results in localized surface plasmon resonance (LSPR) absorption bands of different widths and centered around different wavelengths due to mutual vibration of their free electrons in resonance with given light waves [56]. The LSPR absorption band for small spherical AgNPs is typically situated between 380 to 450 nm [57]. In the present contribution, the UV/Vis absorption spectrum of the dc-APGD treated working solution, which was dominated by the LSPR absorption band with wavelength at its maximum at 404 nm (Figure 2). This confirms the formation of spherical FRU-AgNPs. Additionally, the symmetrical shape of this LSPR absorption band and a low value of its full width at half maximum (FWHM), i.e., 79 nm, suggested that the resultant spherical FRU-AgNPs were monodisperse and non-aggregated (Figure 2) [58].

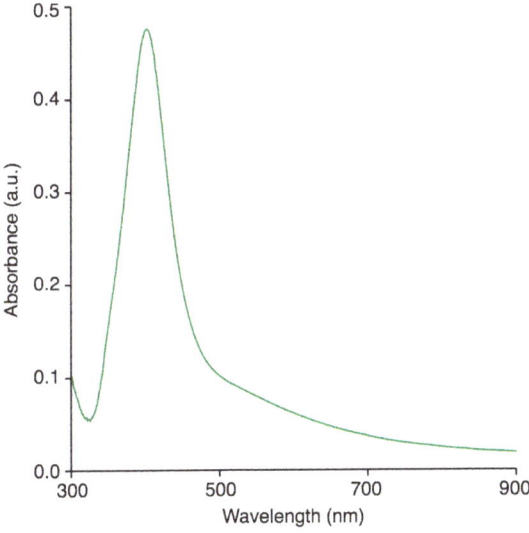

Figure 2. The UV/Vis absorption spectrum of five times diluted colloidal suspension of FRU-AgNPs.

3.2. Granulometric Properties of FRU-AgNPs

Using TEM supported by SAED and EDX as well as DLS, granulometric properties of the fabricated FRU-AgNPs according to their size, shape, elemental composition, and crystalline structure were assessed. Based on TEM measurements, it was established that FRU-AgNPs were approximately spherical (95%) even though the structures of other shapes, i.e., triangular and hexagonal, were also detected (Figure 3). The average size of the resultant FRU-AgNPs along with its size distribution was 14.9 ± 7.9 nm, which means that they were quite uniform with a narrow size distribution (Figure 3). FRU-AgNPs were well dispersed in the aqueous medium, but several aggregates were also observed (Figure 3). The occurrence of aggregates might be related to the sample preparation for TEM measurements (see Section 2.3 for more details).

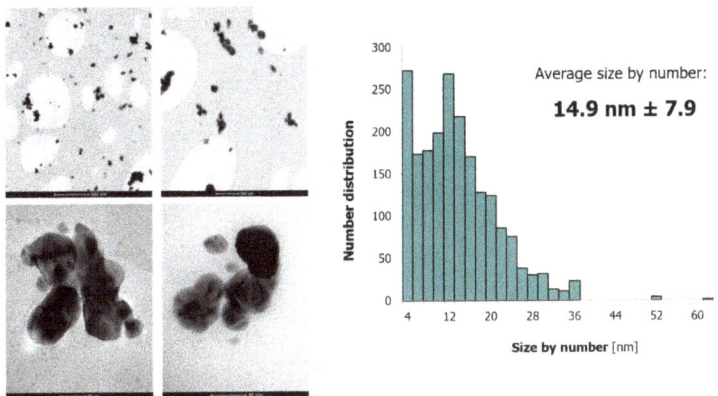

Figure 3. TEM micrographs illustrating shapes and size distribution of FRU-AgNPs.

Figure 4A presents the SAED pattern of the synthesized Ag nanostructures. Based on this, corresponding rings associated with the face-centered cubic (fcc) highly crystalline structure of the produced FRU-AgNPs were determined. Observed d-spacings were 2.38, 2.04, 1.45, and 1.25 Å, which indicates Miller indices of (111), (200), (220), and (311), respectively [18]. To reveal the elemental composition of the synthesized nanomaterial, EDX was applied. Figure 4B shows the respective EDX spectrum. The following elements were identified: Ag (from the synthesized AgNPs), O and C (both from the chemical structure of FRU), and Cu (from the grid onto which the APP-treated working solution was deposited).

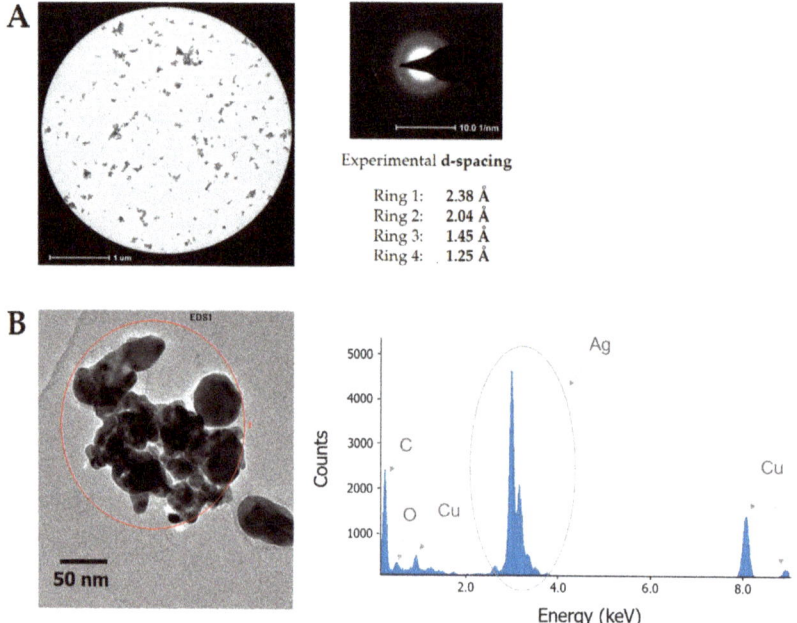

Figure 4. Granulometric properties of Ag nanostructures (**A**) The SAED pattern for the micrograph of FRU-AgNPs and (**B**) the EDX spectrum for the presented FRU-AgNPs.

DLS analyses were performed to corroborate size distribution of FRU-AgNPs calculated on the basis of TEM imaging. Figure 5 presents percentage size distribution by the number of resultant FRU-AgNPs obtained after treatment of the working solution in the applied, dc-APGD-based, continuous-flow reaction-discharge system. Average size of FRU-AgNPs and its distribution was 15.7 ± 2.0 nm and was slightly larger than was determined by using TEM. This discrepancy in the average size, as determined by TEM and DLS, is commonly reported in literature [59]. By applying TEM, it was possible to accurately evaluate the size of the metal core of NPs when compared to DLS in which light is scattered on the analyzed nanomaterial.

The above-listed measurements proved that, by applying dc-APGD operated between the surface of the FLA solution and the pin-type W cathode in the utilized continuous-flow reaction-discharge system, it was possible to obtain uniform and approximately spherical FRU-AgNPs with a narrow size distribution. The proposed system produced 120 mL of colloidal suspensions of FRU-AgNPs per hour. This certainly overcame limitations related to insufficient yield of NPs reported in the case of stationary reaction-discharge systems in which APPs also operated in contact with liquids [10–17]. Subsequently, FAAS was used to determine the concentrations of the purified solutions by dialysis with FRU-AgNPs. The Ag concentration of 52.6 mg·L^{-1} was assessed in the working solution after its dc-APGD treatment and posterior further purification. Considering that the initial concentration of Ag(I) ions in the working solution was 100 mg·L^{-1}, it gave 52.6% efficiency of FRU-AgNPs production by the proposed APP-based system.

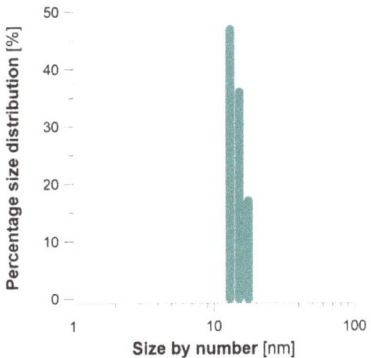

Figure 5. Percentage size distribution by the number of FRU-AgNPs estimated by dynamic light scattering (DLS).

3.3. Stabilization of the Surface of AgNPs by FRU

Efficacy of AgNPs surface stabilization by FRU was examined on the basis of ATR-FTIR spectra of the working solution before and after dc-APGD treatment (Figure 6). For the working solution after dc-APGD treatment, strong absorption bands at 3279 cm^{-1} and 1656 cm^{-1} attributed to ν stretching vibrations of the −O−H group and ν stretching vibrations of the C=O group present in FRU were detected [60]. Slight shifts in the position of strong absorption bands (about 21 cm^{-1}) could be seen when comparing ATR FT-IR spectra of the working solution before and after dc-APGD treatment. Such band shifts might point an interaction of the surface of AgNPs with FRU, which confirms its stabilizing role. Furthermore, the chemical structure of FRU contains a cyclic ring with several −OH groups. The possibility of hydrogen bonding formation between FRU and the surface of Ag nanostructures accounts for efficient application of this monosaccharide as a stabilizer for preventing uncontrolled growth, aggregation, and sedimentation of AgNPs.

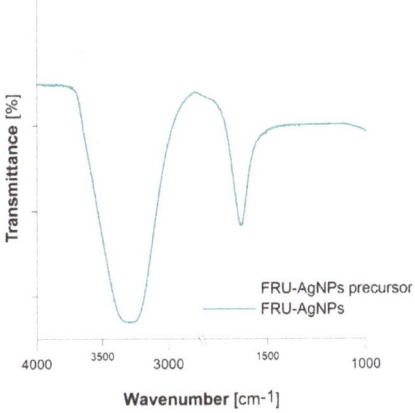

Figure 6. ATR FT-IR spectra of the working solution before (FRU-AgNPs precursor) and after (FRU-AgNPs) dc-APGD treatment.

The further advantage of FRU utilized as a stabilizer is related to its classification as an eco-friendly green capping agent [61]. FRU was previously applied in APP-based synthesis of AgNPs by several research groups [11,16,17]. Richmonds and Sankaran [11] reported a reaction-discharge system with an atmospheric-pressure microplasma (APM) cathode operated in an H-shaped glass cell between the surface of a solution and an Ar nozzle jet [11]. The size of the obtained FRU-AgNPs was 10 nm [11]. Kondeti et al. [16] used a radio-frequency driven APP jet for the production of either raw-AgNPs or FRU-AgNPs. It was found that FRU could be not only the AgNPs-stabilizing surfactant but also the OH scavenger that acted as a reducing agent through the formation of a respective aldehyde and the removal of OH (and H) radicals produced by APP [16]. Chiang et al. [17] also synthesized small FRU-AgNPs (size circa 10 nm) by applying a hybrid microplasma-based electrochemical cell operated at ambient conditions. Importantly for our research, FRU was proven to trigger chemotaxis of plant pathogenic bacteria [62]. Therefore, having in mind future agricultural applications of AgNPs synthesized by the dc-APGD-based reaction-discharge system, this monosugar was selected for the described research and surface stabilization on the fabricated spherical Ag nanostructures.

3.4. Antibacterial Properties of FRU-AgNPs against Bacterial Phytopathogens

Up to the present day, Ag nanostructures have been shown to efficiently inhibit the growth of fungal phytopathogens (such as *Bipolaris sorokiniana*, *Magna porthegrisea* [32], *Colletotrichum* spp. [33], *Fusarium oxysporum* [34], *Alternaria alternata*, *Sclerotinia sclerotiorum*, *Macrophomina phaseolina*, *Rhizoctonia solani*, *Botrytis cinerea*, *Curvularia lunata* [35]) and bacterial phytopathogens (for instance, *Pseudomonas syringae* pv. *syringae*, *Xanthomonas campestris* pv. *vesicatoria* [25], *Xanthomonas perforans* [24], *Pectobacterium* and *Dickeya* spp. [18]). Notably, greater interest has been given to the potential application of AgNPs for the management of plant diseases of fungal origin rather than bacterial, which is putatively due to the necessity of higher effective concentrations [25] or more complex nanocomposites [24] to inactivate the latter phytopathogenic microorganisms. The effectiveness of AgNPs application was demonstrated in greenhouses [24], under field conditions [25] in addition to multiple laboratory screenings. These findings encouraged our group to examine antimicrobial potency of the synthesized FRU-AgNPs against plant pathogenic bacteria subjected to compulsory control measures. Quarantine pests spread efficiently and cause considerable financial damage not only to potato breeding companies but also to single growers. Surveillance for the presence of quarantine microorganisms is compulsory and is conducted by the governmental inspectors. Commonly, besides the destruction of the affected plantation (even entire orchards in the case of Eam), specific monitoring procedures with buffer zones around the infested areas are implemented in addition to raising public awareness by running national and international campaigns. In addition, special warning systems based on climatic data are being developed. For instance, according to the European and Mediterranean Plant Protection Organization (EPPO), in the case of the detection of Eam, an integrated program of chemical control combined with sanitation, pruning, eradication, tree nutrition, and planting of resistant or tolerant cultivars is recommended [63]. Regarding direct control, since streptomycin sprays that suppressed Eam in the USA are not allowed for agricultural use in the European Union, several other chemicals such as flumequine, kasugamycin, fosetyl-Al, or oxonilic acid have been evaluated [63]. Hence, support of research projects resulting in the proposal of novel, effective methods for the eradication of bacteria indexed by EPPO on A1 and A2 lists of pests recommended for the regulation as quarantine pests is of substantial importance.

In this case, the synthesized FRU-AgNPs were established to efficiently inhibit the growth of plant pathogenic bacteria cultivated in liquid media (Table 2). Interestingly, highly virulent Eam, Cm, and Xcc were shown to be more susceptible (MICs of 1.64 mg L^{-1}) to the fabricated Ag nanostructures than the other species tested. On the other hand, Dsol showed the highest resistance with a MIC of FRU-AgNPs being 13.1 mg L^{-1}. It is worth to notice that significant differences in the susceptibility of microorganisms from various species to AgNPs have been reported before [25,32,35]. Higher concentrations of FRU-AgNPs were needed to kill bacterial cells in comparison to inhibition of their growth as might be expected, with a notable exception of Rsol for which both MIC and MBC values were just 6.58 mg L^{-1} of FRU-AgNPs.

Table 2. Minimal inhibitory and bactericidal concentrations of FRU-AgNPs against bacterial phytopathogens.

Bacterial Strain	MIC (mg L^{-1})	MBC (mg L^{-1})
Eam IFB9037	1.64 ± 0.05	3.29 ± 0.09
Cm IFB9038	1.64 ± 0.05	3.29 ± 0.09
Dsol IFB0099	13.1 ± 0.38	26.3 ± 0.75
Rsol IFB8019	6.58 ± 0.19	6.58 ± 0.19
Xcc IFB9022	1.64 ± 0.05	3.29 ± 0.09

Mean values ± standard deviations for three repetitions of the experiment are depicted.

In our previous study, antibacterial properties of AgNPs stabilized either by sodium dodecyl sulphate (SDS) or pectins (PEC) were examined against bacterial phytopathogens belonging to the genera *Dickeya* and *Pectobacterium* [18] including the herein investigated Dsol IFB0099 strain. In reference to this bacterium, PEC-AgNPs and SDS-AgNPs showed higher effectiveness than FRU-AgNPs. Nevertheless, in order to inhibit the growth of Eam, Cm, and Xcc, lower MICs of FRU-AgNPs were needed than in the case of either SDS-AgNPs or PEC-AgNPs towards *Dickeya* or *Pectobacterium* strains (except for *Pectobacterium atrosepticum* IFB5103). In comparison to much more complex DNA-directed AgNPs grown on graphene oxide [24], FRU-AgNPs showed better performance against Xcc than the latter nanomaterial towards a closely related species such as *Xanthomonas perforans* (MIC 1.64 versus 16.0 mg L^{-1}). The reported FRU-AgNPs were also more efficient against Xcc than the silica-silver of nanometric size [25] towards *Xanthomonas campestris* pv. *vesicatoria*. Taking into consideration that the mechanism of antibacterial action of AgNPs is not fully revealed yet [24], additional studies aimed at explaining how the genetic background contributes to the observed variation in the susceptibility of bacteria from different species to AgNPs are necessary. The latter research might provide further details on the interactions on the molecular level between AgNPs and the intracellular bacterial components.

4. Conclusions

Efficient, rapid, eco-friendly, and cost-effective synthesis of spherical and uniform FRU-AgNPs was accomplished by the incorporation of dc-APGD generated between the surface of the FLA solution (containing Ag(I) ions and D-fructose) and the pin-type W cathode in the continuous-flow reaction-discharge system. TEM and DLS measurements provided evidence that the produced Ag nanostructures were of a relatively small size and a narrow size distribution, i.e., 14.9 ± 4.3 and 15.7 ± 2.0 nm, respectively. The formation of metallic Ag of nanometric size was confirmed by SAED and EDX while functionalization of its surface by FRU was demonstrated by ATR FT-IR. Lastly, it was ascertained that FRU-AgNPs exhibit high antimicrobial activities against plant pathogenic bacteria subjected to expensive compulsory control measures under international legislation.

5. Patents

The method for the synthesis of metallic nanostructures is protected by Polish patent application No. P.417933.

Author Contributions: A.D. and A.M.-P. planned all experiments. P.J. carried out FRU-AgNPs synthesis. D.T. recorded UV/Vis absorption spectra. P.C. performed measurements related to morphology of FRU-AgNPs as well as surface functionalization of AgNPs by FRU. P.P. carried out FAAS measurements. A.D. summarized and analyzed all data related to optical and granulometric properties of FRU-AgNPs. A.D. and P.C. summarized the data associated with surface functionalization of AgNPs by FRU. A.M-P. and W.S. with the help of W.B. performed biological experiments associated with antibacterial activity of FRU-AgNPs. P.C. provided graphical support.

A.D. and A.M-P. wrote the presented manuscript. P.J., E.L., P.P. and W.S. corrected the manuscript, supervised all works, and took part in the discussion.

Funding: This work was funded by the National Science Center, Poland (agreements nos. 2014/13/B/ST4/05013 and 2016/21/N/NZ1/02783).

Acknowledgments: The presented work was supported by statutory activity subsidies of the Polish Ministry of Science and Higher Education for the Faculty of Chemistry of Wroclaw University of Science and Technology and Intercollegiate Faculty of Biotechnology University of Gdansk and Medical University of Gdansk (D530-M031-D712-17, 538-M031-B036-18). A.D. is supported by the Foundation for Polish Science (FNP), program START 022.2018.

Conflicts of Interest: The authors declare no conflict of interest.

Abbreviations

AgNPs	silver nanoparticles
APM	atmospheric-pressure micro-plasma
APP	atmospheric pressure plasmas
ATR FT-IR	attenuated total reflection-Fourier transformation infrared spectroscopy
CL	Central Laboratory of Main Inspectorate of Plant Health and Seed Inspection
Cm	*Clavibacter michiganensis*
dc-APGD	direct current atmospheric pressure glow discharge
Dsol	*Dickeya solani*
DLS	dynamic light scattering
Eam	*Erwinia amylovora*
EDX	energy dispersive X-ray scattering
FAAS	flame atomic absorption spectrometry
FLA	flowing liquid anode
EPPO	European and Mediterranean Plant Protection Organization
FRU	fructose
FWHM	full width at half maximum
HV	high voltage
IFB	Intercollegiate Faculty of Biotechnology University of Gdansk and Medical University of Gdansk
LSPR	localized surface plasmon resonance
LMG	Belgian coordinated collections of microorganisms
MBC	minimal bactericidal concentration
McF	McFarland scale
MIC	minimal inhibitory concentration
NCPPB	National collection of plant pathogenic bacteria
NPs	nanoparticles
OD_{600}	optical density at 600 nm
PEC	pectins
PLIs	plasma-liquid interactions
Rsol	*Ralstonia solanacearum*
RONS	reactive oxygen and nitrogen species
SAED	selected area electron diffraction
SDS	sodium dodecyl sulphate
TEM	transmission electron microscopy
Xcc	*Xanthomonas campestris* pv. *campestris*

References

1. Jain, P.K.; Huang, X.; El-Sayed, I.H.; El-Sayed, M.A. Review of some interesting surface plasmon resonance-enhanced properties of noble metal nanoparticles and their applications to biosystems. *Plasmonics* **2007**, *2*, 107–118. [CrossRef]
2. Sau, T.K.; Rogach, A.L.; Jäckel, F.; Klar, T.A.; Feldmann, J. Properties and applications of colloidal nonspherical noble metal nanoparticles. *Adv. Mater.* **2010**, *22*, 1805–1825. [CrossRef] [PubMed]
3. Jain, P.K.; Huang, X.; El-Sayed, I.H.; El-Sayed, M.A. Noble metals on the nanoscale: Optical and photothermal properties and some applications in imaging, sensing, biology, and medicine. *Acc. Chem. Res.* **2008**, *41*, 1578–1586. [CrossRef] [PubMed]
4. Rafique, M.; Sadaf, I.; Rafique, M.S.; Tahir, M.B. A review on green synthesis of silver nanoparticles and their applications. *Artif. Cells Nanomed. Biotechnol.* **2017**, *45*, 1272–1291. [CrossRef] [PubMed]
5. Syafiuddin, A.; Salim, M.R.; Kueh, A.B.H.; Hadibarata, T.; Nur, H. A review of silver nanoparticles: Research trends, global consumption, synthesis, properties, and future challenges. *J. Chin. Chem. Soc.* **2017**, *64*, 732–756. [CrossRef]
6. Wang, H.; Qiao, X.; Chen, J.; Ding, S. Preparation of silver nanoparticles by chemical reduction method. *Colloids Surf. A Physicochem. Eng. Asp.* **2005**, *256*, 111–115. [CrossRef]
7. Iravani, S.; Korbekandi, H.; Mirmohammadi, S.V.; Zolfaghari, B. Synthesis of silver nanoparticles: Chemical, physical and biological methods. *Res. Pharm. Sci.* **2014**, *9*, 385–406. [PubMed]
8. Bar, H.; Bhui, D.K.; Sahoo, G.P.; Sarkar, P.; De, S.P.; Misra, A. Green synthesis of silver nanoparticles using latex of *Jatropha curcas*. *Colloids Surf. A Physicochem. Eng. Asp.* **2009**, *339*, 134–139. [CrossRef]
9. Guzman, M.G.; Dille, J.; Godet, S. Synthesis of silver nanoparticles by chemical reduction method and their antibacterial activity. *Int. J. Chem. Biomol. Eng.* **2009**, *2*, 104–111.
10. Mariotti, D.; Patel, J.; Svrcek, V.; Maguire, P. Plasma-liquid interactions at atmospheric pressure for nanomaterials synthesis and surface engineering. *Plasma Process. Polym.* **2012**, *9*, 1074–1085. [CrossRef]
11. Richmonds, C.; Sankaran, R.M. Plasma-liquid electrochemistry: Rapid synthesis of colloidal metal nanoparticles by microplasma reduction of aqueous cations. *Appl. Phys. Lett.* **2008**, *93*, 131501. [CrossRef]
12. Shirai, N.; Uchida, S.; Tochikubo, F. Synthesis of metal nanoparticles by dual plasma electrolysis using atmospheric dc glow discharge in contact with liquid. *Jpn. J. Appl. Phys.* **2014**, *53*, 46202. [CrossRef]
13. Tochikubo, F.; Shimokawa, Y.; Shirai, N.; Uchida, S. Chemical reactions in liquid induced by atmospheric-pressure dc glow discharge in contact with liquid. *Jpn. J. Appl. Phys.* **2014**, *53*, 126201. [CrossRef]
14. Tochikubo, F.; Shirai, N.; Uchida, S. Liquid-phase reactions induced by atmospheric pressure glow discharge with liquid electrode. *J. Phys. Conf. Ser.* **2014**, *565*, 12010. [CrossRef]
15. Thong, Y.L.; Chin, O.H.; Ong, B.H.; Huang, N.M. Synthesis of silver nanoparticles prepared in aqueous solutions using helium dc microplasma jet. *Jpn. J. Appl. Phys.* **2016**, *55*. [CrossRef]
16. Kondeti, V.S.S.K.; Gangal, U.; Yatom, S.; Bruggeman, P.J. Ag^+ reduction and silver nanoparticle synthesis at the plasma-liquid interface by an RF driven atmospheric pressure plasma jet: Mechanisms and the effect of surfactant. *J. Vac. Sci. Technol. A* **2017**, *35*, 61302. [CrossRef]
17. Chiang, W.-H.; Richmonds, C.; Sankaran, R.M. Continuous-flow, atmospheric-pressure microplasmas: A versatile source for metal nanoparticle synthesis in the gas or liquid phase. *Plasma Sour. Sci. Technol.* **2010**, *19*, 34011. [CrossRef]
18. Dzimitrowicz, A.; Motyka, A.; Jamroz, P.; Lojkowska, E.; Babinska, W.; Terefinko, D.; Pohl, P.; Sledz, W. Application of silver nanostructures synthesized by cold atmospheric pressure plasma for inactivation of bacterial phytopathogens from the genera *Dickeya* and *Pectobacterium*. *Materials* **2018**, *11*, 331. [CrossRef] [PubMed]
19. Dzimitrowicz, A.; Jamroz, P.; Pogoda, D.; Nyk, M.; Pohl, P. Direct current atmospheric pressure glow discharge generated between a pin-type solid cathode and a flowing liquid anode as a new tool for silver nanoparticles production. *Plasma Process. Polym.* **2017**, *14*, 1600251. [CrossRef]
20. Dzimitrowicz, A.; Bielawska-Pohl, A.; diCenzo, G.C.; Jamroz, P.; Macioszczyk, J.; Klimczak, A.; Pohl, P. Pulse-modulated radio-frequency alternating-current-driven atmospheric-pressure glow discharge for continuous-flow synthesis of silver nanoparticles and evaluation of their cytotoxicity toward human melanoma cells. *Nanomaterials* **2018**, *8*, 398. [CrossRef] [PubMed]

21. Vidhu, V.K.; Philip, D. Catalytic degradation of organic dyes using biosynthesized silver nanoparticles. *Micron* **2014**, *56*, 54–62. [CrossRef] [PubMed]
22. He, Y.; Liu, D.; He, X.; Cui, H. One-pot synthesis of luminol functionalized silver nanoparticles with chemiluminescence activity for ultrasensitive DNA sensing. *Chem. Commun.* **2011**, *47*, 10692. [CrossRef] [PubMed]
23. El-Rafie, M.H.; Mohamed, A.A.; Shaheen, T.I.; Hebeish, A. Antimicrobial effect of silver nanoparticles produced by fungal process on cotton fabrics. *Carbohydr. Polym.* **2010**, *80*, 779–782. [CrossRef]
24. Ocsoy, I.; Paret, M.L.; Ocsoy, M.A.; Kunwar, S.; Chen, T.; You, M.; Tan, W. Nanotechnology in plant disease management: DNA-directed silver nanoparticles on graphene oxide as an antibacterial against *Xanthomonas perforans*. *ACS Nano* **2013**, *7*, 8972–8980. [CrossRef] [PubMed]
25. Park, H.-J.; Kim, S.-H.; Kim, H.-J.; Choi, S.-H. A new composition of nanosized silica-silver for control of various plant diseases. *Plant Pathol. J.* **2006**, *22*, 295–302. [CrossRef]
26. Makaremi, M.; Pasbakhsh, P.; Cavallaro, G.; Lazzara, G.; Aw, Y.K.; Lee, S.M.; Milioto, S. Effect of morphology and size of halloysite nanotubes on functional pectin bionanocomposites for food packaging applications. *ACS Appl. Mater. Interfaces* **2017**, *9*, 17476–17488. [CrossRef] [PubMed]
27. Cavallaro, G.; Danilushkina, A.; Evtugyn, V.; Lazzara, G.; Milioto, S.; Parisi, F.; Rozhina, E.; Fakhrullin, R.; Cavallaro, G.; Danilushkina, A.A.; et al. Halloysite nanotubes: Controlled access and release by smart gates. *Nanomaterials* **2017**, *7*, 199. [CrossRef] [PubMed]
28. Velmurugan, P.; Lee, S.-M.; Iydroose, M.; Lee, K.-J.; Oh, B.-T. Pine cone-mediated green synthesis of silver nanoparticles and their antibacterial activity against agricultural pathogens. *Appl. Microbiol. Biotechnol.* **2013**, *97*, 361–368. [CrossRef] [PubMed]
29. Kora, A.J.; Sashidhar, R.B.; Arunachalam, J. Gum kondagogu (*Cochlospermum gossypium*): A template for the green synthesis and stabilization of silver nanoparticles with antibacterial application. *Carbohydr. Polym.* **2010**, *82*, 670–679. [CrossRef]
30. Kumar, R.; Roopan, S.M.; Prabhakarn, A.; Khanna, V.G.; Chakroborty, S. Agricultural waste *Annona squamosa* peel extract: Biosynthesis of silver nanoparticles. *Spectrochim. Acta Part A Mol. Biomol. Spectrosc.* **2012**, *90*, 173–176. [CrossRef] [PubMed]
31. Mukherjee, P.; Roy, M.; Mandal, B.P.; Dey, G.K.; Mukherjee, P.K.; Ghatak, J.; Tyagi, A.K.; Kale, S.P. Green synthesis of highly stabilized nanocrystalline silver particles by a non-pathogenic and agriculturally important fungus *T. asperellum*. *Nanotechnology* **2008**, *19*, 75103. [CrossRef] [PubMed]
32. Jo, Y.-K.; Kim, B.H.; Jung, G. Antifungal activity of silver ions and nanoparticles on phytopathogenic fungi. *Plant Dis.* **2009**, *93*, 1037–1043. [CrossRef]
33. Lamsal, K.; Kim, S.W.; Jung, J.H.; Kim, Y.S.; Kim, K.S.; Lee, Y.S. Application of silver nanoparticles for the control of *Colletotrichum* species *in vitro* and pepper anthracnose disease in field. *Mycobiology* **2011**, *39*, 194–199. [CrossRef] [PubMed]
34. Gopinath, V.; Velusamy, P. Extracellular biosynthesis of silver nanoparticles using *Bacillus* sp. GP-23 and evaluation of their antifungal activity towards *Fusarium oxysporum*. *Spectrochim. Acta Part A Mol. Biomol. Spectrosc.* **2013**, *106*, 170–174. [CrossRef] [PubMed]
35. Krishnaraj, C.; Ramachandran, R.; Mohan, K.; Kalaichelvan, P.T. Optimization for rapid synthesis of silver nanoparticles and its effect on phytopathogenic fungi. *Spectrochim. Acta Part A Mol. Biomol. Spectrosc.* **2012**, *93*, 95–99. [CrossRef] [PubMed]
36. Nene, Y.L.; Thapliyal, P.N. *Fungicides in Plant Disease Control*; International Science Publisher: New York, NY, USA, 1993; ISBN 1881570223.
37. Mansfield, J.; Genin, S.; Magori, S.; Citovsky, V.; Sriariyanum, M.; Ronald, P.; Dow, M.; Verdier, V.; Beer, S.V.; Machado, M.A.; et al. Top 10 plant pathogenic bacteria in molecular plant pathology. *Mol. Plant Pathol.* **2012**, *13*, 614–629. [CrossRef] [PubMed]
38. Kamber, T.; Smits, T.H.M.; Rezzonico, F.; Duffy, B. Genomics and current genetic understanding of *Erwinia amylovora* and the fire blight antagonist *Pantoea vagans*. *Trees* **2012**, *26*, 227–238. [CrossRef]
39. Vanneste, J.L. *Fire Blight: The Disease and Its Causative Agent, Erwinia amylovora*; CABI: Wallingford, UK, 2000; ISBN 9781845932985.
40. Hausbeck, M.K.; Bell, J.; Medina-Mora, C.; Podolsky, R.; Fulbright, D.W. Effect of bactericides on population sizes and spread of *Clavibacter michiganensis* subsp. *michiganensis* on tomatoes in the greenhouse and on disease development and crop yield in the field. *Phytopathology* **2000**, *90*, 38–44. [CrossRef] [PubMed]

41. Hayward, A.C. Biology and epidemiology of bacterial wilt caused by *Pseudomonas solanacearum*. *Annu. Rev. Phytopathol.* **1991**, *29*, 65–87. [CrossRef] [PubMed]
42. Karim, Z.; Hossain, M.; Begum, M. *Ralstonia solanacearum*: A threat to potato production in Bangladesh. *Fundam. Appl. Agric.* **2018**, *3*, 1. [CrossRef]
43. Vicente, J.G.; Holub, E.B. *Xanthomonas campestris* pv. *campestris* (cause of black rot of crucifers) in the genomic era is still a worldwide threat to brassica crops. *Mol. Plant Pathol.* **2013**, *14*, 2–18. [CrossRef] [PubMed]
44. Williams, P.H. Black rot: A continuing threat to world crucifers. *Plant Dis.* **1980**, *64*, 736. [CrossRef]
45. Toth, I.K.; van der Wolf, J.M.; Saddler, G.; Lojkowska, E.; Helias, V.; Pirhonen, M.; Tsror (Lahkim), L.; Elphinstone, J.G. *Dickeya* species: An emerging problem for potato production in Europe. *Plant Pathol.* **2011**, *60*, 385–399. [CrossRef]
46. Slawiak, M.; van Beckhoven, J.R.C.M.; Speksnijder, A.G.C.L.; Czajkowski, R.; Grabe, G.; van der Wolf, J.M. Biochemical and genetical analysis reveal a new clade of biovar 3 *Dickeya* spp. strains isolated from potato in Europe. *Eur. J. Plant Pathol.* **2009**, *125*, 245–261. [CrossRef]
47. Tsror, L.; Erlich, O.; Lebiush, S.; Hazanovsky, M.; Zig, U.; Slawiak, M.; Grabe, G.; van der Wolf, J.M.; van de Haar, J.J. Assessment of recent outbreaks of *Dickeya* sp. (syn. *Erwinia chrysanthemi*) slow wilt in potato crops in Israel. *Eur. J. Plant Pathol.* **2009**, *123*, 311–320. [CrossRef]
48. European and Mediterranean Plant Protection Organization. PM 7/20 (2) *Erwinia amylovora*. *Eppo Bull.* **2013**, *43*, 21–45. [CrossRef]
49. De la Cruz, A.R.; Wiese, M.V.; Schaad, N.W. A semiselective agar medium for isolation of *Clavibacter michiganensis* subsp. *sepedonicus* from potato tissues. *Plant Dis.* **1992**, *76*, 830–834. [CrossRef]
50. Slawiak, M.; Łojkowska, E.; van der Wolf, J.M. First report of bacterial soft rot on potato caused by *Dickeya* sp. (syn. *Erwinia chrysanthemi*) in Poland. *Plant Pathol.* **2009**, *58*, 794. [CrossRef]
51. Motyka, A.; Dzimitrowicz, A.; Jamroz, P.; Lojkowska, E.; Sledz, W.; Pohl, P. Rapid eradication of bacterial phytopathogens by atmospheric pressure glow discharge generated in contact with a flowing liquid cathode. *Biotechnol. Bioeng.* **2018**, *115*, 1581–1593. [CrossRef] [PubMed]
52. French, E.R.; Gutarra, L.; Aley, P.; Elphinstone, J. Culture media for *Pseudomonas solanacearum* isolation, identification and maintenance. *Fitopatologia* **1995**, *30*, 126–130.
53. Agarwal, P.C.; Mortensen, C.N.; Mathur, S.B. Seed-borne diseases and seed health testing of rice. *Phytopathol. Pap.* **1989**, *30*, 1–106.
54. Sledz, W.; Zoledowska, S.; Motyka, A.; Kadzinski, L.; Banecki, B. Growth of bacterial phytopathogens in animal manures. *Acta Biochim. Pol.* **2017**, *64*, 151–159. [CrossRef] [PubMed]
55. Sledz, W.; Los, E.; Paczek, A.; Rischka, J.; Motyka, A.; Zoledowska, S.; Piosik, J.; Lojkowska, E. Antibacterial activity of caffeine against plant pathogenic bacteria. *Acta Biochim. Pol.* **2015**, *62*, 605–612. [CrossRef] [PubMed]
56. Anandalakshmi, K.; Venugobal, J.; Ramasamy, V. Characterization of silver nanoparticles by green synthesis method using *Pedalium murex* leaf extract and their antibacterial activity. *Appl. Nanosci.* **2016**, *6*, 399–408. [CrossRef]
57. Njagi, E.C.; Huang, H.; Stafford, L.; Genuino, H.; Galindo, H.M.; Collins, J.B.; Hoag, G.E.; Suib, S.L. Biosynthesis of iron and silver nanoparticles at room temperature using aqueous *Sorghum bran* extracts. *Langmuir* **2011**, *27*, 264–271. [CrossRef] [PubMed]
58. Smitha, S.; Nissamudeen, K.; Philip, D.; Gopchandran, K.G. Studies on surface plasmon resonance and photoluminescence of silver nanoparticles. *Part A Mol. Biomol. Spectrosc.* **2008**, *71*, 186–190. [CrossRef] [PubMed]
59. Pabisch, S.; Feichtenschlager, B.; Kickelbick, G.; Peterlik, H. Effect of interparticle interactions on size determination of zirconia and silica based systems—A comparison of SAXS, DLS, BET, XRD and TEM. *Chem. Phys. Lett.* **2012**, *521*, 91–97. [CrossRef] [PubMed]
60. Long, D.A. Infrared and Raman characteristic group frequencies. Tables and charts George Socrates John Wiley and Sons, Ltd, Chichester, Third Edition, 2001. Price £135. *J. Raman Spectrosc.* **2004**, *35*, 905. [CrossRef]
61. Mortazavi-Derazkola, S.; Salavati-Niasari, M.; Khojasteh, H.; Amiri, O.; Ghoreishi, S.M. Green synthesis of magnetic Fe_3O_4/SiO_2/HAp nanocomposite for atenolol delivery and in vivo toxicity study. *J. Clean. Prod.* **2017**, *168*, 39–50. [CrossRef]

62. Antunez-Lamas, M.; Cabrera-Ordonez, E.; Lopez-Solanilla, E.; Raposo, R.; Trelles-Salazar, O.; Rodriguez-Moreno, A.; Rodriguez-Palenzuela, P. Role of motility and chemotaxis in the pathogenesis of *Dickeya dadantii* 3937 (ex *Erwinia chrysanthemi* 3937). *Microbiology* **2009**, *155*, 434–442. [CrossRef] [PubMed]
63. *EPPO Quarantine Pest: Data Sheets on Quarantine Pests*; CABI and European Plant Protection Association: Wallingford, UK, 2017.

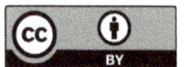

© 2018 by the authors. Licensee MDPI, Basel, Switzerland. This article is an open access article distributed under the terms and conditions of the Creative Commons Attribution (CC BY) license (http://creativecommons.org/licenses/by/4.0/).

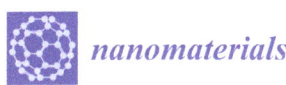

Article

Use of Plasma-Synthesized Nano-Catalysts for CO Hydrogenation in Low-Temperature Fischer–Tropsch Synthesis: Effect of Catalyst Pre-Treatment

James Aluha, Stéphane Gutierrez, François Gitzhofer and Nicolas Abatzoglou *

Department of Chemical and Biotechnological Engineering, Université de Sherbrooke, Sherbrooke (Québec), J1K 2R1 Canada; james.aluha@usherbrooke.ca (J.A.); stephane.gutierrez@usherbrooke.ca (S.G.); francois.gitzhofer@usherbrooke.ca (F.G.)
* Correspondence: nicolas.abatzoglou@usherbrooke.ca; Tel.: +1-819-821-7904

Received: 11 August 2018; Accepted: 4 October 2018; Published: 12 October 2018

Abstract: A study was done on the effect of temperature and catalyst pre-treatment on CO hydrogenation over plasma-synthesized catalysts during the Fischer–Tropsch synthesis (FTS). Nanometric Co/C, Fe/C, and 50%Co-50%Fe/C catalysts with BET specific surface area of ~80 m^2 g^{-1} were tested at a 2 MPa pressure and a gas hourly space velocity (GHSV) of 2000 cm^3 h^{-1} g^{-1} of a catalyst (at STP) in hydrogen-rich FTS feed gas (H$_2$:CO = 2.2). After pre-treatment in both H$_2$ and CO, transmission electron microscopy (TEM) showed that the used catalysts shifted from a mono-modal particle-size distribution (mean ~11 nm) to a multi-modal distribution with a substantial increase in the smaller nanoparticles (~5 nm), which was statistically significant. Further characterization was conducted by scanning electron microscopy (SEM with EDX elemental mapping), X-ray diffraction (XRD) and X-ray photoelectron spectroscopy (XPS). The average CO conversion at 500 K was 18% (Co/C), 17% (Fe/C), and 16% (Co-Fe/C); 46%, 37%, and 57% at 520 K; and 85%, 86% and 71% at 540 K respectively. The selectivity of Co/C for C$_{5+}$ was ~98% with 8% gasoline, 61% diesel and 28% wax (fractions) at 500 K; 22% gasoline, 50% diesel, and 19% wax at 520 K; and 24% gasoline, 34% diesel, and 11% wax at 540 K, besides CO$_2$ and CH$_4$ as by-products. Fe-containing catalysts manifested similar trends, with a poor conformity to the Anderson–Schulz–Flory (ASF) product distribution.

Keywords: nano-catalysts; plasma synthesis; pre-treatment; CO-hydrogenation; low-temperature Fischer–Tropsch

1. Introduction

Carbon is a very fascinating element because in the recent past, there has been substantial evidence showing how the final carbon nanomaterial, its growth process, structural morphology and microstructure can be modified by experimental parameters such as the source of carbon feedstock, gas flow rate, synthesis temperature, and the type of catalyst used, including its composition, shape, and particle size [1]. Due to the exceptional chemical, mechanical, electrical, and thermal properties of carbon, its derivative nanostructures have been utilized in diverse fields [2], including the development of semiconductors and application in electronics [3], production of nano-composite materials [4], and chemically active sensors [5]. Magnetic carbon nanotubes (CNTs) can be found in biomedical applications [6], carbon nanotropes for drug delivery [7], CNTs in field emission devices [8], super-capacitors and batteries for energy storage [9], and high-performance energy conversion in solar cells and fuel cells [10]. In all these emerging fields, the properties of novel nanometric materials exhibit substantial variation from the bulk solid state due to their diminished size, for example, in data storage devices and sensors, finely divided magnetic nanoparticles are most desirable [11].

Today, carbon-supported catalysts are receiving attention, especially in regard to their application in the production of synthetic automobile fuels through the Fischer–Tropsch synthesis (FTS) process [12]. Some authors have indicated that the presence of graphitic carbon in such catalysts seems to enhance the hydrocarbon chain-growth probability [13]. The methods used to prepare these FTS catalysts vary greatly, from incipient wetness impregnation [14] to micro-emulsion [15], sol-gel [16], or colloidal synthesis, coupled with the chemical reduction of the metal salts [17]. Sometimes, a combination of known methods is employed, which may involve precipitation and/or impregnation steps [18], or co-precipitation of the metal salts [19]. Other catalyst preparation methods include electrospinning [20], ion-exchange [21], pulsed electron beam ablation (PEBA) [22], carbon-vapor deposition (CVD) [23], and the spray-drying technology [24]. In other works, the single roller melt-spinning method has been used, which involves in situ carbidation through rapid quenching of skeletal nano-crystalline Fe [25].

The production of FTS catalysts by induction suspension plasma-spray (SPS) technologies have indicated the potential for commercialization [26]. Plasma technologies are becoming attractive due to the shortened catalyst preparation time involved, in addition to the lower energy requirements, production of highly distributed active species, enhanced selectivity, and catalyst lifetime [27]. Other characteristics presented by plasma synthesis include superior catalyst performance, with the activity and selectivity of the catalysts being higher than those for catalysts prepared by impregnation technology [28]. One disadvantage of the wet chemistry techniques that the plasma technologies can easily overcome, is the requirement for stringent control of numerous synthesis parameters and conditions [29], which lowers the process efficiency. This is far and above the need for synthesizing the catalyst support material separately from the active phase that finally demands multi-step activation [30].

Efforts to synthesize FTS catalysts through plasma commenced in the 1980s [31], enabling both single-metal and bimetallic Co-Fe formulations to be produced [32]. Advanced materials such as the photocatalytic Au-Ag core-shell nanoparticles have been synthesized using plasma, whose application today goes beyond the production of FTS catalysts [33]. In fact, plasma techniques can successfully be used both during the catalyst synthesis period [34], and at the pre-treatment stage to activate the catalyst [35]. For example, as used in conventional calcination instead of applying excessively high pre-treatment temperatures such as 973–1473 K [36], the as used in conventional calcination, plasma-glow discharge (PGD) could be applied to lower the pre-treatment temperatures and still produce smaller Co metal nanoparticles (<7 nm) [37], with a significant improvement to metal dispersion as the particle size is shown to be a function of the PGD intensity [38].

Similarly, the dielectric-barrier discharge (DBD) plasma has been seen to promote FTS over Cu/Co-based catalyst, at ambient pressure and much lower temperatures because they strongly suppress CH_4 production [39]. Non-thermal plasma (NTP) reactors, on the other hand, are currently being considered as a viable alternative to the conventional FTS process because they perform reactions rapidly, and may operate at ambient temperature, with or without a catalyst, in minimal space, and at a low cost of maintenance [40]. This is because NTP reactors generate new reactive species through plasma-photon emissions or thermal hot-spots that can initiate catalytic reactions when plasma is combined with the catalyst [41].

Since plasma techniques present many positive effects leading to improved structural properties of FTS catalysts, better metal dispersion, smaller metal cluster size, and more uniform particle size distribution, they also decrease operational temperatures in FTS, with higher CO hydrogenation activity, and better suppression of CH_4 formation and coke deposition [42]. Therefore, the current advancement in the production of synthetic fuels through FTS involves the application of induction SPS technology in producing nanometric C-supported catalysts that inherently consist of active catalytic species for FTS using Fe-based catalysts [26], as well as Co-based, and modified Co-Fe catalysts [43].

This paper is written in the context of earlier work and the novelty of this study encompasses the production of C-supported multi-component FTS catalysts, which further generate structural variations in the catalysts when different pre-treatment procedures are employed. In this investigation, a comparative study was conducted for FTS activity using three different plasma-synthesized catalysts supported on carbon (that is, Co/C, Fe/C, and 50%Co-50%Fe/C formulations). The materials were used to test the effect of (i) temperature, and (ii) the pre-treatment procedure on the FTS product spectrum. An attempt to determine the catalysts' α-values and the H_2 utilization efficiency in the process was made. Since some authors have shown that the selectivity of classical FTS catalysts towards CH_4 is significantly lowered when using a low molar H_2:CO ratio in the gas feed [44], in this study, changing the pre-treatment (or reduction) procedure of plasma-synthesized catalysts has achieved similar results with H_2-rich feeds, which is generally unusual.

2. Materials and Methods

2.1. Materials and Catalyst Synthesis

2.1.1. Materials

The raw materials used in this research included 99.8% Co metal (particle size: 1–10 μm), from Aldrich (Milwaukee, WI, USA); 99.9+% Fe metal (1–10 μm) from Alfa Aesar (Tewksbury, MA USA); the following high purity gases: H_2 (N5.0), CO (N2.5), and Ar (N5.0), from PRAXAIR (Sherbrooke, QC, Canada); mineral oil with catalog name "O122-4, Mineral Oil, Heavy; USP/FCC (Paraffin Oil, Heavy)" from Fisher Scientific (Ottawa, ON, Canada), and 99% squalane solvent from Sigma-Aldrich, (Oakville, ON, Canada).

2.1.2. Catalyst Synthesis by Plasma

The plasma reactor used in catalyst synthesis is a high frequency (HF) 60 kW SPS system operating on a plasma torch supplied by Tekna Inc. (Sherbrooke, QC, Canada), with the PL-50 coil and the subsonic nozzle. In the sheath of the flame, the gas flow rates were set at 75 SLPM for Ar and 10 SLPM for H_2 while the other Ar gas flow rates were 23 SLPM (Central gas) and 10.4 SLPM (Powder). The voltage was set at ~6.6 kV, current 4.4 A, and 0.5 A (grounding) to provide an approximate 29-kW power output.

In catalyst preparation, a mass of 60 g of the metal (Co-only, Fe-only or both in a predetermined ratio, such as 50-50) were mixed with 300 cm^3 of mineral oil by stirring for at least two hours in order to form a homogeneous suspension. This suspension was then injected directly into the plasma at a flow rate of 8.2 $cm^3.min^{-1}$. The plasma equipment is designed in such a way that samples may be collected from both the primary (main) plasma reactor and the secondary (auxiliary) vessel serving to quench the exiting gas [43]. Samples from each of these vessels were collected separately, although they are generally identical in nature by chemical composition. However, certain subtle differences such as particle size may cause their separation into the different vessels. In this study, samples of equal mass were drawn from each vessel and mixed homogeneously before being tested.

2.2. Catalyst Testing and Experimental Methods

2.2.1. Catalyst Activity Testing

The catalysts were tested for Fischer–Tropsch activity in a 0.5 L purpose-made 3-phase-continuously stirred tank slurry reactor (3-φ-CSTSR) supplied by Autoclave Engineers (Erie, PA, USA). The initial results for single metal Co/C and Fe/C catalysts were benchmarked against the commercial Fe/C catalyst and the results can be found in our earlier publication [45]. In addition, details of the testing methodology and instrumentation for the data acquisition defining catalyst activity by CO conversion in FTS can be found in the same article.

In this work, the plasma-synthesized catalysts (7.5 g each) were activated using several reducing media in succession. The pre-treatment was necessary in order to gasify the excess carbon matrix from the metal moieties. The materials were reduced at a constant temperature of 673 K (400 °C) in H_2

flowing at 250 cm^3.min^{-1} for 24 h, followed by CO for 10 h and then H$_2$ again for 10 h. After cooling and purging with inert (Ar), the liquid phase was introduced into the vessel using 250 cm^3 of squalene solvent before CO hydrogenation was then conducted at various temperatures (500, 520, and 540 K) under 2 MPa of pressure. The gas molar ratio used in FTS was H$_2$:CO = 2.2 with the gas composition comprising 65% H$_2$ and 29% CO balanced in Ar, all flowing at 250 cm^3.min^{-1} (STP), giving a gas hourly specific velocity of GHSV = 2000 cm^3.h^{-1}.g^{-1} of the catalyst.

2.2.2. Catalyst Selectivity Determination

Two dedicated offline Varian CP-3800 Gas Chromatographs from Varian, Inc., (Walnut Creek, CA, USA), were used to determine the catalysts' selectivity. By integrating the area under each product peak, one GC was used to calculate the selectivity of the gaseous products (e.g., CO$_2$, CH$_4$, C$_2$H$_6$). After a period of 24 h of catalyst testing, the slurry was sampled, filtered, and injected into the second GC, with selectivity towards each hydrocarbon being determined by peak integration. Full details of the method and approach used to establish the catalyst selectivity can be found in an earlier publication [46]. From the results obtained, plots of selectivity against the hydrocarbon chain length were used to determine the α–values of the catalysts, calculated from their kinetic data using Equations (1) and (2) of the Anderson–Schulz–Flory (ASF) model as done before [47], but in this study, it is done under different FTS reaction conditions.

$$\frac{M_n}{n} = (1-\alpha)^2 \cdot \alpha^{(n-1)} \tag{1}$$

$$\ln\left(\frac{M_n}{n}\right) = n \ln \alpha + \ln\left[\frac{(1-\alpha)^2}{\alpha}\right] \tag{2}$$

where:

M_n = mole fraction of a hydrocarbon with chain length n
n = total number of carbon atoms in the hydrocarbon chain
α = probability of chain growth (α < 1)
(1 − α) = probability of chain termination

2.3. Catalyst Characterization

2.3.1. BET Surface Area Analysis

The fresh samples were characterized by the Brunauer-Emmett-Teller (BET) surface area analysis using an Accelerated Surface Area Porosimeter (ASAP 2020) from Micromeritics Instrument Corp. (Norcross, GA, USA). Full details of the analysis procedure and test conditions for the BET specific surface area determinations are available in an earlier publication [43]. However, in summary, the samples were degassed at 383 K (110 °C) for 16 h until a pressure of less than 10 µm Hg (1 Pa) was obtained in the sample holder, and BET physisorption was carried out using N$_2$ gas under liquid N$_2$ at 77 K (−196 °C).

2.3.2. Microscopic Analysis

The Hitachi S-4700 Scanning electron microscope (SEM) from Hitachi High-Technologies Corp. (Tokyo, Japan) was used to examine the morphological properties of the catalysts, capturing both secondary and backscattered images. An inbuilt X-Max Oxford EDX (energy dispersive X-ray) spectrometer coupled to the SEM (Hitachi, Tokyo, Japan) was used for elemental analysis, while X-ray elemental mapping visually indicated the degree of dispersion of the metals in the carbon matrix. Transmission electron microscopy (TEM) was conducted on a Hitachi H-7500 instrument supplied by Hitachi High-Technologies Corp. (Tokyo, Japan), with sample images captured by means of a bottom-mounted AMT 4k x 4k CCD Camera System Model X41, and the analysis details are available in earlier works [48]. The Nano-measurer version 1.2 "Scion Imager" software was used to analyze the metal nanoparticle size distribution. In order to determine whether a significant difference existed between the various population sets in the particle size analysis, a *t*-test was applied using grouped data of 300 metal nanoparticles each.

2.3.3. X-ray Photoelectron Spectroscopy (XPS)

Elemental composition and the oxidation states of the fresh catalysts were determined by an XPS Kratos Axis Ultra DLD spectrometer from PANalytical B.V. (Almelo, The Netherlands), with sample excitation coming from the monochromatized AlKα line (1486.6 eV) with applied power of 225 W. The analyzer operated in a constant pass energy mode with PE = 160 eV for the survey scans and E_{pass} = 20 eV for the high-resolution scans. The work function of the instrument was calibrated to give a binding energy (BE) of 83.96 eV for the 4f7/2 line of metallic Au. The dispersion of the spectrometer was adjusted to a BE of 93.62 eV for the 2p3/2 line of metallic Cu. The powdered catalysts were mounted on non-conductive adhesive tape. A charge neutralizer was used on all samples to compensate for the charging effect. Charge corrections were done using the graphitic peak set at 284.5 eV.

The Casa XPS software (version 2.3.18) was employed for data analysis. The fitting parameters for the high-resolution Fe 2p and Co 2p spectra were derived from the literature [49]. Since the XPS machine used in the present analysis was similar to the model used in the reference under identical experimental conditions [50], the asymmetric model specified by the XPS reference webpages was used for the fitting parameters of the graphitic C 1s. Data fitting was performed to ensure that the models were within a standard deviation of less than 2, as indicated in our earlier work [48].

2.3.4. X-ray Diffraction (XRD) Analysis

The Philips X'pert PRO Diffractometer from PANalytical B.V. (Almelo, The Netherlands) was used for the powder-XRD analysis in this study. Having been fitted with Ni-filters for the Cu Kα radiation produced at 40 kV and 50 mA with wavelength alpha1 as (λ = 1.540598 Å), the instrument was set in the Bragg-Brentano configuration with a proportional Xe point detector, and the diffractometer was operated on the factory-installed Analytical Data Collector software. The XRD patterns were recorded in the range of 5° and 110° [2θ] for an acquisition time of 4 h per sample. Data collection and analysis was conducted using the Materials Data Inc. software: the MDI JADE 2010 (version 6.7.0 @ 2018-01-31), and the collected data were compared with the Powder Diffraction Files in the Database (version 4.1801) using the PDF-4+ software 2018 (version 4.18.02), published by the International Centre for Diffraction Data (ICDD). A Rietveld quantitative analysis (RQA), which involves quantification of each phase in the material was modeled using the HighScore Plus software (V4.7) in conjunction with the XRD analysis, and details of the methodology used are provided in our earlier works [46]. Characterized by Equation (3), the curve fitting for RQA attempted to determine the amount of each species in the used catalysts [51].

$$W_p = \frac{S_p(ZMV)_p}{\sum_{i=1}^{n} S_i(ZMV)_i} \qquad (3)$$

where

W_p = relative weight fraction of phase p in a mixture of n phases,
S_p = Rietveld scale factor,
Z = number of formula units per cell,
M = mass of the formula unit (in atomic mass units), and
V = the unit cell volume (in Å^3).

3. Results

3.1. Catalyst Testing

3.1.1. Activity Determination by CO and H_2 Conversion

Figure 1 shows that a rise in temperature increased catalyst activity for CO hydrogenation, with FTS operating at 2 MPa pressure and GHSV = 2000 cm^3.h^{-1}.g^{-1} of the catalyst. An identical temperature profile was used in catalyst testing at 500 K for the first 5 h, then ramped and held at 540 K for the next 19 h, and finally dropped to 520 K and held there for another 24 h.

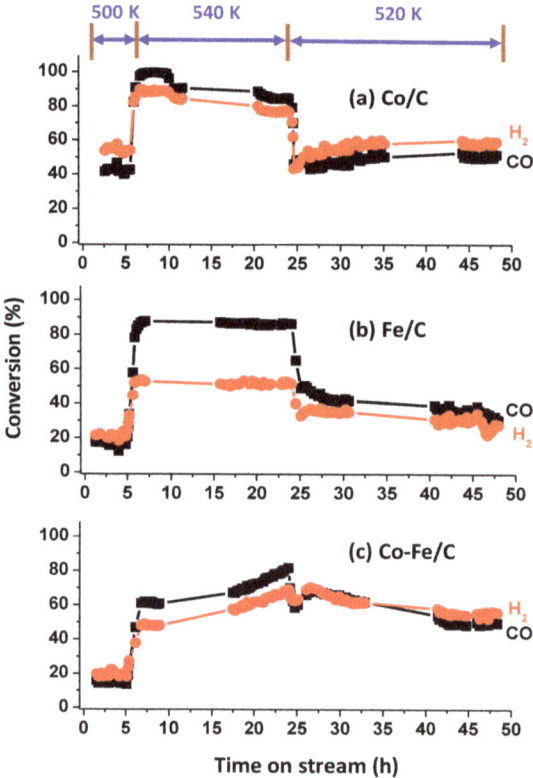

Figure 1. The activity of (**a**) Co/C, (**b**) Fe/C, and (**c**) Co-Fe/C catalysts tested at 500 K, 520 K, and 540 K (pressure = 2 MPa; GHSV = 2000 cm^3 h^{-1} g^{-1} of the catalyst) indicating the CO and H_2 conversions.

The respective CO conversions recorded (at 500 K, 520 K, and 540 K) averaged 18%, 46%, and 85% for the Co/C catalyst; 17%, 37%, and 86% for the Fe/C catalyst; and 16%, 57% and 71% for the Co-Fe/C catalyst. It was expected that in a hydrogen-deficient feed stream, high selectivity towards the production of alkenes is most likely to occur as shown by Equation (4), while in hydrogen-rich feed streams, as is the case in this study (H_2:CO = 2.2), selectivity should lean towards the production of alkanes according to Equation (5). It has been observed that CH_4 production, which is indicated by Equation (6) becomes rampant at elevated temperatures, enhanced by hydrogen-rich feed streams. An active water-gas shift (WGS) catalyst should convert some of the H_2O generated in Equations (4)–(6) into CO_2 and H_2, thereby enriching the H_2 feed stream as given in Equation (7).

$$2n\ H_2 + n\ CO \rightarrow C_nH_{2n} + n\ H_2O \tag{4}$$

$$(2n+1) H_2 + n CO \rightarrow C_nH_{2n+2} + n H_2O \tag{5}$$

$$3 H_2 + CO \rightarrow CH_4 + H_2O \tag{6}$$

$$H_2O + CO \rightarrow CO_2 + H_2 \tag{7}$$

From the gas-product analysis by GC, generally, there was a significant formation of CH_4 observed followed immediately by almost a non-existent (C_2–C_4) portion, with very little of C_2H_6 and C_2H_4 observed (amounting to ~1%, when combined), and no C_3 and C_4 were detected. The other products from C_5 and above were analyzed by the liquid-based GC. Figure 2 provides extra data for the Co/C catalyst, which was tested beyond the 48 h window and it shows that the catalytic activity at 500 K stabilized at a much lower value (~18%) than the initial activity recorded within the first 5 h on stream (~40%). It is suspected that the drop in catalytic activity by the third day was probably not a sign of catalyst deactivation, but rather due to the competition for the active sites by both the feed gas and the accumulated FTS products. This is because by the third day the reactor was already full of the FTS products, as shown in Figure 3 by the massive presence of wax in the reactor. Nonetheless, the catalyst showed a remarkably low production of CO_2 (0.2%) and CH_4 (1.9%), both of which are considered as undesirable by-products. Although the catalyst may have recorded a lower activity after 48 h of operation probably due to the variation in the reactor environment with time-on-stream (TOS), a lower catalytic activity is usually preferred when accompanied by a high selectivity than with a poor selectivity as the unreacted feedstock in the exit gases can always be recycled.

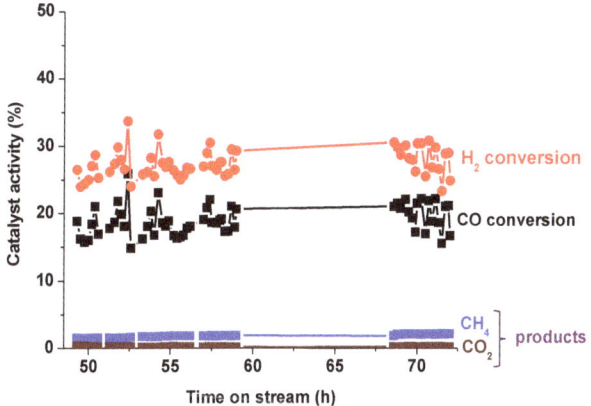

Figure 2. The activity of the Co/C catalyst extended to 72 h on stream at 500 K, 2 MPa and GHSV = 2000 cm^3 h^{-1} g^{-1} of the catalyst.

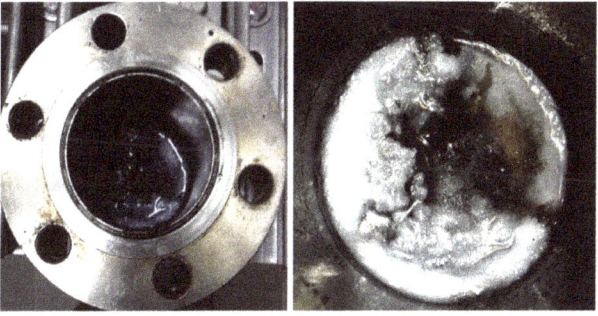

Figure 3. The sample pictures showing a massive wax formation in the reactor after an FTS reaction by carbon-supported catalysts that are evidently black with the wax being conspicuously white.

Since Figure 1 indicates the perpetual switching of the feed-gas consumption as sometimes the CO conversion was higher, equal, or lower than that of H_2, dividing the H_2 conversion by that of CO defined the H_2:CO uptake ratio. See the summary of results in Table 1., which shows the aggregated fractions as light gases (C_2–C_4); gasoline fraction (C_5–C_{12}); diesel (C_{13}–C_{20}), and waxes (C_{21+}).

Table 1. The summarized performance data of the Co/C, Fe/C and 50%Co-50%Fe/C catalysts tested at various temperatures using 2 MPa pressure, and GHSV = 2000 cm^3 h^{-1} g^{-1} of the catalyst.

Catalyst	T (K)	Conversion (mol. %)			Selectivity (mol. % C)							ASF Model	
		H_2	CO	H_2:CO Ratio	CO_2	CH_4	C_2–C_4	C_5–C_{12}	C_{13}–C_{20}	C_{21+}		α-Value	Fit (R^2)
Co/C	500	25.2	17.5	1.5	0.2	1.9	0.2	8.4	61.3	28.1		0.84	0.67
	520	53.4	46.2	1.2	1.7	5.9	0.4	22.2	49.9	19.1		0.89	0.84
	540	76.9	85.0	0.9	13.7	16.4	1.2	24.0	34.2	10.5		0.85	0.90
Co-Fe/C	500	19.5	15.8	1.2	1.3	3.2	0.5	-	-	-		-	-
	520	59.9	57.4	1.0	5.3	8.8	0.9	22.7	43.0	19.3		0.88	0.87
	540	60.2	71.1	0.8	11.0	11.4	1.6	31.7	23.7	20.7		0.85	0.79
Fe/C	500	21.2	17.0	1.3	1.0	2.0	0.3	-	-	-		-	-
	520	31.1	37.3	0.8	5.2	5.1	1.0	9.1	44.8	34.8		0.86	0.31
	540	51.7	86.0	0.6	18.5	11.4	2.1	24.1	31.3	12.8		0.88	0.72

The evident change in the H_2 and CO conversions whose ratio waswhich being either below or above equity was probably due to the formation of different products; for example, more H_2 is required in CH_4 production, which usually occurs at elevated temperatures, according to Equation (6). Increasing temperature lowered the H_2:CO uptake ratio gradually as depicted in Figure 4, as follows: 1.5, 1.2, and 0.9 for the Co/C catalyst (at 500 K, 520 K, and 540 K respectively), 1.3, 0.8, and 0.6 for the Fe/C catalyst and 1.2, 1.0, and 0.8 for the 50%Co-50%Fe/C catalyst. This means that Co/C was the most efficient catalyst in the H_2 utilization and that at lower temperatures, more H_2 was utilized in CO hydrogenation, while at higher temperatures, a significant quantity of CO converted did not incorporate H_2 into the FTS products.

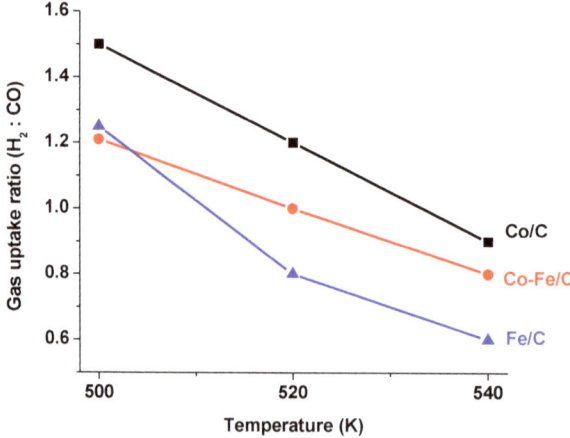

Figure 4. The H_2:CO ratio, r, which indicates that all the catalysts, at higher temperatures, converted more CO to form CO_2 and probably with increased water-gas shift, FTS demanded less H_2.

It was evident that at higher temperatures (540 K), more CO_2 was produced by all the three catalysts (~19% for Fe/C, ~14% for Co/C, and 11% for Co-Fe/C) and presumably with increased water-gas shift, FTS would demand less from the H_2 feed as the system is enriched with the H_2, according to Equation (5). One striking observation made was that since the original intention of this study was to test the catalysts for high-temperature (HT)-FTS, which normally operates above 600 K, but the H_2 utilization was already very poor at 540 K (with large quantities of the CO feed going to CO_2 and CH_4). This led to the conclusion that nanometric plasma-synthesized catalysts are well designed for LT-FTS operations only (below 520 K).

3.1.2. Selectivity Results

As expected, higher temperatures enhanced gasoline production, while lower temperatures enriched the diesel fraction. At 500 K, the Co/C catalyst produced 8% gasoline, 61% diesel, and 28% wax. At 520 K, Co/C produced 22% gasoline, 50% diesel and 19% wax, while at 540 K, it generated 24% gasoline, 34% diesel, and 11% wax.

A pictorial is provided in Figure 5 to demonstrate the shift in the FTS product-distribution towards the left brought about by the influence of temperature, while Figure 6 shows their aggregated fractions. At 500 K, this catalyst produced only about 0.2% CO_2 and 2% CH_4, and approximately 2% CO_2 and 6% CH_4 at 520 K, but a whopping 14% CO_2 and 16% CH_4 at 540 K. On the other hand, at 520 K, the single-metal Fe/C sample produced 9% gasoline, 45% diesel, and 35% wax, while at 540 K, its selectivity was 24% towards gasoline, 31% diesel and 13% wax.

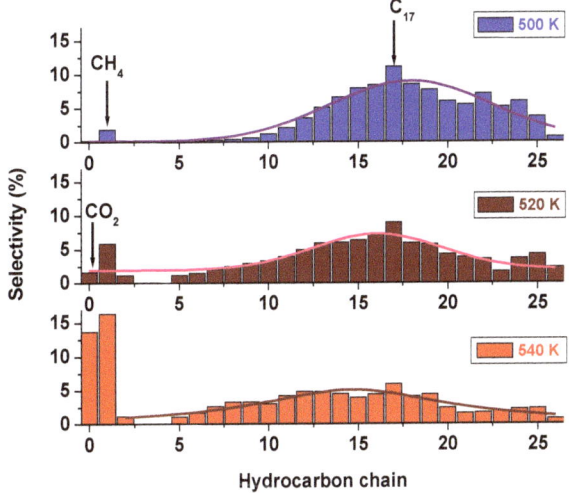

Figure 5. The selectivity plots of the Co/C catalyst tested at 500 K, 520 K and 540 K, 2 MPa pressure, and GHSV = 2000 cm^3 h^{-1} g^{-1} of the catalyst.

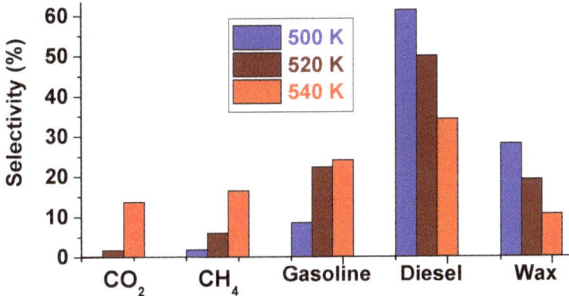

Figure 6. The aggregated product fractions of the Co/C catalyst tested at 500 K, 520 K, and 540 K (pressure = 2 MPa; GHSV = 2000 cm^3 h^{-1} g^{-1} of the catalyst).

Figure 7 depicts similar trends from the Fe-containing formulations, especially the Co-Fe/C bimetallic catalyst, which produced 23% gasoline, 43% diesel, and 19% wax at 520 K; and 32% gasoline, 24% diesel and 21% wax at 540 K, except that the Fe/C catalyst produced significantly more wax (35%) at 520 K than the bimetallic Co-Fe/C sample (19%). In addition, the Fe/C catalyst produced more CO_2 (19%) than the bimetallic Co-Fe/C catalyst (11% CO_2) at 540 K, probably due to the higher WGS activity, but both catalysts generated similar quantities of CH_4 (11%). However, at 520 K, both Fe-containing catalysts showed equal selectivity towards CO_2 (5%), but the bimetallic Co-Fe/C sample produced more CH_4 (9%) than the Fe/C (5%).

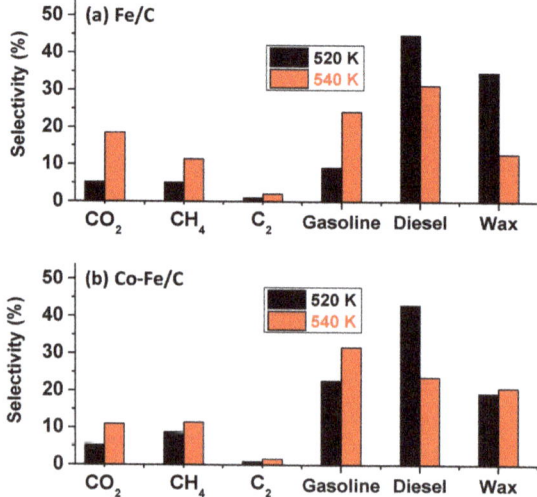

Figure 7. The aggregate selectivity of (**a**) Fe/C and (**b**) Co-Fe/C catalysts tested at 520 K and 540 K (pressure = 2 MPa; GHSV = 2000 cm^3 h^{-1} g^{-1} of the catalyst).

3.1.3. Alpha (α-Value) Determination

From the catalyst selectivity and hydrocarbon distribution, kinetic data applying the Anderson–Schulz–Flory (ASF) model were used to determine the catalysts' α–values. These are interpreted to be the relationship between the rate of chain propagation and the rate of chain termination. Usually the selectivity (Mn), obtained from mass or mol. % contributed by each hydrocarbon is plotted as natural log of (Mn/n) against the hydrocarbon distribution, (with n depicting the number of carbon atoms in each hydrocarbon chain). Figure 8 provides plots of the Co/C catalyst, with Figure 8a showing the full product distribution including CH_4 at 500, 520 and 540 K. Since the sample tested at 500 K showed a significant deviation from the ASF model, this plot was isolated and Figure 8b shows the better fitting plots within the C_5–C_{26} portion (at 520 K, α = 0.89, with a regression fitting, R^2 of 0.84; and at 540 K, α = 0.85 with R^2 = 0.90).

The results of the catalysts with a less perfect fitting to the ASF model are given in Figure 9, where Figure 9a provides the α–values of the bimetallic Co-Fe/C sample tested at 520 K (α = 0.88 with R^2 = 0.87) and at 540 K (α = 0.85, R^2 = 0.79). Figure 9b represents results of the single-metal catalysts fitted in the range of C_{12}–C_{26} in order to enhance the fitting, with the Co/C tested at 500 K (α = 0.84, R^2 = 0.67), and Fe/C tested at 520 K (α = 0.86, R^2 = 0.31), and 540 K (α = 0.88 with R^2 = 0.72). Due to the fact that the catalysts' selectivity data did not seem to conform to the typical linear ASF distribution, an attempt was made to estimate their α–values using the higher molecular weight hydrocarbons from n = 12. The catalysts' estimated α–values were found to be in the range between 0.84–0.89, although with poor linear regression fits.

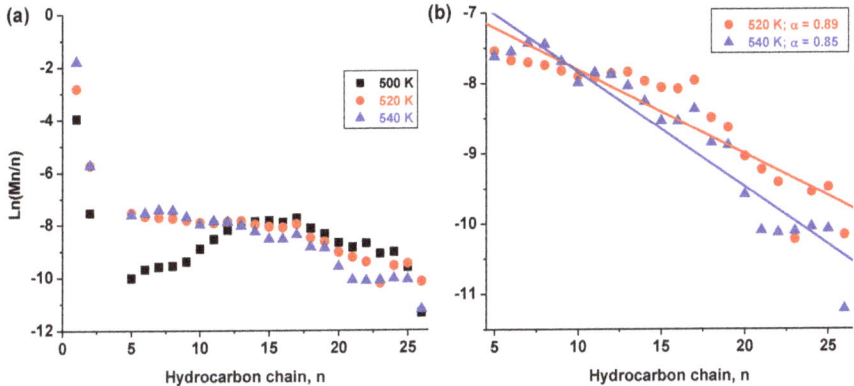

Figure 8. Modeling the ASF kinetics from selectivity data of the Co/C sample (**a**) at 500, 520, and 540 K, and (**b**) at 520 and 540 K.

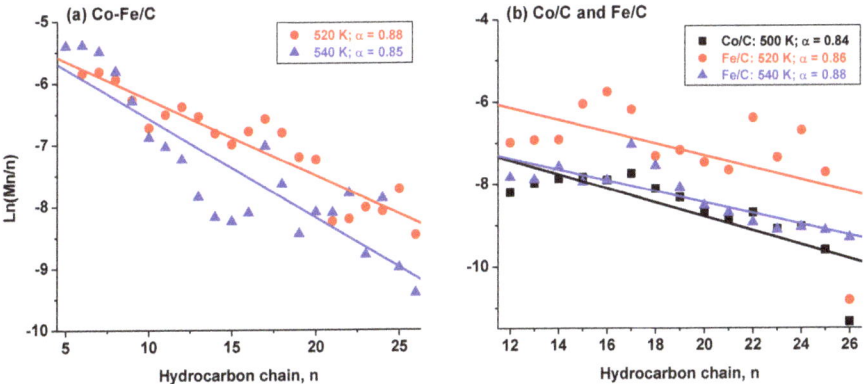

Figure 9. Modelling ASF kinetics using selectivity data of the (**a**) Co-Fe/C and (**b**) single-metal Co/C sample tested at 500 K, and the Fe/C sample tested at 520 K and 540 K.

Table 1 summarizes all the raw data obtained for the catalyst performance in CO hydrogenation including their activity and selectivity, the probability of H_2 utilization as indicated by the ratio of H_2:CO uptake, as well as the estimated α-values with their corresponding linear regression data (R^2). Since the ASF model favours production of the lighter hydrocarbons, formation of longer hydrocarbon chains in significant quantities will likely distort the pattern. In our earlier work, it was observed that various issues can affect conformity to the ASF model especially from poor solubility of the heavier components of the product stream. When some products fail to accumulate in the solvent during sampling, it can lead to a negative deviation from the α-values as predicted by the ASF model [47].

3.2. Catalyst Characterization

3.2.1. BET Surface Area Analysis

Catalyst characterization by BET analysis indicated that all the plasma-produced samples were almost identical, being both nanometric and non-porous in nature, as shown in Table 2. The BET specific surface area was in the range of 73–80 $m^2\ g^{-1}$, and the average pore volume by Barrett-Joyner-Halenda (BJH) model was approximately 0.23 $cm^3\ g^{-1}$, which principally arises from the interstitial volume of the nanometric carbon, while the average pore diameter (by 4V/A) was about 14 nm.

Table 2. The catalyst porosity analysis by the BET method.

Material	BET Specific Surface Area ($m^2\ g^{-1}$)	Average Pore Volume ($cm^3\ g^{-1}$)	Average Pore Diameter, 4V/A (nm)
Co/C	75.7 ± 0.3	0.225	13.6
Co-Fe/C	79.6 ± 0.3	0.225	13.3
Fe/C	73.3 ± 0.2	0.230	14.3

The porosity witnessed here could be associated with the packing of the nano-carbon powder particles since the superimposed isotherms (Type II) as indicated in Figure 10a shows that the samples are indeed non-porous [52]. Figure 10b provides the pore distribution plots proving that the samples are nanometric with limited micro-porosity (below 2 nm), while the augmented meso-porosity in the Co-Fe/C could be due to the larger metal nanoparticle size in the carbon support that subsequently creates sizeable interstitial voids in the nanomaterials. Some authors have found that the catalyst with BET specific surface areas of 40–60 $m^2\ g^{-1}$ had similar average pore volumes in the range of 0.19–0.22 $cm^3\ g^{-1}$, with the average pore diameter of about 14–22 nm [53]. This contrasts with other Fe-based FTS catalysts supported on spherical mesoporous carbon (SMC), exhibiting an order of magnitude higher in porosity, with a pore volume of 2.22 $cm^3\ g^{-1}$ and a BET specific surface area of 767 $m^2\ g^{-1}$ [54].

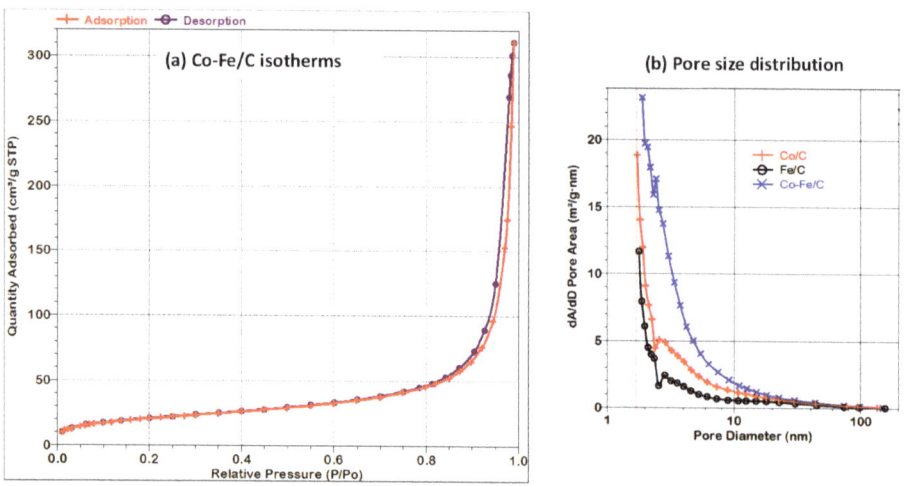

Figure 10. Plots showing (a) the adsorption-desorption isotherms of the fresh Co-Fe/C sample, and (b) the pore size distribution by the BET surface area analysis.

3.2.2. Scanning Electron Microscopy (SEM)

SEM imaging coupled with X-ray analytical methods (EDX mapping and spectroscopy) showed that all the catalysts (fresh and used) comprised uniformly dispersed metal moieties in the carbon support matrix as seen in Figure 11. Elemental analysis by X-ray mapping in the used catalysts confirmed that catalyst synthesis using plasma technology creates well-distributed metal nanoparticles in the materials, irrespective of the metal composition. The waxes generated during FTS were quite revealing as seen in the secondary electron images of Figure 11a.

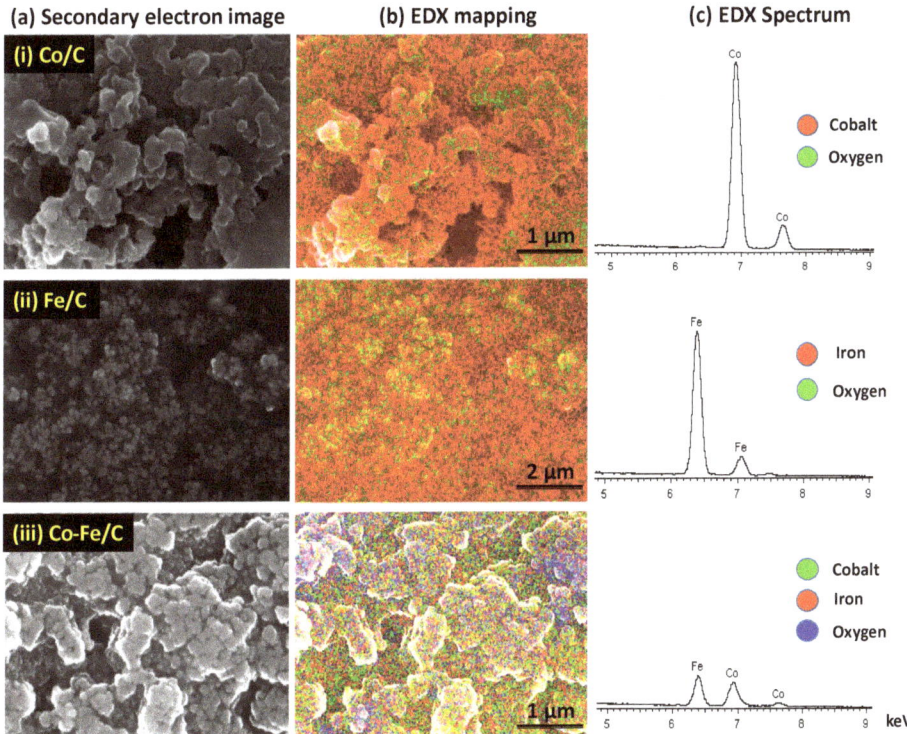

Figure 11. Sample SEM images of the used catalysts: (**i**) Co/C (**ii**) Fe/C and (**iii**) Co-Fe/C displaying (**a**) secondary electron images. (**b**) elemental EDX mapping, and (**c**) EDX spectra.

3.2.3. Transmission Electron Microscopy (TEM)

The analysis of 600 nanoparticles per sample by TEM imaging showed that both the used single metal Co/C and Fe/C catalysts had a bimodal distribution of small nanoparticles in the range below 5 nm and then at approximately 10 nm as shown in Figure 12a for the Co/C catalyst and Figure 12b for the Fe/C catalyst. The used bimetallic Co-Fe/C catalyst displayed a multi-modal nanoparticle distribution since certain catalyst sections were composed of nanoparticles predominantly below 5 nm, while other areas revealed nano-particles with a mean in the range of ~10 nm, as shown in Figure 12c. This occurrence was identical to that in single metal catalysts.

Additionally, the used Co-Fe/C bimetallic catalyst contained much larger nanoparticles, some of which were stretching beyond 20 nm, accompanied by the presence of carbon nanofilaments (CNFs) as seen in Figure 12d. Supplementary images are provided in Figure 13a for the freshly synthesized Co-Fe/C sample through plasma, contrasted with Figure 13b that represents the same, but used catalyst sample after FTS reaction where CO was used in the catalyst pre-treatment procedure. The presence of CNFs are unique to Fe-containing catalysts when reduced in CO, since a H_2 reduction does not produce similar results.

The *t*-test was therefore introduced to determine how significantly different these populations were from each other in each catalyst. It was observed that a freshly synthesized Co/C sample left the plasma reactor with a mono-modal particle-size distribution, as seen in Figure 14a [47], and the same particle-size distribution persisted in the used samples when pre-treated in H_2 only [46]. However, by interrupting the H_2 pre-treatment by a 10-h CO-reduction in-between, (as is the case in this work), a bimodal particle-size distribution emerged as portrayed by Figure 14b.

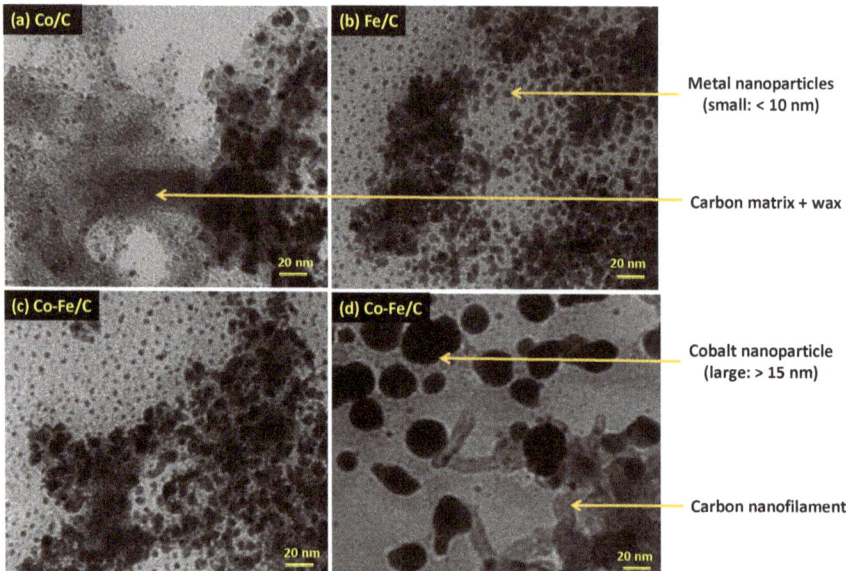

Figure 12. The TEM images of the used (**a**) Co/C (**b**) Fe/C and (**c**) Co-Fe/C catalysts with some sections having nanoparticles predominantly below ~5 nm, or ~10 nm, and (**d**) sections of the Co-Fe/C catalyst with larger nanoparticles ~20 nm and CNFs.

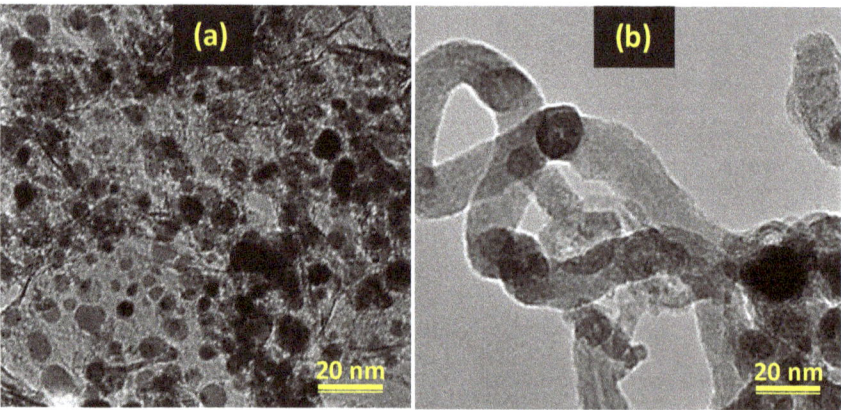

Figure 13. TEM images of the Co-Fe/C catalyst (**a**) freshly synthesized by plasma, and (**b**) after pre-treatment in CO, indicating formation of carbon nanofilaments (CNFs).

It was observed that the t-test for the used Co/C catalyst, which was reduced in both H_2 and CO generated a t-value of 24, indicating that the two distributions were significantly different; with one population having a mean particle size of 6.1 nm, while the other one was 12.3 nm. Since plasma produces materials that are quenched before attaining equilibrium, this implies that strategically, plasma-derived catalyst materials can be manipulated to produce multiple morphologies during catalyst activation, alongside achieving desirable variations in activity and selectivity during the FTS reaction. These attributes can be utilized to modify catalyst performance.

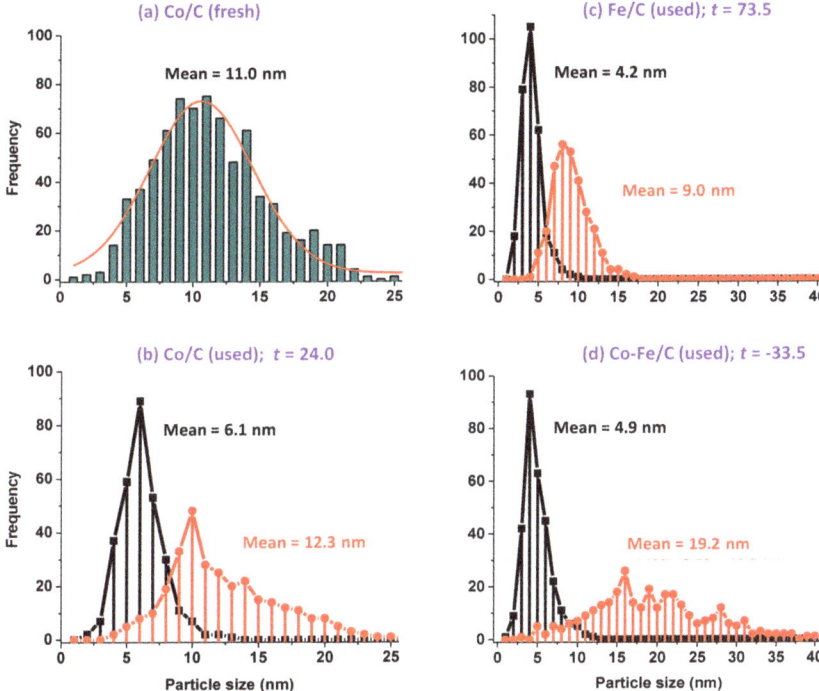

Figure 14. The particle size analysis by TEM imaging showing (**a**) a mono-modal nanoparticle distribution in the fresh Co/C catalyst [47]. (**b**) Bi-modal distribution in the used Co/C. (**c**) Bi-modal distribution in the Fe/C sample, and (**d**) multi-modal distribution in the used Co-Fe/C catalyst.

Similarly, the fresh Fe/C catalyst had a mono-modal nanoparticle-size distribution, but became bimodal after the FTS reaction, (or rather after CO-reduction), as seen in Figure 14c. This finding contrasts remarkably with our earlier work [46], whereby no major disparity was observed in the morphology and particle-size distribution of the fresh and used plasma-synthesized catalysts that were pre-treated in pure H_2 only at the same temperature (673 K) for 24 h, the morphology and particle-size distribution did not vary much. However, in this study, the impact of the CO pre-treatment (10 h) was substantial, producing a clear variation in the particle-size distribution. Since one population of the used catalyst had a mean of 4.2 nm, while the other one had a mean of 9.0 nm, statistically, the two distributions were seen to be significantly different from each other, with a t-value of 74. Moreover, the used bimetallic Co-Fe/C catalyst showed a wide variety of features, ranging from a narrow distribution of nanoparticles with mean 4.9 nm to a broader distribution of nanoparticles ranging from 6.0 nm to 40 nm (mean = 19.2), interjected by the presence of CNFs. Figure 14d shows a t-value of −34 for the Co-Fe/C sample, and Table 3 summarizes all these findings, where s.d. is the standard deviation (σ).

Table 3. Comparing particle size distribution in used catalyst samples by a t-test.

Catalyst	Smaller Particles		Larger Particles		t-Value
	Mean Size (nm)	s.d. (σ)	Mean Size (nm)	s.d. (σ)	
Co/C	6.1	1.7	12.3	4.1	24.0
Fe/C	4.2	0.3	9.0	1.1	73.5
Co/Fe/C	4.9	1.8	19.2	7.2	−33.5

3.2.4. X-ray Photoelectron Spectroscopy (XPS)

An XPS analysis of the fresh single metal catalysts (Co/C and Fe/C) shown in Figure 15a,b, respectively, has been published in an earlier article [48], and are only provided here for the sake of the reader and the completeness of the discussion. The chemical composition of these samples revealed that the predominant species in the Co-based catalyst was metallic (Co^0) with virtually no oxides detected, while the Fe/C sample comprised both the metallic (Fe^0) species and the mixed ionic species (Fe^{2+}/Fe^{3+}) on the surface of the material.

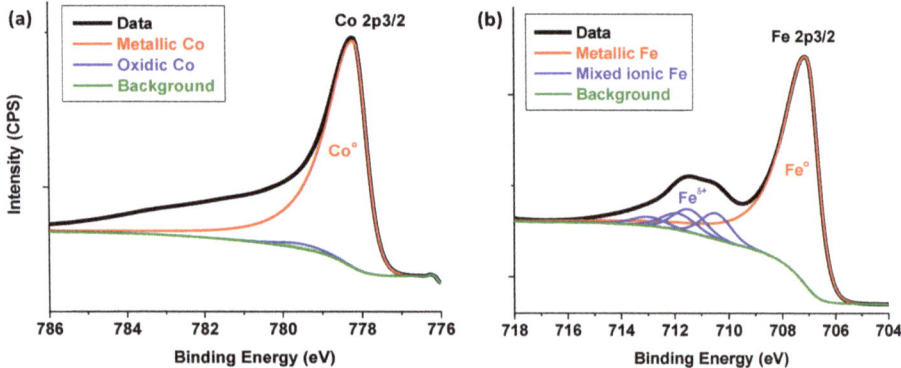

Figure 15. The XPS analysis of the fresh (**a**) Co/C and (**b**) Fe/C catalysts. Reproduced with permission from Reference [48]. Copyright Springer, 2018.

XPS results of the 50%Co-50%Fe/C bimetallic catalyst are presented here for the first time and the intense asymmetric Co 2p3/2 peak at 779 eV shown in Figure 16a signify and confirm the presence of the metallic (Co^0) species. In close proximity is the broad Auger peak at 784 eV for metallic Fe (LMM). On the other hand, the intense Fe 2p3/2 peak at 707 eV in Figure 16b identified the metallic Fe^0 species, while the metallic Co (LMM) Auger peak at around 712 eV was sandwiched between the metallic Fe 2p3/2 at 707 eV and the Fe 2p1/2 at 721 eV. The standard deviation (s.d.) of fitting the envelope to the data was 0.9382, but 0.9379 when the fit included a carbide (Fe_3C) peak at 708 eV, which made the presence of carbides in the samples doubtful since the difference in the s.d. was practically inconsequential.

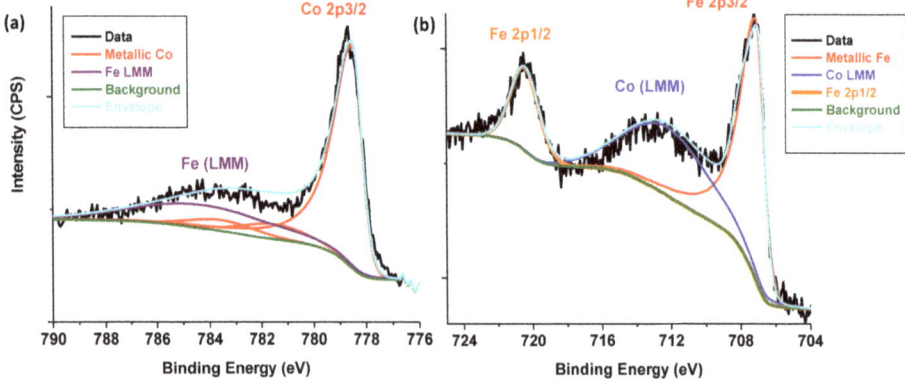

Figure 16. The XPS analysis of (**a**) Co metal, and (**b**) Fe metal in the fresh Co-Fe/C catalyst samples collected from the main plasma reactor.

In observing the C-peak with a binding energy of 284 eV in the bimetallic Co-Fe/C catalyst, two different types of carbon were found in the catalyst, and when quantified as shown in Figure 17, the support was predominantly graphitic-C (G), which comprised about 63–64% and partly amorphous or disordered-C (D) with 36–37%. The G-component was confirmed by the ($\pi \to \pi^*$) transition peak displayed at about 289 eV, seen in Figure 17a, although a bit diminished in Figure 17b.

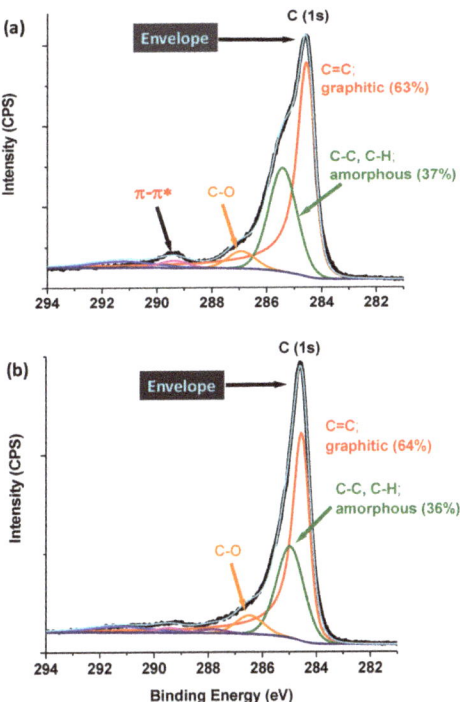

Figure 17. The XPS plots quantifying the C-support in the fresh Co-Fe/C catalyst samples collected from (**a**) the main plasma reactor and (**b**) the secondary plasma reactor.

3.2.5. X-ray Diffraction (XRD)

Several unique challenges exist with XRD analysis of our samples because the isolation of used catalysts from the FTS products is difficult and it prevents proper sample analysis. For example, cleaning the sample from the FTS oils and waxes oxidizes it immediately because the plasma-synthesized samples are potentially pyrophoric and cleaning the samples defeats the purpose of the analysis. Consequently, oily slurries from the FTS reactor were used in the XRD analyses. Figure 18a,c,e indicate the XRD patterns of the freshly synthesized catalyst samples. However, huge broad peaks appear in the XRD spectra of the used samples below a 30° [2θ]-angle, as shown in Figure 18b,d,f, indicating that the samples are highly amorphous, which is not necessarily true. All the used samples largely contained the G(2H)-phase, graphite of the hexagonal crystal structure. This means that during gasification, the D-phase was most likely eliminated.

It has been advanced that the chemical versatility of carbon, especially its high catenation power (to form longer chains and structures) enhances its capacity for sp^2 to sp^3 hybridization and extraordinarily binds to other atoms [2]. In view of this, we suspect that sp-orbital hybridization is the main reason why the metal moieties in the materials get encapsulated by G, in addition to causing the growth of CNFs.

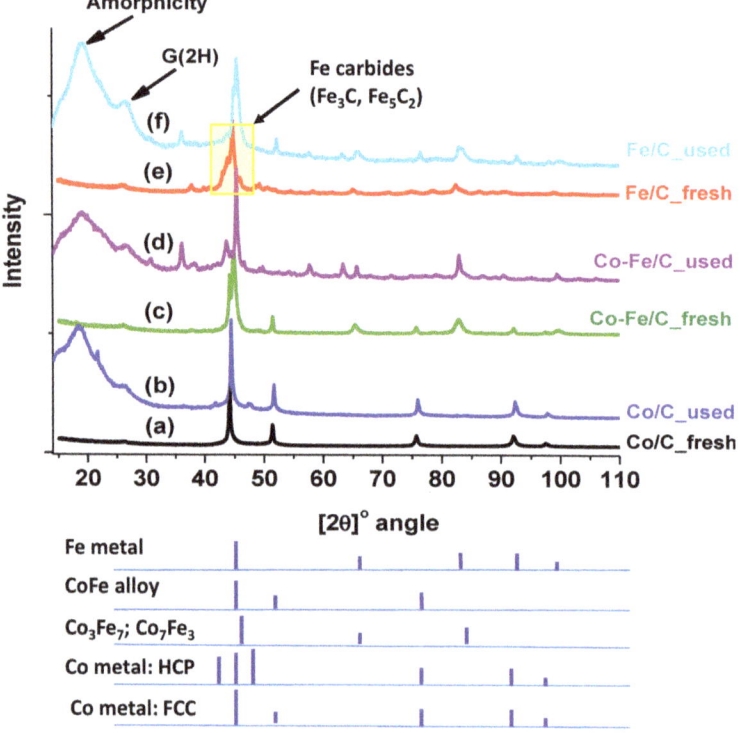

Figure 18. The XRD patterns of the catalyst samples for (a) fresh Co/C (b) used Co/C (c) fresh Co-Fe/C, (d) used Co-Fe/C (e) fresh Fe/C and (f) used Fe/C.

Nonetheless, since some significant differences were conspicuous in the XRD patterns of the fresh and used samples, phase quantification by RQA was attempted, with peak fitting done only for the phases containing Co and Fe, while excluding carbon's G(2H) and the D peaks appearing below 30° [2θ]-angle. After eliminating all amorphicity, Figure 19a–c depict the XRD patterns and their residuals arising from the RQA curve fittings for the used Co/C, Co-Fe/C bimetallic and Fe/C samples, respectively.

Table 4 summarizes the RQA results showing that the single-metal catalysts contained a significant amount of metallic species, where the Co/C sample composed a predominantly face-centered cubic (FCC) crystal structure (62.3%) and some hexagonal closed packed (HCP) crystal structure (37.7%). Both phases appeared in the used sample in the same ratio as the original fresh Co metal that was injected into the plasma, having comprised two phases (62% FCC, and 38% HCP) as analyzed earlier by RQA [45]. In another previous study, it was evident that the HCP phase was vanquished by plasma as observed from both the fresh catalyst and the used sample after pre-treatment in H_2 alone [47]. However, in this work, the HCP phase seems to be regenerated in the used sample after exposure to a CO reduction.

The Fe/C sample on the other hand, contained mainly the α–Fe phase of metallic iron (29%) having the FCC crystal structure. Besides, carbide and oxide phases were identified in the used Fe/C sample (48% Fe_3C and 23% Fe_3O_4; magnetite), both of which were also found in the used bimetallic Co-Fe/C catalyst (31% Fe_3C and 10% Fe_3O_4). Moreover, the Co-Fe/C catalyst contained the following pure metallic phases: the Co^0 (13% FCC) and α–Fe^0 (33% FCC) crystal structures. There were also nano-alloy structures chiefly of the Fe_3Co form detected in the bimetallic sample (14%).

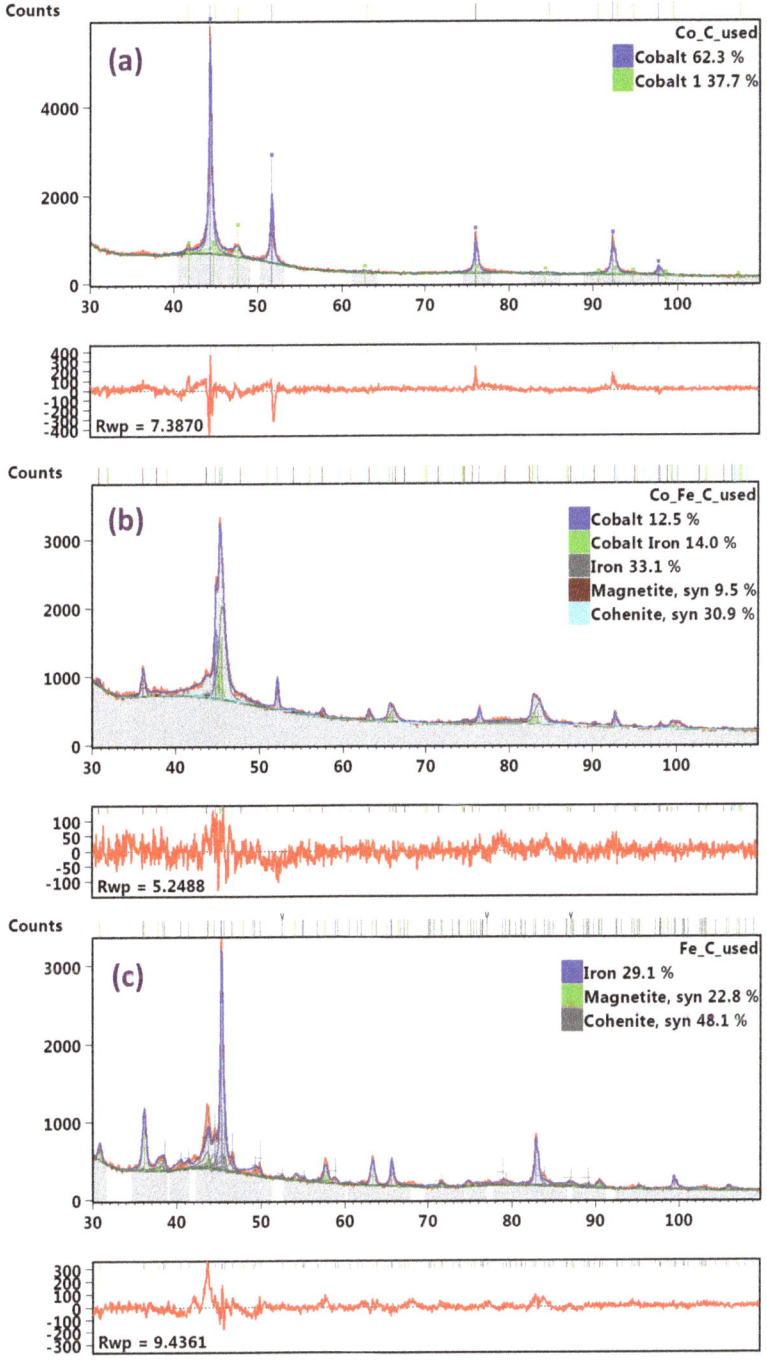

Figure 19. The RQA curve fitting of the used (**a**) Co/C (**b**) Co-Fe/C, and (**c**) Fe/C catalyst samples by XRD analysis.

Table 4. Calculated phase composition of used catalyst samples by RQA from XRD analysis.

Analysis	Property	Co/C		Co-Fe/C		Fe/C	
		Phase	(%)	Phase	(%)	Phase	(%)
XRD (spectral data)	Metallic species	Co (FCC) *	62.3	Co (FCC)	12.5	α-Fe (FCC) *	29.1
		Co (HCP) **	37.7	α-Fe (FCC) *	33.1		
	Nano-alloys	–	–	Fe_3Co	14.0	–	–
	Carbides	–	–	$Fe_3C^{\#}$	30.9	Fe_3C	48.1
	Oxides	–	–	$Fe_3O_4^{\theta}$	9.5	Fe_3O_4	22.8
RQA (statistical data)	$R_{(expected)}$, (R_{exp})	5.6		5.0		6.5	
	$R_{(profile)}$, (R_p)	5.8		4.1		7.3	
	$R_{(weighted\ profile)}$, (R_{wp})	7.4		5.3		9.4	
	GOF^{β}	1.8		1.1		2.1	

FCC = Face-centered cubic crystal structure (*predominant phase); HCP = hexagonal close packed crystal structure (**minor phase); $Fe_3C^{\#}$ = Cohenite; $Fe_3O_4^{\theta}$ = Magnetite; GOF^{β} = goodness of fit $(\chi^2) = (R_{wp}/R_{exp})^2 \approx 1$; R-factors: the Rietveld algorithm optimizes the model function to minimize the weighted sum of squared differences between the observed and computed intensity values; R_p = minimized quantity during fitting procedures (by least-squares); R_{exp} = expected R, or the "best possible "R_{wp}" factor; R_{wp} = weighted profile (R-factor); weighted to emphasize peak intensity over background.

4. Discussion

4.1. Influence of Pre-Treatment Procedure on Catalyst Activity

A comparative study has been conducted for Fischer–Tropsch catalysis using three different plasma-synthesized catalyst formulations supported on carbon (that is, Co/C, Fe/C and the Co-Fe/C). To contextualize the current investigation, earlier studies showed that in order to expose the reactants to the metal nanoparticles in plasma-synthesized catalysts to the reactants, some of the excess C-matrix must be extracted by gasifying the C into CH_4 and other gaseous products [55]. However, in some cases, the over-reduction, particularly of the Fe-based samples, was observed to lower catalytic activity as it ruined the carbidic phase, which is deemed to be the active species in FTS; and incidentally, it was found that the plasma-synthesized Fe catalyst was more sensitive to the reduction procedure (e.g., temperature, time) than the Co-based catalyst [46].

Moreover, when samples were pre-treated in pure H_2 alone (e.g., Co/C at 673 K), the catalyst was observed to deactivate more rapidly with TOS than the samples reduced in CO followed by a H_2 reduction [52]. Furthermore, the samples that were pre-treated in CO followed by a H_2 reduction were observed to be comparatively more effective in CO hydrogenation than those reduced in H_2 alone since a CO-reduction step limited the production of CO_2 as a side FTS product. The CO-reduction step in catalyst pre-treatment has been shown to produce a more stable catalyst over TOS [52], accompanied by a lower H_2O production [56].

In the current investigation, a 3-step reduction was initiated: the first H_2 reduction was to gasify the excess C-matrix around the metal nanoparticles, followed by carburization using a CO-reduction step to activate the catalysts towards a higher selectivity for FTS products, especially in the Fe-based catalysts in order to produce the metal-carbide phase. The final H_2 reduction was to ensure that any possible C-deposits created during CO-reduction were also gasified, while any Co carbides formed in the samples were converted back into the active metallic form [57]. In short, since we know from past studies that H_2-reduction does not affect the morphology of the catalyst [46], this protocol can be viewed as a 44-h H_2-reduction interrupted by a 10-h introduction of CO in the reducing medium after 24 h. It is therefore assumed that higher catalytic activity and the various morphologies generated in the used catalysts came about as a result of the carburization with CO.

Reduction with H_2 at 673 K has been shown to restore the catalyst activity, particularly from depositions of "free" carbon, although bulk-phase carbides existing at temperatures below 550 K could also caused a marked decrease in activity [58]. From Figures 1 and 2, it was observed that after each 24-h experimental run, the samples were still active at every operational temperature, with very little signs of deactivation. The possible deactivation is attributed to the increasing H_2O vapor pressure in the system. This, therefore, means that the carburization step in combination with the H_2-reduction cycles promotes the production of active and stable catalysts online, besides being highly selective for CO hydrogenation towards the formation of C_{5+} fraction.

4.2. Temperature Effect on Hydrogen Utilization Efficiency in CO hydrogenation

Earlier work with the 50%Co-50%Fe/C formulation indicated that the catalyst produces less H_2O in FTS (at 533 K, 2 MPa, and H_2:CO = 2.0) when reduced in CO only than when reduced in H_2 only [56]. Recent work with the Co/C catalyst showed that successive reductions in CO followed by H_2 improves the catalyst performance (at 518 K, 2.2 MPa, and H_2:CO = 1.7), producing relatively less H_2O when compared to the sample that was reduced in H_2 only [52]. In this work, both the above-named catalysts (Co/C, Co-Fe/C) in addition to the Fe/C one have been reduced successively, first in pure H_2, then in pure CO and finally in pure H_2 again. Consequently, a higher degree of H_2-incorporation into the FTS products was evident from these samples at lower FTS temperatures, and an increase in temperature produced a gradual decrease in the H_2:CO uptake ratio. It was observed that a significant quantity of the converted CO formed either CO_2 or CH_4 at the higher temperatures, leading to poor CO hydrogenation towards the C_{5+} fraction.

Some authors have shown that increasing FTS reaction temperature lowers the probability of hydrocarbon growth and, hence, the catalyst's α-value. This means lower C_{5+} selectivity and higher CH_4 production [59], mainly due to higher products desorption rates and lower molecules' residence time on the catalyst surface. Therefore, in agreement, this work shows that at 540 K, the product spectrum was richer in gasoline fraction due to the predominant presence of shorter hydrocarbons. In order to determine the efficiency of the H_2-incorporation in FTS products, the amount of H_2O generated over a period of 24 h in each testing cycle was measured and the H_2 traced back to its origin using Equations (4) and (6). The method used is outlined in a previous manuscript [60], where it was presumed that there was a direct relationship between the amount of H_2O produced and the degree of CO hydrogenation. A summary of these results is provided in Table 5.

Table 5. The calculated catalysts' H_2 utilization efficiency at various temperatures.

Catalyst	T (K)	H_2O		Selectivity (mol. %)		H_2 Efficiency (%)		Ratio
		(cm^3)	moles	C_{5+}	CH_4	C_{5+}	CH_4	(C_{5+}):CH_4
Co/C	500	14.0	0.8	97.8	1.9	15.6	0.5	34.3
	520	41.0	2.3	91.2	5.9	43.7	4.2	10.3
	540	38.0	2.1	68.7	16.4	34.5	12.3	2.8
Co-Fe/C	520	33.0	1.8	85.0	8.8	33.8	5.2	6.4
	540	27.0	1.5	76.1	11.4	26.3	5.9	4.5
Fe/C	520	21.0	1.2	88.7	5.1	22.4	1.9	11.6
	540	15.0	0.8	68.2	11.4	14.3	3.6	4.0

For example, take the case where 14 cm^3 of H_2O was generated by the Co/C catalyst at 500 K. From the selectivity data, which provided the FTS product spectrum, 15.6% of the total H_2 feedstock was utilized in producing C_{5+} while only 0.5% was incorporated in CH_4. This means that for every CH_4 molecule produced, about 35 hydrocarbon monomers, $-[CH_2]-$ were formed; i.e., (C_{5+}):(CH_4) = 35. Thus, in terms of useful product selectivity, although the catalyst activity was relatively low (at ~18% CO conversion), these are proven to be the most efficient FTS reaction conditions with this catalyst. Both the single-metal Co/C and Fe/C catalysts at 520 K were operating at the same H_2 utilization efficiency (~11). The least efficient operation was with the same Co/C catalyst at 540 K; at these conditions, despite the high CO conversion (85%), for every CH_4 molecule produced, only three $-[CH_2]-$ monomers were formed towards the (C_{5+}) hydrocarbon chains. Additionally, these findings imply that the feedstock ratio of H_2:CO = 2.2 was not H_2-efficient at higher temperatures. Studies have shown that increasing the H_2:CO feed ratio decreases the catalyst's α-value because a high H_2 concentration promotes chain-growth termination, which leads to increased CH_4 production and decreased C_{5+} selectivity [59].

Bearing in mind that the original intention of this study was to test the catalysts for HT-FTS, which normally operates above 600 K by gradually increasing the temperature from 500 K, this objective fell short. The reason being by 540 K, the H_2 utilization efficiency for CO hydrogenation was fairly poor, with large quantities of both the CO and H_2 in the feedstock gas going into CO_2 and CH_4, both of which are undesirable in FTS. This observation led to the conclusion that these catalysts are all designed to operate, typically, below 520 K; that is, within the LT-FTS regime only. No further tests were performed beyond 540 K. This was surprising because Fe is known to be a very good HT-FTS catalyst.

4.3. Catalyst Characterization

Since the catalysts produced through plasma have high proportions of graphitic carbon, elemental analysis by conventional methods such as the inductively-coupled plasma mass spectrometry (ICP-MS) are not applicable because it is difficult to grind and completely dissolve G. Nevertheless, an elemental analysis of the single metal catalysts (Co/C and Fe/C) was done by total carbon ignition and found to be roughly 25% atomic % mass-by-mass (at % metal:carbon) [46]. This was confirmed by SEM analysis using EDX semi-quantitative analysis, which indicated a value of 25% (±5). EDX mapping showed that the samples had a homogeneous distribution of the metal moieties in the C-support. The uniform metal dispersion onserved without any indication of metal particle segregation attested attests to the robust nature of the SPS technology in producing high-quality nano-catalyst materials. Catalytic nanoparticles have been shown to be highly reactive [61] and the substantial change in the catalyst morphology and particle size distribution after pre-treatment in CO as indicated by TEM analysis implies that plasma-synthesized materials have a great capacity to be manipulated through different reaction conditions to produce certain desired outcomes in FTS catalysis.

This study has shown that plasma produces metal nanoparticles having a Gaussian-type of particle size distribution with a mean of ~10 nm. However, carburization with CO creates a mechanism that produces bimodal distribution plots in the single metal catalysts. This mechanism is currently not well understood, but it could be related to metal nanoparticles entrapment in the graphitic carbon. Some authors have also succeeded in producing nano-sized FTS catalysts with bimodal pore distribution, where the smaller pores serve as traps for Co nanoparticles, preventing sintering and agglomeration due to confinement effects [62]. A similar phenomenon has been reported for the Fe-based materials where enhanced FTS activity and stability has been recorded through the preferential formation of bimodal crystallite sizes of Fe nanoparticles in bimodal mesoporous structures having average pore sizes of 3.6 and 5.4 nm [63]. Since we noticed an increased concentration of the smaller nanoparticles in our samples (with a mean size of ~5 nm), catalytic activity was also observed to be high. It is suspected that the smaller particles are more active, and therefore, the production of smaller nanoparticles is essential in FTS because they derive their reactivity from the large number of coordinatively unsaturated atoms relative to the total number of metal atoms in their crystallites. It is well known that surface atoms located at the steps, corners, and edges of nanoparticles exhibit the highest catalytic activity due to their low coordination number.

Further, TEM imaging indicated that the bimetallic Co-Fe catalyst had both small (5 nm) and large (10 nm) nanoparticles, besides showing a wide distribution of even bigger nanoparticles including CNFs. In earlier work, we showed that the CO-reduced Co/C catalyst did not display the presence of CNFs [52], and the same has been confirmed in this study. Further, another previous study had indicated the presence of CNFs in all the CO-reduced Co-Fe/C catalysts [56], which is again confirmed in the current work. Therefore, only the Fe species seem to have the capacity to produce CNFs over these catalysts under the prescribed reaction conditions.

A semi-quantitative analysis of the C-support of the fresh catalysts by XPS identified the G-form (~64%) as the predominant phase and that some D-phase comprises ~36%, as shown in Table 6. In a recent publication, we showed that larger metal nanoparticles with a mean size of ~11 nm (compared to ~9 nm) form more D-phase and, hence, have a lower BET specific surface area, because surface area depends on the amount of G-phase in the sample [48]. In the current scenario, the particle size of the fresh Co-Fe/C sample is relatively much larger (14 nm), with a diminished quantity of the G-phase (64%) and, therefore, its BET specific surface area would be expected to be much less, and yet it has the greatest surface area amongst the three. The contradiction may arise due to the fact that the packing of the nano-carbon support particles in the bimetallic Co-Fe/C catalyst seems to create more mesoporous (2–50 nm) spacing than with the single metal catalysts as shown in Figure 10, although their surface areas are within the same range (76 ± 3 $m^2\ g^{-1}$).

Table 6. The summary properties of the fresh catalysts (averaged values).

Catalyst	Mean C Amount (%)		Metal Particle Size (nm)	BET Surface Area ($m^2\ g^{-1}$)
	G-Phase	D-Phase		
Co/C	65	35	11	76
50%Co-50%Fe/C	64	36	14	80
Fe/C	65	35	11	73

In terms of their performance in FTS, all the three catalysts were close at 500 K and, in fact, the Co-Fe bimetallic formulation showed the highest CO conversion at 520 K (with 57%) as compared to the other single metals (46% for Co/C and 37% for Fe/C). When reduced in H_2 alone, it was observed that the 50%Co-50%Fe/C bimetallic was completely inactive at 493 K, while the Co-rich samples (Co/C, and 80%Co-20%Fe) were more active. The Co/C was the most active with over 40% CO conversion [56]. Some authors have observed that in bimetallic formulations, the alloy with an intermetallic ratio of Co:Fe = 1 is not a critical component in enhancing both the FTS activity and selectivity of the carbon-supported catalyst, but rather a Co-rich combination being the most significant, with a metal ratio close to Co_2Fe [64]. However, in the current study, it is shown that in spite of catalyst composition, a CO-reduction step alters the activity of the materials substantially.

From the RQA-XRD analysis, the pronounced presence of the HCP crystal structure (38%) in the used Co/C sample is an interesting observation because HCP as the active phase in the Co catalyst has been shown to exhibit greater intrinsic activity than the FCC [65]. This means that the CO-reduction increased the chance of generating the HCP phase when compared to H_2-reduction. Some authors state that the selective formation of metallic Co in the HCP crystal structure through successive carburization and hydrogenation of a used catalyst is the key to both improved catalytic activity and the effective in situ regeneration [57], as summarized in Equation (8).

$$CoO_{(FCC)} \xrightarrow{CO} Co_2C \xrightarrow{H_2} Co_{(HCP)} \qquad (8)$$

Furthermore, from the XRD analysis, Fe-containing samples were observed to have a concomitant presence of carbide and oxide species in significant quantities. Some authors think that the formation of non-stoichiometric iron-oxide-carbide species which though relatively less stable, is an important combination in Fe-based FTS catalysis [66], and they consider it to be more active and more selective towards olefin formation than the known χ-Fe_5C_2 carbide. This implies that total reduction of the catalyst to metallic state or pure Fe carbides is not beneficial to the FTS process. Our XRD analysis shows that there were rather many phases and probably various active species that were formed either during the plasma synthesis or during CO reduction. Since it was apparent that the catalyst samples did not contain homogeneous active species, it implies that the materials could be applying different FTS reaction mechanisms simultaneously and for that reason, the product spectra did not conform to the linear ASF kinetics. Overall, there are three main interrelated factors in this investigation that could cause the FTS product distributions not fit the usual ASF kinetics:

(i) *Solvent effect*: since some of our earlier works have produced results conforming to the ASF model, the tests had been conducted in hexadecane (C_{16}) solvent, but in this study, squalene (C_{30}) was used instead. It has been argued that when a significant portion of the heavier FTS product components fail to dissolve in the solvent, it lowers its amount in the sample drawn for analysis and this may distort the linearity of the ASF plot [47]. In addition, if polar products such as alcohols are in high proportions, they too may fail to dissolve in the organic medium of the liquid phase. Since C_{17} was the most intense peak, it could be perceived as though the catalysts were most selective towards the production of C_{17}, or that the other products were less soluble in the current solvent.

(ii) *CO-reduction effect on the catalysts*: previous studies with H_2-reduced catalysts indicated near linear plots that conform to the ASF model [47]. However, in this work, the introduction of CO reduction in the catalyst pre-treatment procedure was observed to create a myriad of metal particles and carbon support with different sizes and morphologies, ranging from single-metal zero-valent particles, to metal carbides, bimetallic nano-alloys and carbon nanofilaments. Each one of these moieties in the catalyst could impact the FTS reaction differently.

(iii) *Metal nanoparticle-size effect*: TEM imaging showed that the multi-modal metal nanoparticle-size distributions were generated by CO reduction, and these results were significantly different from those of H_2-reduced catalysts, which showed mono-modal (near Gaussian-type) nanoparticle size distribution. It is suspected that having a substantial variation in the particle-size distribution created energetically diverse active sites, leading to different reaction paths and mechanisms in FTS activity and hence poor conformity to ASF kinetics, which require energetically homogenous active sites.

TEM analysis showed a multi-modal distribution of the metal nanoparticles in the three catalysts. In the literature [67], it has been shown that (i) crystallite size impacts FTS activity for Co crystallites smaller than 10 nm, and (ii) increasing the Co crystallite size leads to higher CO hydrogenation towards C_{5+} selectivity, extending past the 6–8 nm region. Our tested catalysts, which contain a high percentage of nanoparticles below 5 nm were highly active for FTS. Obtaining C-supported FTS catalysts with extremely small nanoparticles is not unusual; some authors have achieved Co nanoparticles with 2–6 nm (TEM analysis), using the microemulsion method, and the nanoparticles are mostly confined inside the CNTs [68]. In this work, small metal nanoparticles have been achieved through plasma synthesis and CO reduction without the use of CNTs, because the nanoparticles are confined in the G-support matrix.

Moreover, the high H_2:CO ratio of 2.2 used in this study could have contributed to the high catalytic activity because some authors have linked catalyst reactivity to H_2 exposure since CO molecules dissociate more efficiently on the larger Co nanoparticles (15 nm) than on the smaller ones (4 nm), and higher exposure of Co nanoparticles to H_2 has been found to enhance CO dissociation rates [69]. Therefore, since higher H_2 concentration tends to favor chain termination reactions, it leads to the formation of shorter-chain hydrocarbons, which enrich the gasoline fraction [70]. Optimally, it has been observed that an FTS catalyst must have metal nanoparticles within a narrow range of about 6–8 nm [71], and this assertion has been supported by kinetic studies indicating that the FCC structure of Co metal favors the H-assisted CO dissociation mechanism [72], and we find our samples to be highly dominated by the presence of FCC crystal structures.

4.4. Benefits of Using Plasma Technology in Synthesizing FTS Catalysts

In Fe-catalyzed FTS, the reaction mechanism depends on the presence of Fe carbides [66], and currently in industry, the Fe carbides are generated mainly by carburizing the Fe oxides with CO [73]. In this work, the carbides were produced in plasma. Earlier, we attempted to benchmark our plasma-synthesized Fe-based catalyst with the commercial nano-hematite (Fe-NanoCat®) by carburizing the nano-hematite using CO. Although the Fe-NanoCat® catalyst was still very active for CO hydrogenation in FTS, it showed excessive nano-particle agglomeration, while the plasma-derived samples did not [46]. On the other hand, metallic Co, which is the predominant phase in our samples is considered to be the most active FTS species in Co-based catalysts [65], and these too were generated through plasma.

Therefore, the benefits of plasma technology in regard to catalyst synthesis over other conventional methods such as precipitation or impregnation methods, include the following:

- *SPS technology shrinks synthesis steps*: Since plasma technology is a single-step method, it diminishes the number of operational factors and repetitive control parameters involved at each stage (e.g., synthesis pressure, temperature, pH, time, purity), besides lowering the labor and materials costs, which makes catalyst production process much easier, and this greatly increases the probability of reproducing the material [45].
- *Plasma synthesis is a robust and adaptable method*: Plasma produces high-quality catalysts, which are both nanometric and non-porous in nature as revealed by BET surface area measurements. From a microscopic (SEM) analysis using EDX mapping, the materials show high metal particle dispersion with uniform distribution in the carbon matrix and all the samples are remarkably identical in morphology in spite of their compositions [60]. Moreover, SPS technology provides such versatility that one recipe can be used to produce a variety of catalytic formulations and this makes the synthesis method highly reliable [43].
- *Plasma fosters the design of functional nanomaterials*: Since the FTS reaction involves the production of a mixture of large polymeric molecules such as waxes that easily cause catalyst deactivation, the nanometric and non-porous nature of these materials make them ideal for circumventing mass transfer and diffusion limitations during FTS.
- *Production of ready-to-use catalysts*: Catalysts produced through plasma do not require elaborate improvement procedures or sophisticated pre-treatment methods before their application in the FTS process, and can be promoted with other metals both during production [60], and after plasma synthesis [74]. In this work, we show that identical materials can be modified through strategic pre-treatments in order to produce a diversity of morphologies and by varying the reaction conditions, different FTS products can be obtained.
- *In situ production of graphitic carbon support*: With SPS technology, the metallic active phases (Co^0 for Co-based catalysts and Fe_xC for Fe-based catalysts) are produced concomitantly with the C-support in the plasma [46]. This contrasts with traditional approaches where if a C-support is utilized, for example, activated carbon, carbon nanotubes or CNFs [75], the support must be produced in another process first before metal deposition.
- *Superior catalytic performance*: In this work, the catalysts did not show many signs of deactivation after 24 h of FTS. In earlier works, catalysts produced through plasma showed superior catalytic performance (~4 times more active) when compared to those prepared by precipitation or impregnation methods under identical FTS reaction conditions [45]. Plasma-synthesized metal nanoparticles do not seem to agglomerate during the FTS reaction like catalysts prepared by precipitation or impregnation methods when subjected to high-temperature treatment [46]. Besides, the catalysts do not deactivate due to carburization when reduced in CO [56]. In fact, this work proves that CO reduction has a positive effect on catalytic performance.

5. Conclusions

The results of a comparative study for three catalysts (single-metal Co/C, Fe/C and the bimetallic 50%Co-50%Fe/C) are presented. The catalysts were synthesized through plasma and with a BET specific surface area of ~80 $m^2 \cdot g^{-1}$; they are remarkably identical in morphology too (as seen from SEM imaging coupled with EDX elemental mapping). They show a high metal particle dispersion and a uniform distribution since the metal nanoparticles do not show any segregation in the carbon matrix. The catalysts were tested on bench-scale for the production of synthetic automobile fuels in typical FTS process conditions (500–540 K; 2 MPa pressure; $H_2:CO = 2.2$; GHSV = 2000 cm^3 h^{-1} g^{-1} of the catalyst).

XRD analysis revealed the presence of Co^0 with an FCC and HCP crystal structure (62% and 38% respectively) in the used Co/C sample, while cohenite (Fe$_3$C) and magnetite (Fe$_3$O$_4$) phases were evident in the used Fe/C and bimetallic Co-Fe samples. The FCC metallic phase (α–Fe) dominated in both the fresh and used Fe-containing samples, which was confirmed by XPS analysis. Semi-quantitative analysis of fresh catalysts by XPS showed that the carbon support matrix was ~65% G and ~35% D. Further, TEM imaging revealed that the metal nanoparticles do not sinter even when exposed to high-temperature treatments (in excess of 673 K) before and during the FTS reaction; the main reason being that the nanoparticles are "caged" in the graphitic-C framework, which prevents particle interaction and agglomeration. Moreover, the catalysts did not seem to deactivate as a result of carburization or oxidation as shown through XPS and XRD analyses.

Catalyst modification by consecutive reduction at 673 K using H_2 (24 h), CO (10 h), and then H_2 again (10 h), activated and improved the FTS activity remarkably. This yielded catalyst stability and high selectivity for CO hydrogenation over TOS, but with low conformity to the Anderson–Schulz–Flory (ASF) distribution. Although having low reliability due to imperfect linear regression fittings, the estimated α–values in this study were in the range of 0.84–0.89. However, earlier works had shown similar values, but with much higher linear regression fittings. Reduced conformity to the ASF distribution could be attributed to several interrelated issues including: (i) solvent effects, where a large portion of the product stream fails to dissolve in the liquid phase for analysis; (ii) CO-reduction effect on the catalyst, which generates substantial variation in the metal nanoparticle-size distribution; and (iii) metal particle-size effect, which lead to the creation of energetically diverse active sites, and since ASF kinetics require energetically homogenous active sites, catalyst samples in this work may have fashioned several different reaction paths and mechanisms.

Generally, higher temperatures enhanced the yield of the gasoline fraction, accompanied by a decrease in hydrogen utilization efficiency (lower $H_2:CO$ uptake ratio). On the other hand, lower temperatures enriched the diesel fraction, with a better hydrogen utilization efficiency since a higher H_2 percentage was incorporated in C_{5+} molecules. The Co/C catalyst gave up to 98% C_{5+} selectivity at 500 K (Table 5). An attempt to raise the FTS temperature beyond 540 K generated excessive CO_2 and CH_4, both of which are undesirable because they lowered the C_{5+} selectivity to ~70–80%. It was observed, therefore, that the catalysts are better fitted for LT-FTS operations. TEM imaging showed bimodal nanoparticle size distribution in the used catalysts after CO reduction possibly by a reaction mechanism that increases the number of smaller nanoparticles with mean size of ~4–6 nm. The smaller nanoparticles are presumed to be highly energetic and, therefore, catalytically more active than the original plasma-synthesized nanoparticles with mean size of ~9–11 nm.

Author Contributions: (1) Conceptualization: J.A., and N.A.; (2) Methodology: F.G. (expertise in Plasma Technology), J.A. (Experimental set-up, Data collection and Data analysis), S.G. (XRD analysis and RQA modelling); (3) Writing-Original Draft Preparation: J.A.; (4) Writing-Review & Editing: J.A., N.A., and F.G.; (5) Supervision: N.A., and F.G.; (6) Funding Acquisition: N.A.

Funding: This research was funded by Canadian BiofuelNet National Centre of Excellence (NCE) grants [(NSERC grant# 419517-2011 and SSHRC grant #: 900-2011-0001)]. BiofuelNet is a member of the Networks of Centres of Excellence of Canada program that focuses on the development of advanced biofuels.

Acknowledgments: We are grateful to Kossi Béré for the technical support in using the induction plasma system for catalyst synthesis, and we thank the CCM (Centre de Caractérisation des Matériaux, Université de Sherbrooke) staff for facilitating the characterization of the catalysts: Carl St.-Louis for BET surface area analysis, Sonia Blais for XPS, and Charles Bertrand for Microscopy (SEM/EDX mapping and TEM analysis).

Conflicts of Interest: The authors declare no conflict of interest. The funders had no role in the design of the study; in the collection, analyses, or interpretation of data; in the writing of the manuscript, and in the decision to publish the results.

Abbreviations

The following abbreviations have been used in this manuscript:

ASF	Anderson–Schulz–Flory distribution
BET	Brunauer-Emmett-Teller method for specific surface area analysis
BJH	Barrett-Joyner-Halenda (porosity analysis model)
CNFs	Carbon nanofilaments
CNTs	Carbon nanotubes
CVD	Carbon-vapor deposition
D	Disordered or amorphous carbon
DBD	Dielectric-barrier discharge (plasma)
EDX	Energy dispersive X-ray spectroscopy
FCC	Face centred cubic crystal structure
FTS	Fischer–Tropsch synthesis
G	Graphitic carbon
G(2H)	Graphite of the hexagonal crystal structure
GC	Gas chromatography
GHSV	Gas hourly space velocity
HCP	Hexagonal closed packing crystal structure
LT-FTS	Low-temperature Fischer–Tropsch synthesis
NTP	Non-thermal plasma reactor
PEBA	Pulsed electron beam ablation
PGD	Plasma-glow discharge
r	Measured feedstock gases consumed in FTS reaction (% by %) as a ratio (H_2:CO)
RQA	Rietveld quantitative analysis
SLPM	Standard litres per minute
STP	Standard temperature and pressure
SEM	Scanning electron microscopy
SPS	Suspension plasma-spray technology
TEM	Transmission electron microscopy
TOS	Time-on-stream
WGS	Water-gas shift
XPS	X-ray photoelectron spectroscopy
XRD	X-ray diffraction analysis
3-φ-CSTSR	Three-phase continuously-stirred-tank slurry reactor

References

1. Raghubanshi, H.; Dikio, E.D. Synthesis of helical carbon fibers and related materials: A review on the past and recent developments. *Nanomaterials* **2015**, *5*, 937–968. [CrossRef] [PubMed]
2. Nasir, S.; Hussein, M.Z.; Zainal, Z.; Yusof, N.A. Carbon-based nanomaterials/allotropes: A glimpse of their synthesis, properties and some applications. *Materials* **2018**, *11*, 295. [CrossRef] [PubMed]
3. Avouris, P.; Chen, Z.; Perebeinos, V. Carbon-based electronics. *Nat. Nanotechnol.* **2007**, *2*, 605–615. [CrossRef] [PubMed]
4. Sun, X.; Suarez, A.I.O.; Meijerink, M.; van Deelen, T.; Ould-Chikh, S.; Zečević, J.; de Jong, K.P.; Kapteijn, F.; Gascon, J. Manufacture of highly loaded silica-supported cobalt Fischer–Tropsch catalysts from a metal organic framework. *Nat. Commun.* **2017**, *8*, 1680. [CrossRef] [PubMed]
5. Zaporotskova, I.V.; Boroznina, N.P.; Parkhomenko, Y.N.; Kozhitov, L.V. Carbon nanotubes: Sensor properties. A review. *Mod. Electron. Mater.* **2016**, *2*, 95–105. [CrossRef]
6. Samadishadlou, M.; Farshbaf, M.; Annabi, N.; Kavetskyy, T.; Khalilov, R.; Saghfi, S.; Akbarzadeh, A.; Mousavi, S. Magnetic carbon nanotubes: Preparation, physical properties, and applications in biomedicine. *Artif. Cells Nanomed. Biotechnol.* **2018**, *46*, 1314–1330. [CrossRef] [PubMed]
7. Tripathi, A.C.; Saraf, S.A.; Saraf, S.K. Carbon nanotropes: A contemporary paradigm in drug delivery. *Materials* **2015**, *8*, 3068–3100. [CrossRef]

8. Wong, Y.M.; Wei, S.; Kang, W.P.; Davidson, J.L.; Hofmeister, W.; Huang, J.H.; Cui, Y. Carbon nanotubes field emission devices grown by thermal CVD with palladium as catalysts. *Diam. Relat. Mater.* **2004**, *13*, 2105–2112. [CrossRef]
9. Sun, L.; Wang, X.; Wang, Y.; Zhang, Q. Roles of carbon nanotubes in novel energy storage devices. *Carbon* **2017**, *122*, 462–474. [CrossRef]
10. Dai, L.; Chang, D.W.; Baek, J.-B.; Lu, W. Carbon nanomaterials for advanced energy conversion and storage. *Small* **2012**, *8*, 1130–1166. [CrossRef] [PubMed]
11. Petit, C.; Taleb, A.; Pileni, M.-P. Self-organization of magnetic nanosized cobalt particles. *Adv. Mater.* **1998**, *10*, 259–261. [CrossRef]
12. Zhu, C.; Zhang, M.; Huang, C.; Zhong, L.; Fang, K. Carbon-encapsulated highly dispersed FeMn nanoparticles for Fischer–Tropsch synthesis to light olefins. *New J. Chem.* **2018**, *42*, 2413–2421. [CrossRef]
13. Chen, W.; Kimpel, T.F.; Song, Y.; Chiang, F.-K.; Zijlstra, B.; Pestman, R.; Wang, P.; Hensen, E.J.M. Influence of carbon deposits on the cobalt-catalyzed Fischer–Tropsch reaction: Evidence of a two-site reaction model. *ACS Catal.* **2018**, *8*, 1580–1590. [CrossRef] [PubMed]
14. Lögdberg, S.; Yang, J.; Lualdi, M.; Walmsley, J.C.; Järås, S.; Boutonnet, M.; Blekkan, E.A.; Rytter, E.; Holmen, A. Further insights into methane and higher hydrocarbons formation over cobalt-based catalysts with γ-Al_2O_3, α-Al_2O_3 and TiO_2 as support materials. *J. Catal.* **2017**, *352*, 515–531. [CrossRef]
15. Zamani, Y. Fischer–Tropsch synthesis over nano-sized iron-based catalysts: Investigation of promoter and temperature effects on products distribution. *Pet. Coal* **2015**, *57*, 71–75.
16. Sarkari, M.; Fazlollahi, F.; Atashi, H.; Mirzaei, A.A.; Hecker, W.C. Using different preparation methods to enhance Fischer–Tropsch products over iron-based catalyst. *Chem. Biochem. Eng. Q.* **2013**, *27*, 259–266.
17. Delgado, J.A.; Claver, C.; Castillón, S.; Curulla-Ferré, D.; Godard, C. Effect of the polymeric stabilizer in the aqueous phase Fischer–Tropsch synthesis catalyzed by colloidal cobalt nanocatalysts. *Nanomaterials* **2017**, *7*, 58. [CrossRef] [PubMed]
18. Riedel, T.; Schaub, G. Low-temperature Fischer–Tropsch synthesis on cobalt catalysts - Effects of CO_2. *Top. Catal.* **2003**, *26*, 145–156. [CrossRef]
19. Cai, Z.; Li, J.; Liew, K.; Hu, J. Effect of La_2O_3-dopping on the Al_2O_3 supported cobalt catalyst for Fischer–Tropsch synthesis. *J. Mol. Catal. A Chem.* **2010**, *330*, 10–17. [CrossRef]
20. Klaigaew, K.; Samart, C.; Chaiya, C.; Yoneyama, Y.; Tsubaki, N.; Reubroycharoen, P. Effect of preparation methods on activation of cobalt catalyst supported on silica fiber for Fischer–Tropsch synthesis. *Chem. Eng. J.* **2015**, *278*, 166–173. [CrossRef]
21. Tang, Q.; Wang, Y.; Zhang, Q.; Wan, H. Preparation of metallic cobalt inside nay zeolite with high catalytic activity in Fischer–Tropsch synthesis. *Catal. Commun.* **2003**, *4*, 253–258. [CrossRef]
22. Ali, A.; Henda, R.; Aluha, J.; Abatzoglou, N. Co-doped ZnO thin films grown by pulsed electron beam ablation as model nano-catalysts in Fischer–Tropsch synthesis. *AIChE J.* **2018**, *64*, 3332–3340. [CrossRef]
23. Xiong, H.; Motchelaho, M.A.M.; Moyo, M.; Jewell, L.L.; Coville, N.J. Correlating the preparation and performance of cobalt catalysts supported on carbon nanotubes and carbon spheres in the Fischer–Tropsch synthesis. *J. Catal.* **2011**, *278*, 26–40. [CrossRef]
24. Zhao, G.; Zhang, C.; Qin, S.; Xiang, H.; Li, Y. Effect of interaction between potassium and structural promoters on Fischer–Tropsch performance in iron-based catalysts. *J. Mol. Catal. A Chem.* **2008**, *286*, 137–142. [CrossRef]
25. Xu, K.; Sun, B.; Lin, J.; Wen, W.; Pei, Y.; Yan, S.; Qiao, M.; Zhang, X.; Zong, B. ε-iron carbide as a low-temperature Fischer–Tropsch synthesis catalyst. *Nat. Commun.* **2014**, *5*, 1–7. [CrossRef] [PubMed]
26. Blanchard, J.; Abatzoglou, N.; Eslahpazir-Esfandabadi, R.; Gitzhofer, F. Fischer–Tropsch synthesis in a slurry reactor using a nano-iron carbide catalyst produced by a plasma spray technique. *Ind. Eng. Chem. Res.* **2010**, *49*, 6948–6955. [CrossRef]
27. Liu, C.-J.; Vissokov, G.P.; Jang, B.W.L. Catalyst preparation using plasma technologies. *Catal. Today* **2002**, *72*, 173–184. [CrossRef]
28. Rutkovskii, A.E.; Vishnyakov, L.R.; Chekhovskii, A.A.; Kirkun, N.I. Use of plasma technology in creating catalysts on carriers. *Powder Metall. Met. Ceram.* **2000**, *39*, 207–209. [CrossRef]
29. Gardezi, S.A.; Landrigan, L.; Joseph, B.; Wolan, J.T. Synthesis of tailored eggshell cobalt catalysts for Fischer–Tropsch synthesis using wet chemistry techniques. *Ind. Eng. Chem. Res.* **2012**, *51*, 1703–1712. [CrossRef]

30. Xie, W.; Zhang, Y.; Liew, K.; Li, J. Effect of catalyst confinement and pore size on Fischer–Tropsch synthesis over cobalt supported on carbon nanotubes. *Sci. China Chem.* **2012**, *55*, 1811–1818. [CrossRef]
31. Khodakov, A.Y.; Chu, W.; Fongarland, P. Advances in the development of novel cobalt Fischer–Tropsch catalysts for synthesis of long-chain hydrocarbons and clean fuels. *Chem. Rev.* **2007**, *107*, 1692–1744. [CrossRef] [PubMed]
32. Dalai, A.K.; Bakhshi, N.N.; Esmail, M.N. Characterization studies of plasma-sprayed cobalt and iron catalysts. *Ind. Eng. Chem. Res.* **1992**, *31*, 1449–1457. [CrossRef]
33. Müller, A.; Peglow, S.; Karnahl, M.; Kruth, A.; Junge, H.; Brüser, V.; Scheu, C. Morphology, optical properties and photocatalytic activity of photo- and plasma-deposited Au and Au/Ag core/shell nanoparticles on titania layers. *Nanomaterials* **2018**, *8*, 502. [CrossRef] [PubMed]
34. Dalai, A.K.; Bakhshi, N.N.; Esmail, M.N. Conversion of syngas to hydrocarbons in a tube-wall reactor using Co-Fe plasma-sprayed catalyst: Experimental and modeling studies. *Fuel Process. Technol.* **1997**, *51*, 219–238. [CrossRef]
35. Chu, W.; Xu, J.; Hong, J.; Lin, T.; Khodakov, A. Design of efficient Fischer–Tropsch cobalt catalysts via plasma enhancement: Reducibility and performance (review). *Catal. Today* **2015**, *256*, 41–48. [CrossRef]
36. Keyvanloo, K.; Huang, B.; Okeson, T.; Hamdeh, H.H.; Hecker, W.C. Effect of support pretreatment temperature on the performance of an iron Fischer–Tropsch catalyst supported on silica-stabilized alumina. *Catalysts* **2018**, *8*, 77. [CrossRef]
37. Chu, W.; Wang, L.-N.; Chernavskii, P.A.; Khodakov, A.Y. Glow-discharge plasma-assisted design of cobalt catalysts for Fischer–Tropsch synthesis. *Angew. Chem. Int. Ed.* **2008**, *47*, 5052–5055. [CrossRef] [PubMed]
38. Hong, J.; Chu, W.; Chernavskii, P.A.; Khodakov, A.Y. Cobalt species and cobalt-support interaction in glow discharge plasma-assisted Fischer–Tropsch catalysts. *J. Catal.* **2010**, *273*, 9–17. [CrossRef]
39. Al-Harrasi, W.S.S.; Zhang, K.; Akay, G. Process intensification in gas-to-liquid reactions: Plasma promoted Fischer–Tropsch synthesis for hydrocarbons at low temperatures and ambient pressure. *Green Process. Synth.* **2013**, *2*, 479–490. [CrossRef]
40. Govender, B.B.; Iwarere, S.A.; Ramjugernath, D. The application of non-thermal plasma catalysis in Fischer–Tropsch synthesis at very high pressure: The effect of cobalt loading. In Proceedings of the World Congress on Engineering and Computer Science (WCECS 2017), San Francisco, NC, USA, 25–27 October 2017; Volume II. ISBN 978-988-14048-4-8; ISSN 12078-10958 (Print); ISSN 12078-10966 (Online).
41. Van Durme, J.; Dewulf, J.; Leys, C.; van Langenhove, H. Combining non-thermal plasma with heterogeneous catalysis in waste gas treatment: A review. *Appl. Catal. B* **2008**, *78*, 324–333. [CrossRef]
42. Taghvaei, H.; Heravi, M.; Rahimpour, M.R. Synthesis of supported nanocatalysts via novel non-thermalplasma methods and its application in catalytic processes. *Plasma Process Polym.* **2017**, *16*, 1–20.
43. Aluha, J.; Bere, K.; Abatzoglou, N.; Gitzhofer, F. Synthesis of nano-catalysts by induction suspension plasma technology (SPS) for Fischer–Tropsch reaction. *Plasma Chem. Plasma Process.* **2016**, *36*, 1325–1348. [CrossRef]
44. Davis, B.H. Fischer–Tropsch synthesis: Comparison of performances of iron and cobalt catalysts. *Ind. Eng. Chem. Res.* **2007**, *46*, 8938–8945. [CrossRef]
45. Aluha, J.; Boahene, P.; Dalai, A.; Hu, Y.; Bere, K.; Braidy, N.; Abatzoglou, N. Synthesis and characterisation of nanometric Co/C and Fe/C catalysts for Fischer–Tropsch synthesis: A comparative study using a fixed-bed reactor. *Ind. Eng. Chem. Res.* **2015**, *54*, 10661–10674. [CrossRef]
46. Aluha, J.; Braidy, N.; Dalai, A.; Abatzoglou, N. Low-temperature Fischer–Tropsch synthesis using plasma-synthesised nanometric Co/C and Fe/C catalysts. *Can. J. Chem. Eng.* **2016**, *94*, 1504–1515. [CrossRef]
47. Aluha, J.; Hu, Y.; Abatzoglou, N. Effect of CO concentration on the α-value of plasma-synthesized Co/C catalyst in Fischer–Tropsch synthesis. *Catalysts* **2017**, *7*, 69. [CrossRef]
48. Aluha, J.; Blais, S.; Abatzoglou, N. Phase quantification of carbon support by X-ray photoelectron spectroscopy (XPS) in plasma-synthesized Fischer–Tropsch nanocatalysts. *Catal. Lett.* **2018**, *148*, 2149–2161. [CrossRef]
49. Biesinger, M.C.; Payne, B.P.; Grosvenor, A.P.; Lau, L.W.M.; Gerson, A.R.; Smart, R.S.C. Resolving surface chemical states in XPS analysis of first row transition metals, oxides and hydroxides: Cr, Mn, Fe, Co and Ni. *Appl. Surf. Sci.* **2011**, *257*, 2717–2730. [CrossRef]
50. Biesinger, M.C. Carbon. In *X-ray Photoelectron Spectroscopy (XPS) Reference Pages*; 2018; Available online: http://www.xpsfitting.com/search/label/carbon (accessed on 11 August 2018).

51. Rietveld, H.M. A profile refinement method for nuclear and magnetic structures. *J. Appl. Cryst.* **1969**, *2*, 65–71. [CrossRef]
52. Aluha, J.; Abatzoglou, N. Activation and deactivation scenarios in a plasma-synthesized Co/C catalyst for Fischer–Tropsch synthesis. *Can. J. Chem. Eng.* **2018**, *96*, 2127–2137. [CrossRef]
53. Özkara-Aydınoğlu, Ş.; Ataç, Ö.; Gül, Ö.F.; Kınayyiğit, Ş.; Şal, S.; Baranak, M.; Boz, İ. α-olefin selectivity of Fe–Cu–K catalysts in Fischer–Tropsch synthesis: Effects of catalyst composition and process conditions. *Chem. Eng. J.* **2012**, *181–182*, 581–589. [CrossRef]
54. Chen, Q.; Liu, G.; Ding, S.; Sheikh, M.C.; Long, D.; Yoneyama, Y.; Tsubaki, N. Design of ultra-active iron-based Fischer–Tropsch synthesis catalysts over spherical mesoporous carbon with developed porosity. *Chem. Eng. J.* **2018**, *334*, 714–724. [CrossRef]
55. Blanchard, J.; Abatzoglou, N. Nano-iron carbide synthesized by plasma as catalyst for Fischer–Tropsch synthesis in slurry reactors: The role of iron loading and K, Cu promoters. *Catal. Today* **2014**, *237*, 150–156. [CrossRef]
56. Aluha, J.; Abatzoglou, N. Synthetic fuels from 3-φ Fischer–Tropsch synthesis using syngas feed and novel nanometric catalysts synthesised by plasma. *Biomass Bioenerg.* **2016**, *95*, 330–339. [CrossRef]
57. Kwak, G.; Kim, D.-E.; Kim, Y.T.; Park, H.-G.; Kang, S.C.; Ha, K.-S.; Juna, K.-W.; Lee, Y.-J. Enhanced catalytic activity of cobalt catalysts for Fischer–Tropsch synthesis via carburization and hydrogenation and its application to regeneration. *Catal. Sci. Technol.* **2016**, *6*, 4594–4600. [CrossRef]
58. Anderson, R.B.; Hall, W.K.; Krieg, A.; Seligman, B. Studies of the Fischer–Tropsch synthesis. V. Activities and surface areas of reduced and carburized cobalt catalysts. *J. Am. Chem. Soc.* **1949**, *71*, 183–188. [CrossRef]
59. Todic, B.; Nowicki, L.; Nikacevic, N.; Bukur, D.B. Fischer–Tropsch synthesis product selectivity over an industrial iron-based catalyst: Effect of process conditions. *Catal. Today* **2016**, *261*, 28–39. [CrossRef]
60. Aluha, J.; Abatzoglou, N. Promotional effect of Mo and Ni in plasma-synthesized Co-Fe/C bimetallic nano-catalysts for Fischer–Tropsch synthesis. *J. Ind. Eng. Chem.* **2017**, *50*, 199–212. [CrossRef]
61. Navalón, S.; García, H. Nanoparticles for catalysis. *Nanomaterials* **2016**, *6*, 123. [CrossRef] [PubMed]
62. Ishihara, D.; Tao, K.; Yang, G.; Han, L.; Tsubaki, N. Precisely designing bimodal catalyst structure to trap cobalt nanoparticles inside mesopores and its application in Fischer–Tropsch synthesis. *Chem. Eng. J.* **2016**, *306*, 784–790. [CrossRef]
63. Cho, J.M.; Han, G.Y.; Jeong, H.-K.; Roh, H.-S.; Bae, J.-W. Effects of ordered mesoporous bimodal structures of Fe/KIT-6 for CO hydrogenation activity to hydrocarbons. *Chem. Eng. J.* **2018**, *354*, 197–207. [CrossRef]
64. Dlamini, M.W.; Kumi, D.O.; Phaahlamohlaka, T.N.; Lyadov, A.S.; Billing, D.G.; Jewell, L.L.; Coville, N.J. Carbon spheres prepared by hydrothermal synthesis - a support for bimetallic iron cobalt Fischer–Tropsch catalysts. *ChemCatChem* **2015**, *7*, 3000–3011. [CrossRef]
65. Jacobs, G.; Ma, W.; Gao, P.; Todic, B.; Bhatelia, T.; Bukur, D.B.; Davis, B.H. The application of synchrotron methods in characterizing iron and cobalt Fischer–Tropsch synthesis catalysts. *Catal. Today* **2013**, *214*, 100–139. [CrossRef]
66. Bengoa, J.F.; Alvarez, A.M.; Cagnoli, M.V.; Gallegos, N.G.; Marchetti, S.G. Influence of intermediate iron reduced species in Fischer–Tropsch synthesis using Fe/C catalysts. *Appl. Catal. A.* **2007**, *325*, 68–75. [CrossRef]
67. Botes, F.G.; Niemantsverdriet, J.W.; van de Loosdrecht, J. A comparison of cobalt and iron based slurry phase Fischer–Tropsch synthesis. *Catal. Today* **2013**, *215*, 112–120. [CrossRef]
68. Trépanier, M.; Dalai, A.K.; Abatzoglou, N. Synthesis of CNT-supported cobalt nanoparticle catalysts using a microemulsion technique: Role of nanoparticle size on reducibility, activity and selectivity in Fischer–Tropsch reactions. *Appl. Catal. A.* **2010**, *374*, 79–86. [CrossRef]
69. Tuxen, A.; Carenco, S.; Chintapalli, M.; Chuang, C.-H.; Escudero, C.; Pach, E.; Jiang, P.; Borondics, F.; Beberwyck, B.; Alivisatos, A.P.; et al. Size-dependent dissociation of carbon monoxide on cobalt nanoparticles. *J. Am. Chem. Soc.* **2013**, *135*, 2273–2278. [CrossRef] [PubMed]
70. Madon, R.J.; Iglesia, E. The importance of olefin readsorption and H_2/CO reactant ratio for hydrocarbon chain growth on ruthenium catalysts. *J. Catal.* **1993**, *139*, 576–590. [CrossRef]
71. Bezemer, G.L.; Bitter, J.H.; Kuipers, H.P.C.E.; Oosterbeek, H.; Holewijn, J.E.; Xu, X.; Kapteijn, F.; van Dillen, A.J.; de Jong, K.P. Cobalt particle size effects in the Fischer–Tropsch reaction studied with carbon nanofiber supported catalysts. *J. Am. Chem. Soc.* **2006**, *128*, 3956–3964. [CrossRef] [PubMed]

72. Liu, J.-X.; Su, H.-Y.; Sun, D.-P.; Zhang, B.-Y.; Li, W.-X. Crystallographic dependence of CO activation on cobalt catalysts: HCP versus FCC. *J. Am. Chem. Soc.* **2013**, *135*, 16284–16287. [CrossRef] [PubMed]
73. Ding, M.; Yang, Y.; Wu, B.; Xu, J.; Zhang, C.; Xiang, H.; Li, Y. Study of phase transformation and catalytic performance on precipitated iron-based catalyst for Fischer–Tropsch synthesis. *J. Mol. Catal. A Chem.* **2009**, *303*, 65–71. [CrossRef]
74. Aluha, J.; Abatzoglou, N. Gold-promoted plasma-synthesized Ni-Co-Fe/C catalyst for Fischer–Tropsch synthesis. *Gold Bull.* **2017**, *50*, 147–162. [CrossRef]
75. Blanchard, J.; Oudghiri-Hassani, H.; Abatzoglou, N.; Jankhah, S.; Gitzhofer, F. Synthesis of nanocarbons via ethanol dry reforming over a carbon steel catalyst. *Chem. Eng. J.* **2008**, *143*, 186–194. [CrossRef]

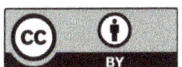

© 2018 by the authors. Licensee MDPI, Basel, Switzerland. This article is an open access article distributed under the terms and conditions of the Creative Commons Attribution (CC BY) license (http://creativecommons.org/licenses/by/4.0/).

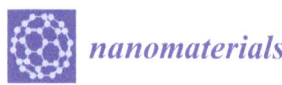

Article

Synthesis of Pd-Fe System Alloy Nanoparticles by Pulsed Plasma in Liquid

Shota Tamura [1], Tsutomu Mashimo [1,*], Kenta Yamamoto [1], Zhazgul Kelgenbaeva [1], Weijan Ma [1], Xuesong Kang [1], Michio Koinuma [2], Hiroshi Isobe [3] and Akira Yoshiasa [3]

[1] Institute of Pulsed Power Science, Kumamoto University, Kumamoto 860-0862, Japan; 171d9101@st.kumamoto-u.ac.jp (S.T.); yamaken030806@gmail.com (K.Y.); jaza-86@mail.ru (Z.K.); 167d9102@st.kumamoto-u.ac.jp (W.M.); kangxuesong126@gmail.com (X.K.)
[2] Faculty of Engineering, Kumamoto University, Kumamoto 860-0862, Japan; koinuma@chem.chem.kumamoto-u.ac.jp
[3] Faculty of Science, Kumamoto University, Kumamoto 860-0862, Japan; isobe@sci.kumamoto-u.ac.jp (H.I.); yoshiasa@sci.kumamoto-u.ac.jp (A.Y.)
* Correspondence: mashimo@gpo.kumamoto-u.ac.jp; Tel.: +81-96-342-3295

Received: 29 November 2018; Accepted: 12 December 2018; Published: 18 December 2018

Abstract: We synthesized Pd-Fe series nanoparticles in solid solution using pulsed plasma in liquid with Pd-Fe bulk mixture electrodes. The Pd-Fe atomic percent ratios were 1:3, 1:1, and 3:1, and the particle size was measured to be less than 10 nm by high-resolution transmission electron microscopy (HR-TEM). The nanoparticles showed face-centered cubic structure. The lattice parameter increased with increasing Pd content and followed Vegard's law, and energy-dispersive X-ray spectra were consistent with the ratios of the starting samples, which showed a solid solution state. The solid solution structure and local structure were confirmed by HR-TEM and X-ray absorption fine structure.

Keywords: Pd-Fe alloy; nanoparticle; pulsed plasma in liquid

1. Introduction

Pd is well-known as a hydrogen storage metal [1–3]. Pd-Fe alloy can be used to catalyze fuel cells and improve their conversion of chemical to electric energy. Furthermore, Pd-Fe alloy nanoparticles may increase the conversion rate of fuel cells. Research has shown that oxygen reduction of Pd-Fe catalyst is very stable in alkaline solution [4–6]. Mashimo's laboratory has already synthesized Pt-Fe alloy nanoparticles [7]. Pd-Fe alloy nanoparticles in solid solution are expected to show excellent catalytic properties because of the interaction of 3d and 4d electrons. Pd-Fe alloy is half immiscible at room temperature.

Our previous studies have shown that pulsed plasma in liquid (PPL) is a good alternative method for synthesizing various nanomaterials [8]. This process is relatively cheap and environmentally friendly. The short duration (several microseconds) and quenching of the surrounding cool liquid limit the size of the crystals, which enables the synthesis of very small and/or metastable particles. We have synthesized nanoparticles of such materials as single elements [9], carbon-coated metals [10], fullerene [9], and onion-like carbon [11], and compound nanoparticles of oxides, carbides, and sulfides [12–14].

In this study, we seek to synthesize Pd-Fe alloy nanoparticles with atomic percent ratios of 1:3, 1:1, and 3:1 using PPL with Pd-Fe bulk mixture electrodes of the same composition. We expect that using melted Pd-Fe bulk electrodes will yield Pd-Fe solid solution nanoparticles because Pd and Fe ions exist in the environment of the pulsed plasma, so Pd-Fe clusters may easily form.

2. Materials and Methods

A schematic of the experimental setup is shown in Figure 1. Metal electrodes (cathodes and anodes) were submerged in a liquid connected to the power source. The impulse plasma was produced by the spark discharge between two electrodes. The gap between the two electrodes was approximately 0.2 mm, and the electrical current pulses that produced the pulsed plasma had a duration of about 20 µs. One of the electrodes was kept vibrating, so that the discharging could proceed continuously.

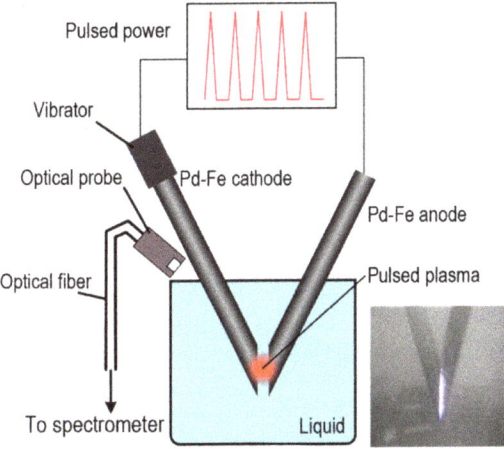

Figure 1. Schematic of pulsed-plasma-in-liquid method.

In the plasma discharge experiment, we prepared two alloy bulk electrodes, each with a rod that was 4 mm in diameter and composed of pure Pd and Pd-Fe with atomic percent ratios of 1:3, 1:1, and 3:1. We first set the Pd-Fe electrodes into a 200-mL 99% ethanol solution and applied a pulsed voltage of 60.5 V for 60 min. Although the input voltage was set, the voltage applied to the electrodes varied with the discharge. Figure 2 shows the variation in output current. The current pulses were each about 10 µs with a rise time of less than 5 µs at intervals of about 100 µs. The current range was about 1.0–2.0 A. After the experiment, the samples were separated from the liquid into floating (upper) and sedimented (bottom) parts using a centrifuge, and then dried. Then we used an electric stove to dry these two parts for 4 h.

During the synthesis, atomic emission spectra of the plasma discharge were collected by an ALS SEC2000 UV-V optical spectrometer placed close to the plasma discharge zone outside the quartz beaker. Emission spectrum peaks were identified according to the NIST1 database [15].

The X-ray diffraction (XRD) patterns for the samples were measured with a Rigaku RINT-2500 VHF diffractometer, using CuKα radiation at 40 kV and 200 mA. We used high-resolution transmission electron microscopy (HR-TEM) (Philips Tecnai F20) to observe the morphology and microstructure of prepared samples. Elemental analysis was performed using a JEOL JSM-7600F energy-dispersive X-ray (EDX) spectroscope at 15 kV with a point resolution of 1.0 nm. We measured the X-ray absorption fine structure (XAFS) spectra near the Pd K-edge in transmission mode (with a beam size of 1.2 × 0.3 mm) at beamline NW10A AR, KEK, Tsukuba, Japan. Synchrotron radiation was monochromatized by a Si (311) double-crystal monochromater. X-ray energy calibration was performed by setting the copper metal pre-edge absorption peak to 8978.8 eV. Mirrors were used to eliminate higher harmonics. The radial structural function was obtained by performing a Fourier transform over the range $2.5 < k < 10.5$ Å^{-1}. We used an analytical edge XAFS (EXAFS) formula to carry out Fourier filtering and non-linear least-squares fitting of structural parameters.

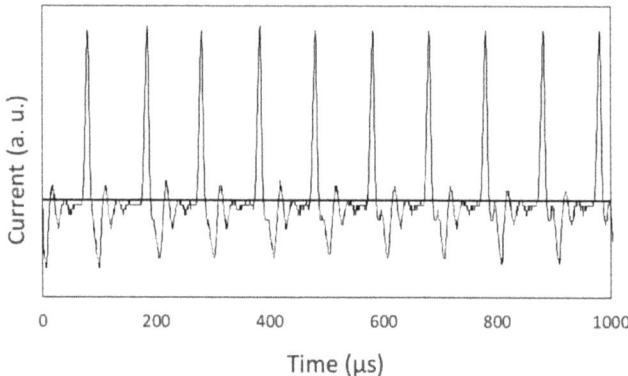

Figure 2. Waveform of output current.

3. Results and Discussion

3.1. X-ray Diffraction

Figure 3 shows the XRD patterns of the floated (upper) (a) and sedimented (bottom) (b) samples of Pd-Fe alloy together with those of single-element Pd and Fe nanoparticles obtained by PPL. As the Pd concentration in samples increases, their XRD peaks become much more similar to those of Pd. Both the 1:1 and 3:1 Pd-Fe nanoparticles of the bottom and upper samples show the face-centered cubic (FCC) Pd phase in which all peaks are around 41 degrees, not the body-centered cubic (BCC) phase of Fe, which almost comes out at 45 degrees, while the 1:3 Pd-Fe shows both BCC and FCC phases. Each peak of the Pd phase shifts to larger 2θ, and those of the Fe phase shifts to smaller 2θ. As shown in Table 1, the lattice constants of the upper Pd-Fe alloy nanoparticles are slightly larger than those of the bottom ones. This may be caused by the larger surface area of the upper nanoparticles. The lattice parameter of the nanoparticles is smaller than that of pure Pd (3.9048 Å). This is because the ion radius of Pd is larger than that of Fe.

Table 1. Calculated lattice parameters of FCC phase of Pd-Fe alloy nanoparticles.

Lattice Parameter (Å)	Upper	Bottom
Pd	3.9676(39)	3.9506(37)
Pd_3Fe	3.8553(102)	3.8540(1)
PdFe	3.8140(4)	3.8168(13)
$PdFe_3$	3.8001(57)	3.7851(30)

Figure 4 shows the lattice parameter versus composition. The lattice parameter increases with Pd ratio, which follows Vegard's law. This shows that the synthesized Pd-Fe samples consist of solid solution nanoparticles with FCC structure.

We estimated the production rate of PdFe nanoparticles to be about 1.1 g per hour by measuring the weight of the electrodes.

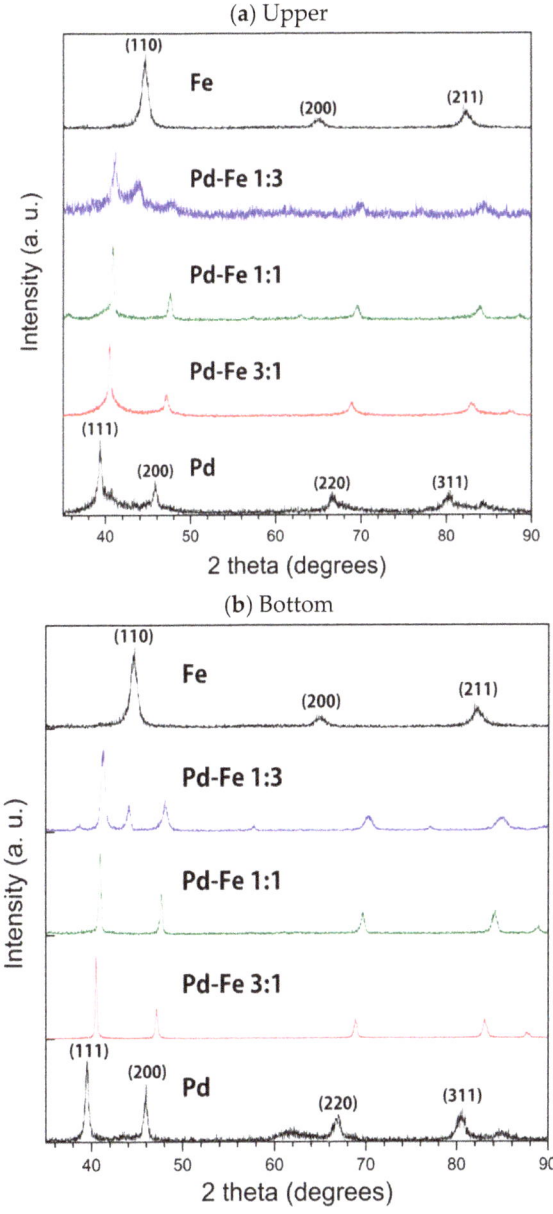

Figure 3. XRD patterns of Pd-Fe alloy nanoparticles and of elemental Pd and Fe nanoparticles in upper (**a**) and bottom (**b**) samples.

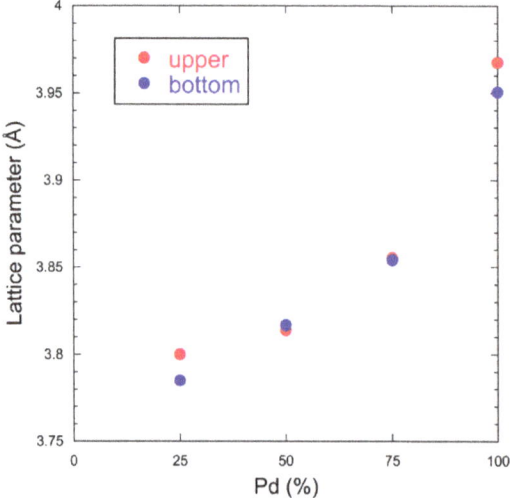

Figure 4. Lattice parameter versus Pd ratio of Pd-Fe alloy nanoparticles and pure Pd (100%) nanoparticles. The Pd-Fe nanoparticles have atomic percent ratios of 1:3, 1:1, and 3:1.

3.2. High-Resolution Transmission Electron Microscopy with Energy Dispersive X-ray Spectrometry

Figure 5 shows the HR-TEM images of the upper and bottom samples of the 1:1 Pd-Fe alloy nanoparticles with the particle size distributions. We see from these figures that the average particle diameter of the upper is less than 4 nm and that of the bottom is less than 6 nm. Figure 6 shows the expanded HR-TEM images of selected areas and each corresponding fast Fourier transform (FFT) for the interplanar spacing of the 111 face, with average values of 2.270 Å (upper) and 2.089 Å (bottom). In this figure, we can see lattice ordering on the nano scale.

Figure 7a–c represents the HR-TEM EDX spectrum of the obtained nanoparticle when Pd:Fe = 1:3, 1:1, and 3:1, respectively. We measured the elemental composition at the point in each particle indicated by a red circle (<10 nm) in the high-angle annular dark-field scanning transmission electron microscopy (HAADF-STEM) image. The Pd-to-Fe atomic percent ratios for the 1:3, 1:1, and 3:1 samples were 1.3:3.2, 3.8:3.0, and 12.5:3.5, respectively, which are comparable to those of the starting bulk mixture electrode.

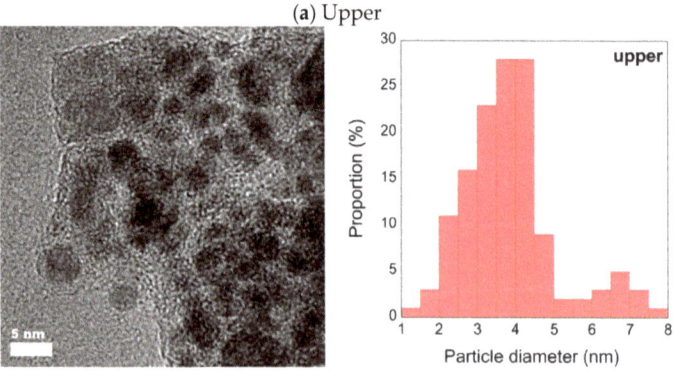

Figure 5. *Cont.*

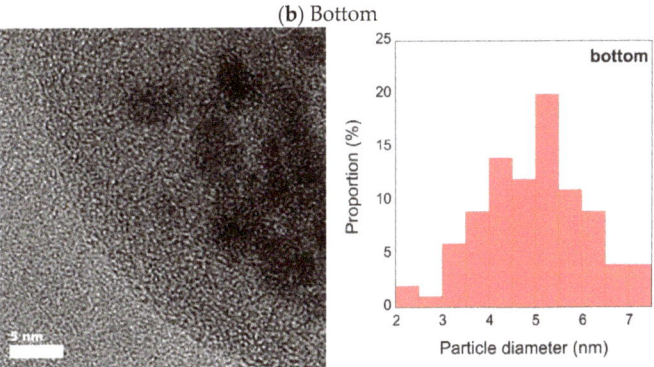

Figure 5. HR-TEM images of upper (**a**) and bottom (**b**) 1:1 Pd-Fe sample with particle diameter distribution.

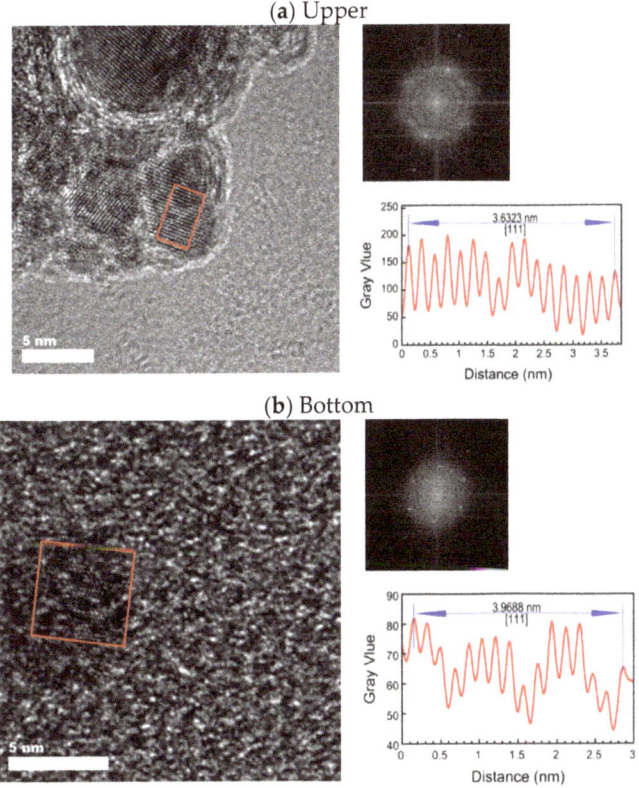

Figure 6. HR-TEM images of upper (**a**) and bottom (**b**) 1:1 Pd-Fe alloy nanoparticles with FFT pattern and surface spacing in the region enclosed in red.

From the XRD and HR-TEM results, we conclude that Pd-Fe solid solution nanoparticles with any composition ratios can be synthesized by PPL using Pd-Fe bulk mixture electrodes.

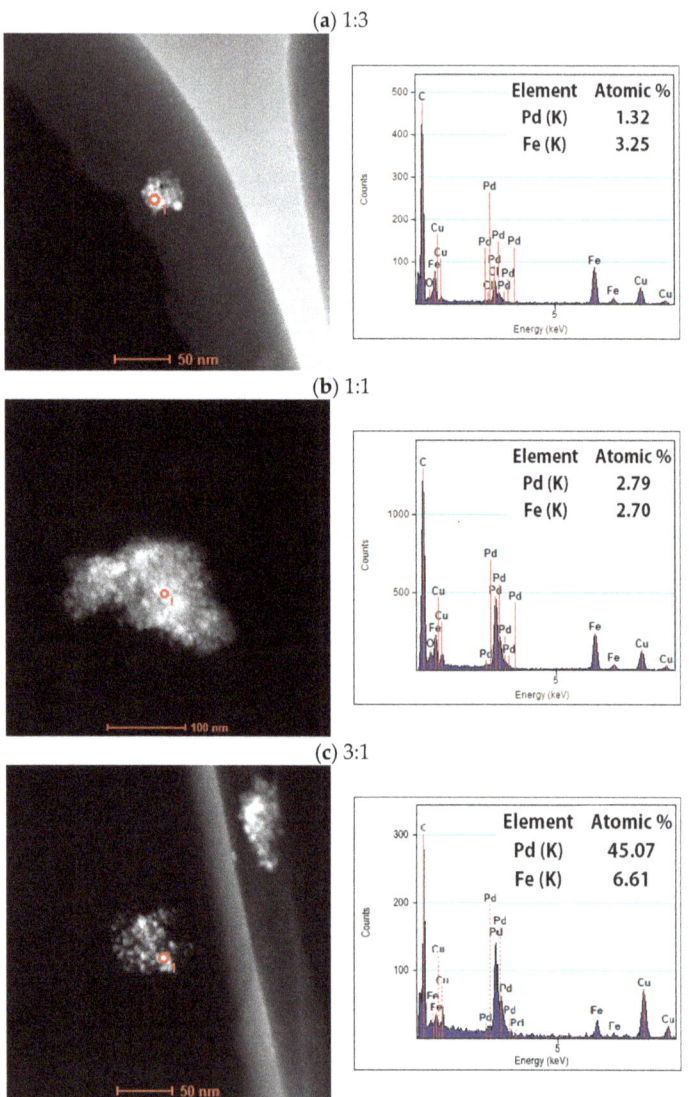

Figure 7. HAADF-STEM image and EDX analysis of upper 1:3 (**a**); 1:1 (**b**); and 3:1 (**c**) Pd-Fe alloy nanoparticles.

3.3. X-ray Absorption Near Edge Structure

In Figure 8, the Pd K-edge X-ray absorption near-edge-structure (XANES) patterns of the synthesized nanoparticles are compared with those of the Pd foil. The Pd-Fe samples show a pattern similar to that of the Pd metal foil, though the amplitude of the sinusoidal structure decreases with increasing iron content. This indicates an increase in irregularity due to solid solution of different atomic sizes for iron. Figure 9 shows the first-derivative XANES spectra of the samples in Figure 8. The maximum peak in the first-derivative XANES spectrum in Figure 9, which corresponds to the energy with the largest slope in Figure 8, represents the threshold energy of the absorption edge. No chemical shifts of the threshold energies for Pd-Fe nanoparticles appear in Figure 8 or Figure 9. These results indicate that the samples keep the FCC structure and metallic character of Pd.

From extended x-ray absorption fine structure (EXAFS) we obtained the radial distribution function and the interatomic distance from the X-ray absorbing atom to the adjacent atoms. Figure 10 shows the FFTs of the EXAFS oscillation function $k^3\chi(k)$ showing the distances from the X-ray absorbing Pd atoms to the adjacent Pd and Fe atoms. The first and second peaks indicate the first set of nearest Pd-Fe and Pd-Pd distances, respectively. The shape of the Pd-Pd peak for pure Pd becomes asymmetric because of the backscattering amplitude. The Pd-Fe peak height increases and the Pd-Pd peak height decreases with increasing iron content.

Table 2 shows the local Pd-Pd and Pd-Fe interatomic distances determined from the EXAFS analyses. The Pd-Pd and Pd-Fe distances are 2.76 and 2.62 Å, respectively, indicating the distances for the coordination number of 12 in FCC structure. The Pd and Fe are mixed at the atomic level, which proves that the obtained sample is a Pd-Fe solid solution.

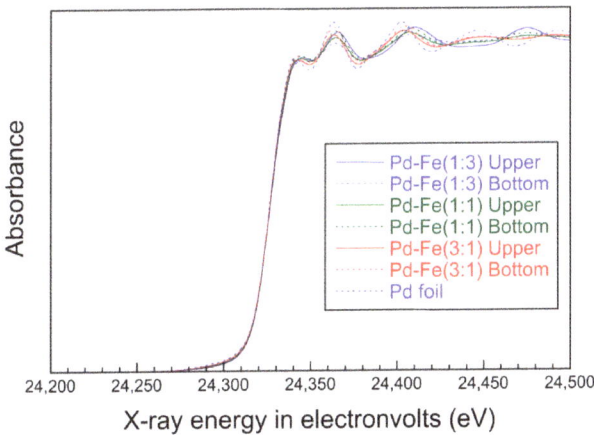

Figure 8. Normalized XANES of Pd parts of nanoparticles.

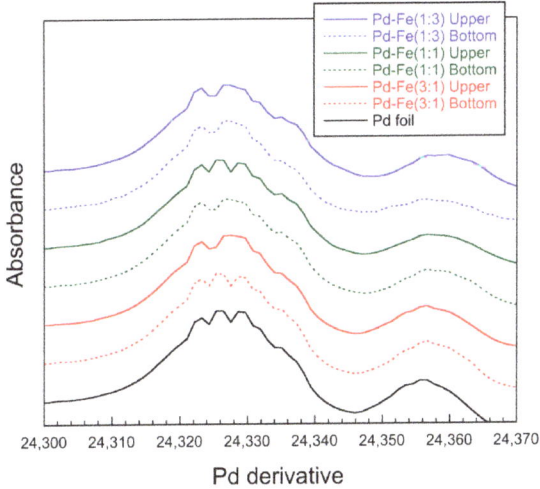

Figure 9. Derivative XANES of Pd parts of nanoparticles.

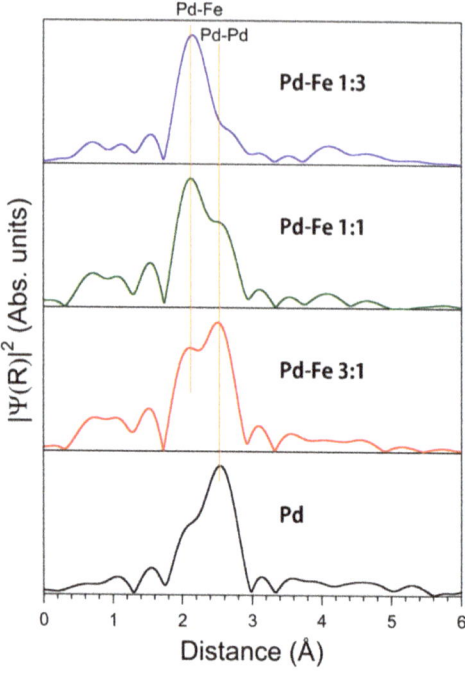

Figure 10. Fourier transforms of the Pd K-edge EXAFS oscillation function $k^3\chi(k)$. No phase shift corrections are made. The first sets of nearest peaks represent the Pd-Fe and Pd-Pd distances.

Table 2. Local bonding distances (Å) in Pd-Fe alloy nanoparticles determined by EXAFS.

Sample	Pd-Pd Distance (Å)	Pd-Fe Distance (Å)
Pd Upper	2.76(1)	-
Pd$_3$Fe Upper	2.76(1)	2.62(2)
PdFe Upper	2.74(2)	2.61(2)
PdFe$_3$ Upper	2.75(2)	2.63(1)

3.4. Atomic Emission Spectrum and Nanoparticle Formation Mechanism

Figure 11 shows the atomic optical emission spectra from the plasma discharge between the Pd-Fe electrodes submerged in ethanol. The main signals in the spectra belong to Fe (Fe$^+$) and Pd (Pd$^+$). The Pd lines are weak. The PdII lines may be too weak to be measured. The first and second ionization energies of Pd and Fe are 804.4, 1870 and 762.5, 1561.9 kJ/mol, respectively. We cannot observe the spectra of diatomic species such as OH, N2, CH, and C2. From the spectra of the Pd-Fe nanoparticles, we infer their formation mechanism via PPL as follows: Any raw materials, even those with high melting/boiling points, can be ionized by the high plasma temperature (2000–2500 °C). Therefore, Pd-Fe is ionized in the first stage, and positively charged Pd$^+$ and Fe$^+$ ions appear and disperse throughout the liquid. Then, Pd$^+$ and Fe$^+$ ions gather and form Pd-Fe nanoparticles under quenching by the surrounding cool liquid (Figure 12). The short pulse duration and rapid quenching prevent particle growth; therefore, the nanoparticles synthesized by PPL are very small.

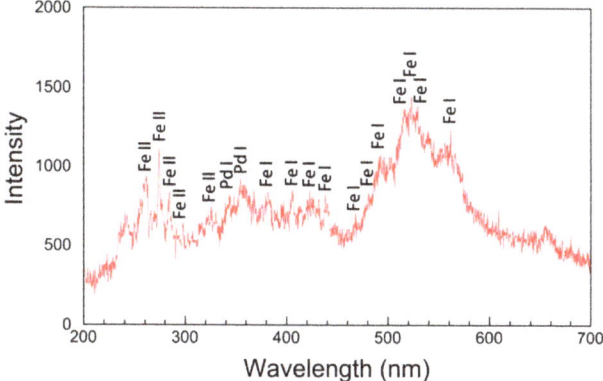

Figure 11. Optical emission spectrum from pulsed plasma in ethanol solution with Pd-Fe electrodes.

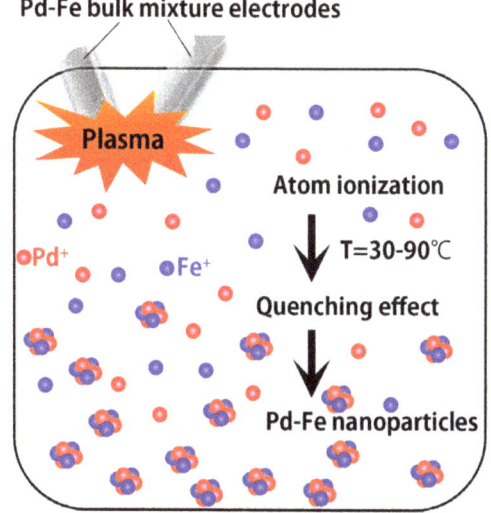

Figure 12. Illustration of Pd-Fe alloy nanoparticle formation via pulsed plasma in water.

4. Conclusions

We have succeeded in synthesizing Pd-Fe series nanoparticles in solid solution with Pd:Fe composition ratios of 1:3, 1:1, and 3:1 by the PPL method using Pd-Fe alloy electrodes with the same compositions. The resulting 1:1 and 3:1 Pd-Fe particles are FCC while the 1:3 Pd-Fe particles are a mixture of BCC and FCC. The lattice parameter increases with increasing Pd concentration and follows Vegard's law. The EDX and XAFS results also confirm the solid solution state. The sizes of the solid solution alloy particles are less than 10 nm. We expect synthesized Pd-Fe solid solution nanoparticles to show comparable or better catalytic properties than Pd nanoparticles.

Author Contributions: Conceptualization, T.M.; methodology, T.M.; formal analysis, M.K., H.I. and A.Y.; investigation, S.T., K.Y., Z.K., W.M., X.K. and A.Y.; data curation, S.T., T.M.; writing—original draft preparation, S.T.; writing—review and editing, T.M., A.Y.; visualization, S.T., X.K.; supervision, T.M.; funding acquisition, T.M.

Funding: This research received no external funding.

Acknowledgments: We greatly appreciate the valuable assistance of M. Tsushida and Kenta Yamamoto with the experiments. The authors thank Mark Kurban, from Edanz Group (www.edanzediting.com/ac) for editing a draft of this manuscript.

Conflicts of Interest: The authors declare no conflict of interest.

References

1. Gelatt, C.D.; Ehrenreich, H.; Weiss, J.A. Transition-metal hydrides: Electronic structure and the heats of formation. *Phys. Rev. B* **1978**, *17*, 1940–1957. [CrossRef]
2. Vuillemin, J.J.; Priestly, M.G. De Haas-Van Alphen effect and Fermi surface in palladium. *Phys. Rev. Lett.* **1965**, *14*, 307–309. [CrossRef]
3. Perkas, N.; Teo, J.; Shen, S.; Wang, Z.; Highfield, J.; Zhong, Z.; Gedanken, A. Supported Ru catalysts prepared by two sonication-assisted methods for preferential oxidation of CO in H2. *Phys. Chem. Chem. Phys.* **2011**, *13*, 15690–15698. [CrossRef] [PubMed]
4. Ke, X.; Cui, G.-F.; Shen, P.-K. Stability of Pd-Fe Alloy Catalysts. *Wuli Huaxue Xuebao Acta Phys. Chim. Sin.* **2009**, *25*, 213–217.
5. Shao, Mi.; Sasaki, K.; Adzic, R.R. Pd-Fe Nanoparticles as Electrocatalysts for Oxygen Reduction. *J. Am. Chem. Soc.* **2006**, *128*, 3526–3527. [CrossRef] [PubMed]
6. Zhu, B.W.; Lim, T.T. Catalytic Reduction of Chlorobenzenes with Pd/Fe Nanoparticles: Reactive Sites, Catalyst Stability, Particle Aging, and Regeneration. *Environ. Sci. Technol.* **2007**, *41*, 7523–7529. [CrossRef] [PubMed]
7. Tamura, S.; Kelgenbaeva, Z.; Yamamoto, K.; Chen, L.; Mashimo, T. Preparation of FePt Nanoparticles by Pulsed Plasma in Liquid Method. *Eng. Mater.* **2017**, *730*, 248–252. [CrossRef]
8. Omurzak, E.; Jasnakunov, J.; Mairykova, N.; Abdykerimova, A.; Maatkasymova, A.; Sulaimankulova, S.; Matsuda, M.; Nishida, M.; Ihara, H.; Mashimo, T. Synthesis Method of Nanomaterial by Pulsed Plasma in Liquid. *J. Nanosci. Nanotechnol.* **2007**, *7*, 3157–3159. [CrossRef] [PubMed]
9. Kelgenbaeva, Z.; Omurzak, E.; Takebe, S.; Sulaimankulova, S.; Abdullaeva, Z.; Iwamoto, C.; Mashimo, T. Synthesis of pure iron nanoparticles at liquid-liquid interface using pulsed plasma. *J. Nanopart. Res.* **2014**, *16*, 2603. [CrossRef]
10. Abdullaeva, Z.; Omurzak, E.; Iwamoto, C.; Chen, L.; Mashimo, T. Onion-like carbon-encapsulated Co, Ni, and Fe magnetic nanoparticles with low cytotoxicity synthesized by a pulsed plasma in a liquid. *Carbon* **2012**, *550*, 1776–1785. [CrossRef]
11. Omurzak, E.; Abdullaeva, Z.; Iwamoto, C.; Ihara, H.; Sulaimankulova, S.; Mashimo, T. Synthesis of Hollow Carbon Nano-Onions Using the Pulsed Plasma in Liquid. *J. Nanosci. Nanotechnol.* **2015**, *15*, 3703–3709. [CrossRef] [PubMed]
12. Omurzak, E.; Mashimo, T.; Iwamoto, C.; Matsumoto, Y.; Sulaimankulova, S. Synthesis of Blue Amorphous TiO_2 and Ti_nO_{2n-1} by the Impulse Plasma in Liquid. *J. Nanosci. Nanotechnol.* **2009**, *9*, 6372–6375. [CrossRef] [PubMed]
13. Chen, L.; Mashimo, T.; Omurzak, E.; Okudera, H.; Iwamoto, C.; Yoshiasa, A. Pure Tetragonal ZrO_2 Nanopartiles Synthesized by Pulsed Plasma in Liquid. *J. Phys. Chem. C* **2011**, *15*, 9370–9375. [CrossRef]
14. Omurzak, E.; Mashimo, T.; Sulaimankulova, S.; Takebe, S.; Chen, L.; Abdullaeva, Z.; Iwamoto, C.; Oishi, Y.; Ihara, H.; Okudera, H.; et al. Wurtzite-type ZnS nanoparticles by pulsed electric discharge. *Nanotechnology* **2011**, *22*, 365602. [CrossRef] [PubMed]
15. Ralchenko, Y.; Kramida, A.E.; Reader, J.; NIST ASD Team. *NIST Atomic Spectra Database*; Version 5; National Institute of Standards and Technology. 2011. Available online: http://physics.nist.gov/asd (accessed on 20 August 2018).

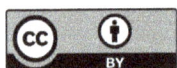

© 2018 by the authors. Licensee MDPI, Basel, Switzerland. This article is an open access article distributed under the terms and conditions of the Creative Commons Attribution (CC BY) license (http://creativecommons.org/licenses/by/4.0/).

MDPI
St. Alban-Anlage 66
4052 Basel
Switzerland
Tel. +41 61 683 77 34
Fax +41 61 302 89 18
www.mdpi.com

Nanomaterials Editorial Office
E-mail: nanomaterials@mdpi.com
www.mdpi.com/journal/nanomaterials

www.ingramcontent.com/pod-product-compliance
Lightning Source LLC
LaVergne TN
LVHW071954080526
838202LV00064B/6747